Fibromyalgia Syndrome and Widespread Pain

From Construction to Relevant Recognition

Fibromyalgia Syndrome and Widespread Pain

From Construction to Relevant Recognition

Editors

Winfried Häuser, MD

Professor
Department of Psychosomatic Medicine and Psychotherapy
Consultant
Technische Universität München
Munich, Germany

Serge Perrot, MD, PhD

Professor
Pain Physician and Rheumatologist
Head of Pain Center
Cochin University Hospital
Paris Descartes University
Paris, France

Wolters Kluwer

Philadelphia • Baltimore • New York • London
Buenos Aires • Hong Kong • Sydney • Tokyo

International Association for the Study of Pain
IASP
Working together for pain relief

Acquisitions Editor: Keith Donnellan
Product Development Editor: Sean McGuire
Production Project Manager: Linda Van Pelt
Design Coordinator: Elaine Kasmer
Manufacturing Coordinator: Beth Welsh
Marketing Manager: Stacy Malyil
Prepress Vendor: Newgen Knowledge Works Pvt. Ltd., Chennai, India

9 8 7 6 5 4 3 2 1

Printed in China

Library of Congress Cataloging-in-Publication Data
Names: Hauser, Winfried, author, editor. | Perrot, Serge, 1960- author, editor. | International Association for the Study of Pain, issuing body.
Title: Fibromyalgia syndrome and widespread pain : from construction to relevant recognition / Winfried Hauser, Serge Perrot.
Description: First edition. | Philadelphia : Wolters Kluwer Health, [2019] | Includes bibliographical references.
Identifiers: LCCN 2018017921 | ISBN 9781975102852 (paperback)
Subjects: | MESH: Fibromyalgia
Classification: LCC RC927.3 | NLM WE 544 | DDC 616.7/42—dc23
LC record available at https://lccn.loc.gov/2018017921

LWW.com

CCS0618

PREFACE

Fibromyalgia syndrome is a controversial condition, built over centuries and based on numerous putative pathophysiologies. It had been considered primarily a muscular disorder; then a psychological disorder; later a central dysfunctional condition; and recently a pain condition related to nociplastic mechanisms.

In fact none of these pathophysiologic concepts are satisfactory, and the recent findings of small fiber polyneuropathies in some patients with fibromyalgia syndrome have demonstrated that it is a never-ending story, grouping numerous subentities.

The recent American College of Rheumatology 2010, and the 2011 and 2016 criteria have provided some improvement in classification and diagnostic approaches. A number of clinicians and researchers believe that fibromyalgia syndrome and chronic widespread pain deserve a conceptualization, not only for scientific but also for therapeutic purposes.

In this International Association for the Study of Pain (IASP) book, we would like to consider all concepts of chronic widespread pain and fibromyalgia syndrome with pathophysiologic and therapeutic approaches, with validated data, and with relevant concepts. We will try to demonstrate that different approaches and concepts are different pieces of a puzzle that we are building together, but not exclusively.

The aim of this book is to propose an international textbook on chronic widespread pain and fibromyalgia syndrome, under the auspices of IASP, grouping clinicians from different specialties and researchers from different fields.

With this book, we hope that beyond prejudice and misconceptions, clinicians and also researchers will find interesting approaches and start future collaborations and further studies, mainly for the benefit of our patients.

Prof. Dr. Winfried Häuser
Prof. Dr. Serge Perrot

CONTRIBUTORS

Jacob N. Ablin, MD
Senior Lecturer
Internal Medicine
Sackler Faculty of Medicine
Tel Aviv University
Chief
Internal Medicine
Tel Aviv Sourasky Medical Center
Tel Aviv, Israel

Anne-Françoise Allaz, MD
Professor
Department of General Internal Medicine and Rehabilitation
Geneva University
Head
Beau-Séjour Division of Rehabilitation and Internal Medicine
University Hospitals
Geneva, Switzerland

Fabiola Atzeni, MD, PhD
Professor
Department of Clinical and Experimental Medicine
Senior Consultant
Rheumatology Unit
University of Messina
Messina, Italy

Didier Bouhassira, MD, PhD
Professor
Director
Inserm U987
Centre d'Evaluation et de Traitement de la Douleur
Ambroise Paré Hospital
Boulogne-Billancourt, France

Christine Cedraschi, PhD
Senior Lecturer
Faculty of Medicine
University of Geneva
Psychologist
Division of General Internal Medicine & Multidisciplinary Pain Center
Division of Clinical Pharmacology and Toxicology
Geneva University Hospitals
Geneva, Switzerland

Daniel J. Clauw, MD
Professor
Anesthesiology, Medicine & Psychiatry
University of Michigan Medical School
Director
Chronic Pain & Fatigue Research Center
Michigan Medicine
University of Michigan
Ann Arbor, Michigan

Benjamin Coleman, BA
Postbaccalaureate Fellow
National Institute of Neurological Disorders and Stroke
National Institutes of Health
Bethesda, Maryland

Mary-Ann Fitzcharles MB, ChB
Professor
Rheumatology and Pain Management
McGill University
Senior Physician
Rheumatology and Pain Medicine
Montreal General Hospital
Montreal, Quebec, Canada

Björn Gerdle, MD, PhD
Professor
Department of Medicine and Health
Linköping University
Consultant
Pain and Rehabilitation Centre
University Hospital
Linköping, Sweden

Winfried Häuser, MD
Professor
Department of Psychosomatic Medicine and Psychotherapy
Consultant
Technische Universität München
Munich, Germany

Anna K. Koch, PhD
Scientific Assistant
Department of Internal and Integrative Medicine
Kliniken Essen-Mitte
Faculty of Medicine
University of Duisburg-Essen
Essen, Germany

Eva Kosek, MD, PhD
Professor
Department of Clinical Neuroscience
Karolinska Institutet
Stockholm
Senior Consultant
Stockholm Spine Center
Löwenströmska Hospital
Upplands Väsby, Sweden

Jost Langhorst, MD
Professor and Head
Department of Integrative Gastroenterology
Kliniken Essen-Mitte
Faculty of Medicine
University of Duisburg-Essen
Essen, Germany

Françoise Laroche, MD, PHD
Professor
Chief
Department of Pain
Saint-Antoine Hospital
University Paris Sorbonne
Paris, France

Britt Larsson, MD, PhD
Professor
Department of Medicine and Health
Linköping University
Consultant
Pain and Rehabilitation Centre
University Hospital
Linköping, Sweden

Kathy Longley
Fibromyalgia Patient Representative
Medical Writer and Editor
Bristol, UK

Ignazio Francesco Masala, MD
Consultant
Trauma and Orthopedic Unit
Santissima Trinità Hospital
Cagliari, Italy

Serge Perrot, MD, PhD
Professor
Pain Physician and Rheumatologist
Head of Pain Center
Cochin University Hospital
Paris Descartes University
Paris, France

Traian Popa, MD, PhD
Senior Research Fellow
National Institute of Neurological Diseases and Stroke
National Institutes of Health
Bethesda, Maryland

Piercarlo Sarzi-Puttini, MD
Professor
Department of Medicine
University of Milan
Chief
Rheumatology Unit
ASST Fatebenepratelli—Sacco
Milan, Italy

Joseph Snow, PhD, ABPP-Cn
Staff Scientist
Clinical Neuropsychologist
National Institutes of Health
National Institute of Mental Health
Office of the Clinical Director
Bethesda, Maryland

Claudia Sommer, MD
Professor
Senior Physician
Department of Neurology
University of Würzburg
Würzburg, Germany

Rossella Talotta, MD
Senior Physician
Department of Rheumatology
Luigi Sacco University-Hospital
Milan, Italy

Nurcan Üçeyler, MD
Professor
Senior Physician
Department of Neurology
University of Würzburg
Würzburg, Germany

Christin Veasley, BSc
Co-founder and Director
Chronic Pain Research Alliance
Milwaukee, Wisconsin

Brian Walitt, MD
Staff Clinician
National Institutes of Nursing Research
National Institutes of Health
Bethesda, Maryland

Andreas Winkelmann, MD
Senior Physician
Department of Orthopedic Surgery
Physical Medicine and Rehabilitation
Medical Center of University München
Munich, Germany

Frederick Wolfe, MD
Professor
University of Kansas School of Medicine
Director
National Data Bank for Rheumatic
Diseases
Wichita, Kansas

CONTENTS

SECTION THREE: **Epidemiology and Social Impact**

SECTION FOUR: **Diagnosis**

SECTION FIVE: **Pathophysiologic Concepts**

SECTION SIX: Management Approaches in Fibromyalgia Syndrome

SECTION SEVEN: Conclusion and Future Research Agenda

SECTION 1

The Concepts of Fibromyalgia Syndrome

CHAPTER 1

History of Fibromyalgia Syndrome: Social and Medical Construction—From the Ancient Ages to Neurosciences

Serge Perrot

Summary Points

- The story of fibromyalgia syndrome (FMS) is very long, starting from the ancient times, with Hippocrates.
- The story of FMS has followed the current state of the science, from muscle pathophysiology to psychiatry, from neurosciences to genetics.
- FMS is a disrupting condition that does not fit with the Cartesian model, but should be accepted as a disease of adaptation and of coping strategies, and a functional disease.
- The story is not finished with new hypotheses on infectious causes, or on peripheral neuropathies.

FM is considered as a recent disease,[29] and some physicians remain doubtful about its reality. In 1926, Hunter[21] had already stated that "it requires a little courage to present a paper on this subject, for fibrositis, or myalgia, has no generally recognised pathology and the term has in the past been used very loosely to cover many pathologic conditions." In fact, the name "fibromyalgia syndrome" is recent, proposed by Hench[19] in 1976, but the story began long before this labeling. Over time, its story has been influenced by current concepts, from muscle disorder to psychology, from genetic predisposition to hormonal dysfunction, and finally with important findings related to the neurosciences, from small fibers to brain. We will follow this story along the ages and sciences to better understand this complex pain disorder, between soma and psyche, and between medicine and psychosociology.

This story aims to demonstrate that patients have existed all throughout the centuries, with numerous approaches and pathophysiologic explanations. The term "fibromyalgia syndrome" is perhaps one milestone of this long story, linked to the current 21st-century visions of a condition that we consider as an example of difficult links between body and mind. It is obvious that FMS is a disrupting condition, for both patients and researchers, raising important questions on the links between body and mind: Is it a disease or a syndrome? Are there specific causes? Is it in the body or in the brain? Is it real or artificial? In all cases, science should be open, without prejudices but always validated, and always dedicated to the cure of our patients, whatever the explanation. This is why FMS should be recognized as a challenge, for patients, for medical science, and also for our modern society.

AT THE BEGINNING: GREEK AND ROMAN LITERATURE

"Joint Pain Is Driven by the Brain"

The history of pain medicine and rheumatology is very old, and it is possible to find interesting concepts and descriptions of pain in the ancient Greek literature. In 410 BC, Hippocrates (430 to 380 BC) described the "Rheuma Theory": a mechanism of pain where the brain sends liquid to the lower limb, and when there is more liquid, there is more pain. *Rheuma* means fluid in Greek, and in fact, the Rheuma theory explains the influence of the brain on the body.[17]

It is interesting to note that this concept is close to the recent concepts of central sensitization. Hippocrates was one of the first to consider that pain is not a punishment but a natural phenomenon. He also described the use of nonpharmacologic tools to relieve pain: cold and hot application, and plasters.[17]

After Hippocrates, Theophrastus (372 BC to 287 BC), a Greek physician who was one of Aristotle's disciples, described widespread pain conditions. Theophrastus published the "characters," where he described a feature of general pain in muscles and tendons, as a special condition that he called "lassitude."

Four hundred years later, Galien (131 BC to 201 AD) also tried to classify pain symptoms. He stated that the brain is the center of pain and all sensations. In his system, pain was the result of soul disorders and passions.

THE VERY FIRST MEDICAL DESCRIPTION OF FIBROMYALGIA SYNDROME IN RENAISSANCE TIMES

Guillaume de Baillou (1538 to 1616) was a physician (Dean of the University of Paris, medical faculty, 1580), and founder of modern epidemiology who revived Hippocratic medical practice in Renaissance Europe. He was the first to define the term "rheumatism" in its modern sense. In 1592, he published a book, "Liber de rheumatismo," in which there are some descriptions of muscular pain close to FMS.

STARTING TO ESTABLISH PATHOPHYSIOLOGY: FIBROMYALGIA SYNDROME AS A MUSCLE DISORDER

In the 19th century, the first pathophysiologic approaches emerged, and FMS was described as "muscular rheumatism." In the 19th century, concomitantly, several European authors described similar clinical syndromes with widespread pain localized in the muscles.

The Tender Points

The tender points were described by Valleix[39] in France, in 1841. In 1858, in Great Britain, Inman[22] described a muscular localized pain independent of innervation and also described "referred pain." In Germany in 1903, Froriep[13] described nodules in the muscles with pain induced by pressure. Later, in 1952, Travell[37] coined the word "myofascial" and the myofascial pain syndrome.

Toward the Description of Fibrositis

Balfour,[2] a surgeon in Edinburgh was the first, in 1815, to describe the "muscular rheumatism": "A special pain, usually driven by an inflammatory action, involving fibrous and white tissues, belonging to muscles and joints, like tendons, aponevroses." He called this widespread pain "fibrosistitis."

After that, there have been several descriptions of widespread pain, related to muscle pathophysiology. In 1904, Gowers[15] introduced the term "fibrositis." After the description of fibrositis, Telling[35] described nodular fibromyositis and was the first to try to unify different disorders with different names, describing the same pathophysiologic entity (Fig. 1.2).

However, subsequent studies of muscle biopsies have failed to find local abnormalities, and the term "fibrositis" is therefore considered a misnomer.[5] Only muscle microcirculation and metabolic abnormalities have been found.[4]

THE END OF THE 19TH AND THE START OF THE 20TH CENTURY: THE GOLDEN ERA OF PSYCHOLOGY

The end of the 19th century and the start of the 20th century can be considered as the era of psychology, also with the specific rise of psychoanalysis.

Neurasthenia

A very interesting condition, surprisingly very close to the American College of Rheumatology (ACR) 2010 criteria of FMS has been described in 1869 under the name of neurasthenia, described by Beard[3] (Table 1.1, Fig. 1.1).

TABLE 1.1 Criteria for neurasthenia described by Beard

- Cephalalgia
- Insomnia, nightmares
- Rachialgia, coccygodynia
- Fatigue, mainly in the morning, with muscular atrophia
- Dyspepsia
- Sexual disorders and dysfunction
- Psychological asthenia
- Memory loss

From Beard G. Neurasthenia or nervous exhaustion. *Boston Med Surg J.* 1869;3:217–220.

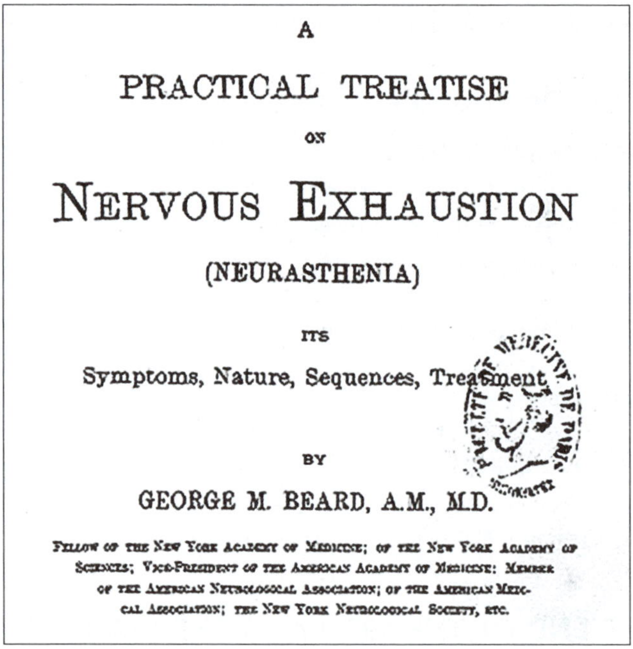

A

PRACTICAL TREATISE

ON

NERVOUS EXHAUSTION

(NEURASTHENIA)

ITS

Symptoms, Nature, Sequences, Treatment

BY

GEORGE M. BEARD, A.M., M.D.

FELLOW OF THE NEW YORK ACADEMY OF MEDICINE; OF THE NEW YORK ACADEMY OF SCIENCES; VICE-PRESIDENT OF THE AMERICAN ACADEMY OF MEDICINE: MEMBER OF THE AMERICAN NEUROLOGICAL ASSOCIATION; OF THE AMERICAN MEDICAL ASSOCIATION; THE NEW YORK NEUROLOGICAL SOCIETY, ETC.

FIGURE 1.1 Neurasthenia.

From Beard G. Neurasthenia or nervous exhaustion. *Boston Med Surg J.* 1869;3:217–220.

Psychogenic and Psychosomatic Rheumatism

In this line, FMS was considered a psychological disorder, with several new labels: myofibrositis mimicking other diseases[27] or psychogenic rheumatism.[7]

Post-Traumatic Pain

The Second World War was a period in which several descriptions were reported in male soldier patients.[7,31] This is very close to another syndrome, described 50 years later, in 1991, the Gulf War syndrome (review by Thomas[36] in 2006).

A Somatoform Disorder

Recent studies have not confirmed that FMS is a primary psychological disorder. Indeed, there are more anxiety and more depression in FMS, but also in all other chronic syndromes compared to healthy controls.[20] Anxiety and depression increase when related to medical symptoms without identified pathology.[24] There is no proven specific psychological feature or trait associated with FMS,[11] whereas cognitive dysfunction and inefficient coping are severe.[14]

The recent term "somatic symptom disorder" has been introduced to merge somatoform disorder and somatization disorder by the *Diagnostic and Statistical Manual of Mental Disorders* (*DSM-5*) classification in 2014. A *somatoform disorder* is defined as medically unexplained somatic symptoms that persist for at least 6 months and lead to a significant impairment of the ability to function in everyday life. In fact, FMS is not synonymous with somatoform disorder; the clinical features of FMS and persistent somatoform pain disorder overlap in individuals with chronic widespread pain without specific somatic disease factors.[18]

FROM THE 1950s, THE STRESS THEORY: FIBROMYALGIA SYNDROME AS A STRESS-INDUCED DISORDER WITH CHANGES IN THE STRESS HORMONES REACTION

Many years after the theory of stress originated by the famous endocrinologist Hans Selye, in the 1950s, there have been several studies on endocrine abnormalities of the hypothalamic–pituitary–adrenal (HPA) axis in FMS, and this concept is probably valid for some subgroups of patients. These theories describe endocrine abnormalities of the HPA axis that result in a blunted adrenal cortisol response to adrenocorticotropic hormone (ACTH) with significant reduction in basal cortisol compared with healthy controls in females with FMS.[34]

Other theories have looked at insulin-like growth factor (IGF1) and growth hormone (GH) levels in FMS patients.

They have found low IGF1 in one-third of patients, resulting in decreased nocturnal GH secretion.[23]

TIME FOR RECOGNITION: RECOGNITION OF THE DISEASE AND DIAGNOSTIC CRITERIA

Between the 1970s and the 1990s, recognition of the disease was an important step for patients and for physicians: The disease received a name, diagnostic criteria, and assessment tools.

Naming the Disease and Official Integration in the Disease Classification

In 1976, Hench[19] described the term "fibromyalgia syndrome" as a nonarticular rheumatism. In 1990, the World Health Organization recognized FMS. In 1987, the American Medical Association (AMA) recognized FMS as a true illness and a major cause of disability.

In 1992, at the Second World Congress on Myofascial Pain and Fibromyalgia in Copenhagen, a consensus statement on FMS was created and published in *The Lancet* under the name "Copenhagen Declaration 1992."[30]

In 1992, FMS was integrated into the *International Classification of Diseases* (*ICD-10*) in the chapter on nonarticular rheumatic diseases, with unknown etiology, under the code M79-0.

Concomitantly, Several Classification Criteria Have Been Proposed

In 1972, the first criteria to be proposed were published by Smythe.[32]

In the 1980s, another researcher, Yunus, further clarified FMS by proposing the need for a unified classification system as well as the first diagnostic criteria. He was

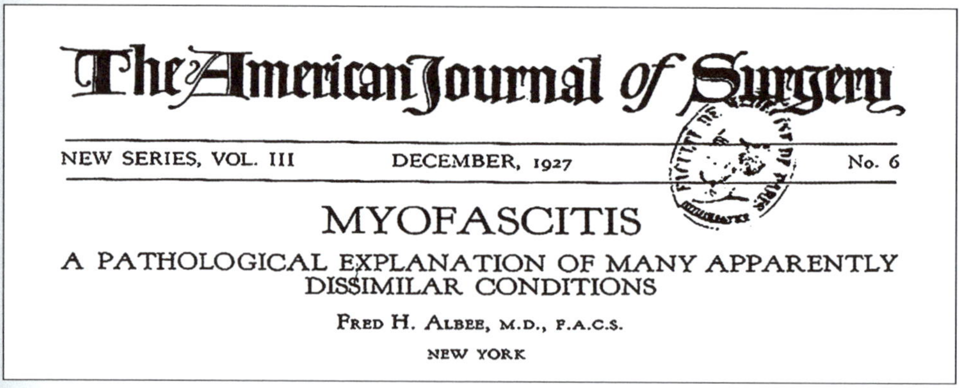
The American Journal of Surgery

NEW SERIES, VOL. III   DECEMBER, 1927   No. 6

MYOFASCITIS

A PATHOLOGICAL EXPLANATION OF MANY APPARENTLY DISSIMILAR CONDITIONS

FRED H. ALBEE, M.D., F.A.C.S.

NEW YORK

FIGURE 1.2 Myofasciitis.

From Albee FH. Myofascitis. *Am J Surg*. 1927;6:523–533.

the first to popularize the word "fibromyalgia syndrome," and in 1981, the Yunus criteria were released.[43]

Wolfe et al.[42] in 1990 published the most famous criteria under the name of "ACR 1990 Classification Criteria" (Fig. 1.3), initially not dedicated for diagnosis but for classification, and requiring a tender point examination. The value of 11 of 18 tender points was discussed, and important symptoms such as fatigue, sleep disturbances, and cognitive dysfunction were not included; thus, new research and criteria emerge: the new ACR 2010 criteria, revised in 2011 and in 2016, were proposed.[41] Aside fatigue and cognitive disorders that were included, one major change with these new criteria was that a diagnosis of FMS does not exclude the presence of other clinically important illnesses.

Several Tools to Assess Fibromyalgia Syndrome

The first tool to assess FMS, the Fibromyalgia Impact Questionnaire (FIQ), was developed in the late 1980s by Burckhardt et al.[8] at Oregon in Portland. Since then, FIQ has been extensively used as one of the main indexes of therapeutic efficacy in FMS.

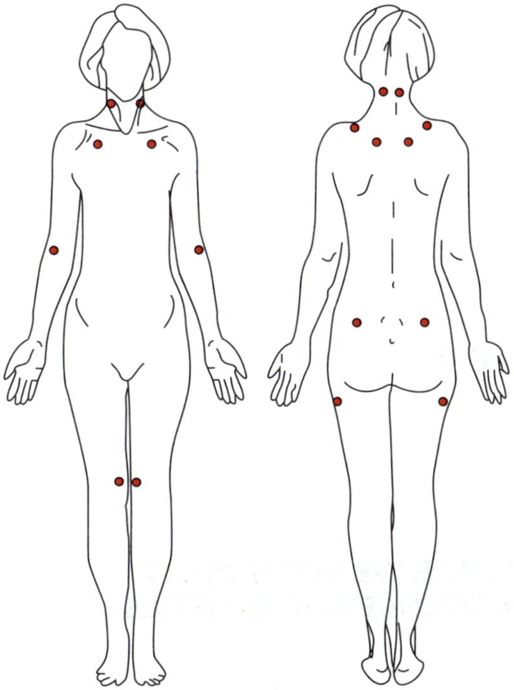

FIGURE 1.3 American College of Rheumatology 1990 tender points.

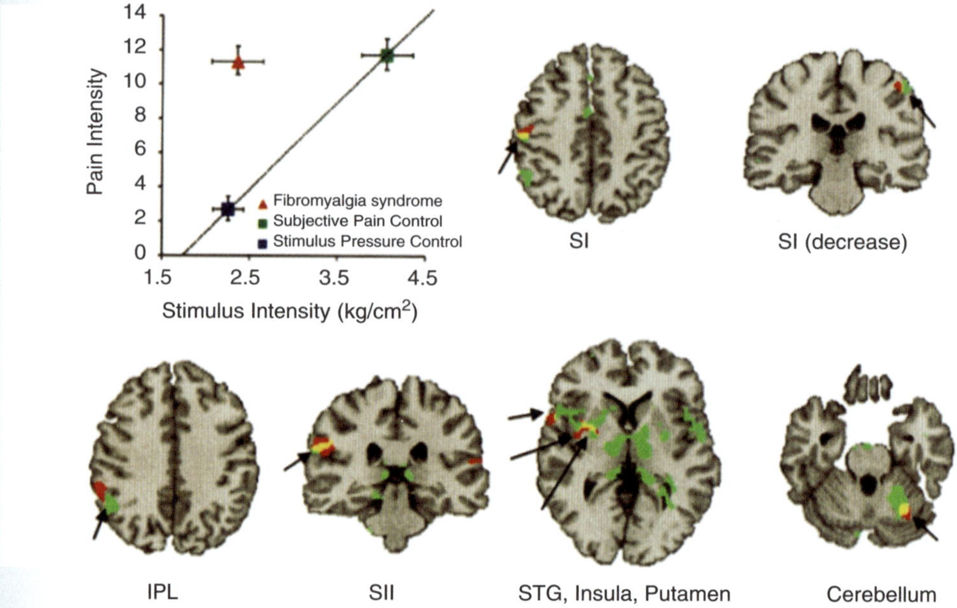

FIGURE 1.4 Brain.

SI, primary somatosensory cortex; IPL, inferior parietal lobule; SII, secondary somatosensory cortex; STG, superior temporal gyrus.

From Gracely RH, Petzke F, Wolf JM, Clauw DJ. Functional magnetic resonance imaging evidence of augmented pain processing in fibromyalgia. *Arthritis Rheum.* 2002;46(5):1333–1343.

Some Tools to Screen for Fibromyalgia Syndrome

As diagnostic criteria may be difficult to use in clinical practice, and for a more generalized use, some screening tools have been developed, such as the Fibromyalgia Rapid Screening Tool (FiRST), a six-item questionnaire.[28]

Recommendations

After the recognition of the syndrome, time for official guidelines and recommendations has come with international recommendations, such as the EULAR,[26] the Canadian,[12] or the German recommendations.[33]

WHERE ARE WE NOW? ALL IS NEUROSCIENCE AND GENETICS

The 21st century can be considered the century of neurosciences, as there have been major findings in that scientific arena.

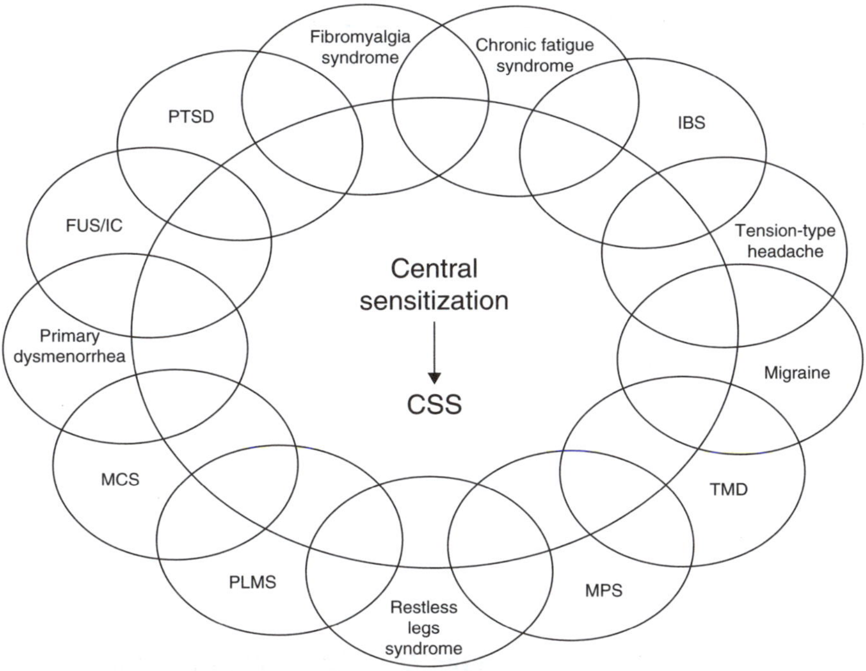

FIGURE 1.5 Central sensitivity syndromes.

FUS/IC, female urethral syndrome/interstitial cystitis; IBS, irritable bowel syndrome; MCS, multiple chemical sensitivity; MPS, myofascial pain syndrome; PLMS, periodic limb movement disorder; PTSD, posttraumatic stress disorder; TMD, temporomandibular disorder.

From Yunus MB. Fibromyalgia and overlapping disorders: the unifying concept of central sensitivity syndromes. *Semin Arthritis Rheum*. 2007;36(6):339–356.

Central Sensitization and Central Nervous System Imaging: Fibromyalgia Syndrome Is Real

The concept of central sensitization and central nervous system (CNS) imaging has represented an important step for physicians in that it demonstrates that specific changes are observed in the FMS patients' brains (Figs. 1.4 and 1.5).[10,40] These findings were important for many physicians, including rheumatologists and orthopedists, leading to the conclusion that finally FMS was real.[6]

Is Fibromyalgia Syndrome a Neurologic Condition?

Concomitantly, other authors have suggested that FMS could be part of neuropathic disorders, and several works have investigated peripheral nervous system changes in FMS, finding some abnormalities in the small nerve fibers in a subgroup of patients.[38]

Is Fibromyalgia Syndrome a Dysfunctional Pain Syndrome?

Not yet validated, but in discussion, the classification of pain disorders may incorporate a new class of pain syndromes, the dysfunctional/functional pain syndromes, including FMS, irritable bowel syndrome, restless leg syndrome, and cystalgia. Even if there are common mechanisms with neuropathic pain, this new class may definitely differentiate FMS from neuropathic pain syndromes, where a lesion of the neurologic system is mandatory. This is close to another classification, proposed by Yunus,[43] the concept of central sensitization syndromes.

In the 21st Century, Is Everything Genetically Driven?

As in many diseases, a genetic predisposition has been evoked in FMS. Much research, especially in Israel, has tried to identify genetic factors that may predispose one to FMS.[9] Most of the targets that have been studied are related to serotonin receptors and transporters, enzymes like COMT, and dopamine receptors, but most results are disappointing.[25]

CONCLUSION: FIBROMYALGIA SYNDROME—A NEVER-ENDING STORY?

In conclusion, the history of FMS is a story of controversies: the fight between subjectivity and cartesianism, and between old mind and body concepts. FMS represents the emblematic condition of unexplained medical symptoms far from well-defined diseases with objective biomarkers. It is the far end of medicine, sociology, and psychology, addressing difficult questions to medical science. This exciting scientific history is not finished, but we do hope that this history will come to a time when patients will no longer be stigmatized. Even if no one denies that patients exist, there are still many "fibroskeptical" physicians and, as in the 1920s, the question "is fibromyalgia syndrome real?" remains. It is time that medicine recognizes these patients and their conditions, without any prejudice and with the best scientific evidence.

REFERENCES

1. Albee FH. Myofascitis. *Am J Surg.* 1927;**6**:523–533.
2. Balfour W. Observations on the pathology and cure of rheumatism. *Edinb Med Surg J.* 1815; **11**:168–187.
3. Beard G. Neurasthenia or nervous exhaustion. *Boston Med Surg J.* 1869;**3**:217–220.
4. Bengtsson A. The muscle in fibromyalgia. *Rheumatology.* 2002;**41**:721–724.
5. Bennett RM. Fibrositis: misnomer for a common rheumatic disorder. *West J Med.* 1981;**134**:405–413.
6. Bernstein J. Not the last word: fibromyalgia is real. *Clin Orthop Relat Res.* 2016;**474**(2):304–309.
7. Boland EW. Psychogenic rheumatism: the musculoskeletal expression of psychoneurosis. *Ann Rheum Dis.* 1947;**6**(4):195–203.

8. Burckhardt CS, Clark SR, Bennett RM. The fibromyalgia impact questionnaire: development and validation. *J Rheumatol.* 1991;**18**:728–733.
9. Buskila D, Sarzi-Puttini P. Biology and therapy of fibromyalgia. Genetic aspects of fibromyalgia syndrome. *Arthritis Res Ther.* 2006;**8**(5):218.
10. Cagnie B, Coppieters I, Denecker S, Six J, Danneels L, Meeus M. Central sensitization in fibromyalgia? A systematic review on structural and functional brain MRI. *Semin Arthritis Rheum.* 2014;**44**:68–75.
11. Ekselius L, Bentsson A, von Knorring L. Personality traits as determined by means of the Karolinska scales of personality in patients with fibromyalgia. *J Musculoskel Pain.* 1998;**6**:35–49.
12. Fitzcharles MA, Ste-Marie PA, Goldenberg DL et al. 2012 Canadian guidelines for the diagnosis and management of fibromyalgia syndrome: executive summary. *Pain Res Manag.* 2013;**18**:119–126.
13. Froriep R. *Ein Beitrag zur Pathologie des Rheumatismus.* Weimar; 1843.
14. Glass JM. Review of cognitive dysfunction in fibromyalgia: a convergence on working memory and attentional control impairments. *Rheum Dis Clin North Am.* 2009;**35**(2):299–311.
15. Gowers W. A lecture on lumbago: its lessons and analogues. *Br Med J.* 1904;**1**:117–121.
16. Gracely RH, Petzke F, Wolf JM., Clauw DJ. Functional magnetic resonance imaging evidence of augmented pain processing in fibromyalgia. *Arthritis Rheum.* 2002;**46**(5):1333–1343.
17. Grossman BJ. Rheumatoid arthritis from prehistory to Hippocrates. *Proc Inst Med Chic.* 1966;**26**:114–115.
18. Häuser W, Bialas P, Welsch K, Wolfe F. Construct validity and clinical utility of current research criteria of *DSM-5* somatic symptom disorder diagnosis in patients with fibromyalgia syndrome. *J Psychosom Res.* 2015;**78**(6):546–552.
19. Hench PK. Non-articular rheumatism. *Arthritis Rheum.* 1976; **19**:1088.
20. Henningsen P, Zimmermann T, Sattel H. Medically unexplained physical symptoms, anxiety, and depression: a meta-analytic review. *J Psychosom Med.* 2003;**65**:528–533.
21. Hunter C. An address on fibrositis (myalgia, chronic muscular rheumatism). *Can Med Assoc J.* 1926;**16**:1319–1324.
22. Inman T. Remarks on myalgia or muscular pain. *Br Med J.* 1858;**1**:407–408, 866–868.
23. Jones KD, Deodhar P, Lorentzen A, Bennett RM, Deodhar AA. Growth hormone perturbations in fibromyalgia: a review. *Semin Arthritis Rheum.* 2007;**36**:357–379.
24. Katon W, Sullivan M, Walker E. Medical symptoms without identified pathology: relationship to psychiatric disorders, childhood and adult trauma, and personality traits. *Ann Intern Med.* 2001;**134**:917–925.
25. Lee YH, Choi SJ, Ji JD, Song GG. Candidate gene studies of fibromyalgia: a systematic review and meta-analysis. *Rheumatol Int.* 2012;**32**(2):417–426.
26. Macfarlane GJ, Kronisch C, Dean LE, et al. EULAR revised recommendations for the management of fibromyalgia. *Ann Rheum Dis.* 2017;**76**(2):318–328.
27. Murray G. Myofibrositis as simulator of other maladies. *Lancet.* 1929;**1**:113–116.
28. Perrot S, Bouhassira D, Fermanian J. Cercle d'Etude de la Douleur en Rhumatologie. Development and validation of the Fibromyalgia Rapid Screening Tool (FiRST). *Pain.* 2010;**150**(2):250–256.
29. Perrot S. Fibromyalgia syndrome: a relevant recent construction of an ancient condition? *Curr Opin Support Palliat Care.* 2008;**2**:122–127.
30. Quintner J. Fibromyalgia: the Copenhagen Declaration. *Lancet.* 1992;**340**:1103.
31. Savage O. Rheumatic diseases in the forces. *Br Med J.* 1942;**2**:336–338.
32. Smythe HA. Non-articular rheumatism and the fibrositis syndrome. In: Hollander JL, McCarty DJ, ed. *Arthritis and Allied Conditions.* 8th ed. Philadelphia, PA: Lea and Febiger; 1972:874–884.
33. Sommer C, Alten R, Bär KJ, et al. Drug therapy of fibromyalgia syndrome: updated guidelines 2017 and overview of systematic review articles. *Schmerz.* 2017;**31**(3):274–278.
34. Tak LM, Cleare AJ, Ormel J, et al. Meta-analysis and meta-regression of hypothalamic-pituitary-adrenal axis activity in functional somatic disorders. *Biol Psychol.* 2011;**87**(2):183–194.

35. Telling W. Nodular fibromyositis—an everyday affliction and its indentity with so-called muscular rheumatism. *Lancet.* 1911;**1**:154–158.
36. Thomas HV, Stimpson NJ, Weightman A, Dunstan F, Lewis G. Pain in veterans of the Gulf War of 1991: a systematic review. *BMC Musculoskelet Disord.* 2006(Sep **20**);7:74.
37. Travell J, Rinzler SH. The myofascial genesis of pain. *Postgrad Med.* 1952;**11**(5):425–434.
38. Üçeyler N, Zeller D, Kahn AK, et al. Small fibre pathology in patients with fibromyalgia syndrome. *Brain.* 2013;**136**:1857–18567.
39. Valleix FLI. *Traité des névralgies ou affections douloureuses des nerfs.* Paris: J.-B. Baillière; 1841.
40. Walitt B, Ceko M, Gracely JL, Gracely RH. Neuroimaging of central sensitivity syndromes: key insights from the scientific literature. *Curr Rheumatol Rev.* 2016;**12**(1):55–87.
41. Wolfe F, Clauw DJ, Fitzcharles MA, et al. 2016 Revisions to the 2010/2011 fibromyalgia diagnostic criteria. *Semin Arthritis Rheum.* 2016;**46**:319–329.
42. Wolfe F, Smythe HA, Yunus MB, et al. The American College of Rheumatology 1990 criteria for the classification of fibromyalgia. Report of the Multicenter Criteria Committee. *Arthritis Rheum.* 1990;**33**:160–172.
43. Yunus M, Masi A, Calabro J, Miller K, Feigenbaum S. Primary fibromyalgia (fibrositis): clinical study of 50 patients with matched-controls. *Semin Arthritis Rheum.* 1981;**11**:151–171.
44. Yunus MB. Fibromyalgia and overlapping disorders: the unifying concept of central sensitivity syndromes. *Semin Arthritis Rheum.* 2007;**36**(6):339–356.

CHAPTER 2

Fibromyalgia Syndrome: Aspects of the Social Construction of Organized Distress

Frederick Wolfe

Summary Points

- Fibromyalgia syndrome (FMS) is an arbitrarily and broadly defined disorder of widespread pain and multiple symptoms that is strongly influenced in its expression and prevalence by culture, context, and social forces.
- It has no binding definition and no way of objective testing for it.
- Its success came through patient support groups that utilized extensive electronic communication and active political promotion, huge support from the pharmaceutical industry, and proselytizing research physicians.
- Support from the public and physicians is tenuous, and the future of the illness remains to be seen.

From individuals with various symptoms, including pain and fatigue, a group syndrome of physician-defined organized distress (FMS) emerged in the last part of the 20th century. Related to neurasthenia of the 19th and early 20th centuries, it had roots, at least in part, in psychogenic mass sociogenic illness (MSI), and it grew by imitation. Its success came through patient support groups that utilized extensive electronic communication and active political promotion, huge support from the pharmaceutical industry, and proselytizing research physicians. Support from the public and physicians is tenuous, and the future of the illness remains to be seen.

FMS is an arbitrarily and broadly defined disorder of widespread pain and multiple symptoms that is strongly influenced in its expression and prevalence by culture, context, and social forces.[3,22,36,37,44,51] It "has no binding definition . . . and no way of objectively testing for it."[34] There are two conspicuous views of FMS, and they are substantially in disagreement. The first view, which has gradually become ascendant, holds that FMS is a *disease* whose pathogenesis primarily involves neurobiologic dysregulation that results in "central augmentation–" . . . "enhanced sensitivity to sensory stimuli, widespread pain, fatigue, sleep dysfunction, among other symptoms."[38] In addition, external factors such as stress and psychological factors can play a (usually) limited role in the development and severity of FMS. This reductionist view of FMS is not merely part of a scientific controversy, but forms the underpinnings of a movement that has substantial social, political, and economic consequences. Most accounts under this view present snippets of text as evidence of the existence of FMS in past centuries ("it was always present"), ranging from the Gilgamesh (2100 BC) and the book of Job from the 6th century BC to more recent but always isolated events.[33,42]

The alternative constructionist or nominalist view[39] holds that neurobiologic alteration is a mechanism, not a disease, and is present in most human pain conditions. The key factors in FMS development and sustenance are culture, context, and individual differences.[36,37,39,17,28] FMS criteria, which characterized and subsequently identified the disorder, were constructed by physicians, not discovered by them. We label FMS as an arbitrarily defined disorder, as the original 1990 definition from which the FMS movement grew was arbitrary and was only one of a several possible available definitions.[52] FMS symptoms (but not FMS) first appear historically, in many isolated cases, in the 19th century within the concept of neurasthenia—a wildly popular disorder associated with hysteria and paralysis—that has virtually disappeared from general medical practice[36,37,17,45] and briefly in allied disorders such as "Railway Spine."[11,23] As a now generally accepted and separate disorder, FMS (re)appears in the second half of the 20th century. No set of criteria adequately separates FMS from similar "functional" disorders. And it is not possible to tell when FMS begins and ends.[53]

A key observation that further undermined FMS as a distinct and separate entity was the 2013 demonstration by Wolfe et al.[48] that FMS was a dimensional (or continuum disorder). Using the polysymptomatic distress (PSD) (or fibromyalgianess) scale of the American College of Rheumatology (ACR) 2010 FMS criteria (and its 2011 modification for survey and clinical research) as a measure of the degree of FMS symptoms and symptom intensity,[49,50] they showed that FMS symptoms are present in persons with pain who do not meet the FMS criteria. Such observations led to confirmatory studies of FMS symptoms in pain patients who do not meet FMS criteria.[8,9,24] FMS symptoms—fatigue, sleep disturbance, cognitive symptoms, and widening of body pain—can be thought of as the "normal" and usual way that humans respond to pain and distress, while diagnosed FMS represents the severe end of the spectrum of PSD. Observed neurobiologic alterations cannot be considered to be abnormalities if they are present almost universally. Instead, they represent neurobiologic mechanisms by which the FMS phenotype is expressed and presented.

The complexity of human illness in most instances arises from a wide range of genetic, metabolic, behavioral, and environmental risk factors.[27] In thinking about FMS, it is useful to consider it, at least in part, as a psychogenic disorder. Psychogenic symptoms are those that arise by action of the unconscious mind. For such disorders, "there is nothing imaginary or simulated about the patient's perception of his or her illness. Although the symptom may be psychogenic, the pain or the grinding fatigue is very real."[37] In a recent article, the distinguished oncologist and author Groopman,[20] who did not consider himself "suggestible," describes his development of pain following an incorrect diagnosis of multiple metastases. "After the incident with the deceptive bone scan," he wrote, "I experienced how powerful the mind can be in generating bodily symptoms." Psychogenic pain does not imply a psychological or psychiatric disorder. FMS exists as a psychogenic group illness in which people with high levels of PSD band together in what may be called organized distress. They share common beliefs, economic and political goals, and supporters.

There is a conceptual link between the organized distress of FMS and MSI. MSI is a "constellation of symptoms suggestive of organic illness, but without an identifiable cause, that occurs between two or more people who share beliefs related to those symptoms."[6] "It mirrors prominent social concerns, changing in relation to context and circumstance that typically indicates the presence of psychogenic symptoms." However, "there is no particular predisposition to mass sociogenic illness and it is a behavioural reaction that anyone can show in the right circumstances." MSIs are usually short-lived, but can be precursors to long-term illnesses. With respect to FMS, an important MSI was known as Royal Free Disease in 1955,[31] which seems to have been the initiator of "benign myalgic encephalomyelitis" (also known as chronic fatigue or chronic fatigue syndrome), which in turn is related to FMS in common symptoms and overlapping diagnoses, beliefs, and political and social goals. MSIs represent "psychic epidemics,"—"an illness attribution that spreads epidemically, then is forgotten."[35]

Although there has been some change in society's view of FMS, many, perhaps most people believe it to be a "psychological" illness. Psychological differs from psychogenic. In this setting, "psychological" is an epithet: Psychological illnesses are "not real," "in the head," "self induced," associated with mental disease; and persons with them can be thought of as undeserving, not worthy, malingerers, or worse.[43] FMS is in part a "contested" disorder because of this potential link with psychological illness.[14] Often, such incorrect concerns are not always wrong, as they are compounded by the repeated observation of increased levels of psychological and psychogenic symptoms and the increased proportion of diagnosed psychological disease in those with FMS.[7,30] FMS has extremely low prestige among physicians.[1,21] It also comes under attack because it "has no binding definition . . . and no way of objectively testing for it."[34] With respect to causation and severity, "I am the evidence" rules among those with the disorder.[16] Persons with FMS ask others to believe them with regard to severity and consequences that cannot be validated externally. Writing of beliefs about "neurasthenics," Wessely, citing literature, described them this way: "Patients were 'the terror of the busy physician,' 'occupied by their symptoms beyond reason,' 'going from physician to physician,' where they 'write down their sensations in long memoranda which they hasten to read and to explain."[46] Almost the same phrases could be used to describe some FMS patients.[32]

Using neurasthenia as the model ("once neurasthenia was viewed as psychiatric, a principal social function was lost. . . . and it "disappeared"[45]), FMS should have disappeared, too. Instead, it became a movement of organized distress.[3,19] From the patients' perspective, the goals of the movement were to demonstrate that the (a) symptoms were real, not psychological, (b) FMS was a "disease"—a real disease, (c) organic based on neurobiologic abnormalities, (d) worthy of receiving disability benefits, and (e) worthy of respect.[14] To accomplish these goals, patient organizations were formed. Using Internet and print-based tools,[4,5,12,26] patient groups influenced legislators, media, professional physician organizations, and the US National Institutes of Health, and they were successful in obtaining funding from pharmaceutical companies. In addition to patient organizations, the activities of pharmaceutical companies and physician groups and research physicians played an important role in legitimizing the disorder.[3,15] The rise and dominance of the Internet led to the easy access and internationalization of medical information and publications. Thus, it became possible that research and treatments that were not available or allowed in some countries to become widely disseminated and influential.

The benefit of FMS diagnosis to patients with FMS symptoms is to assert the organicity and realness of their disorder, and to oppose the demeaning characterizations noted previously. For such patients, FMS, spreading by imitation, is a desirable diagnosis.[18] A key measure of success of the movement was the recruitment of patients into the diagnosis. Because pain and symptoms can be characterized by many different diagnoses, the goal of advocates was to get patients and physicians to adopt the FMS diagnosis rather than to use other diagnostic explanations. There is evidence that they have been successful. For example, the prevalence of FMS among US military families rose with "the advent of federally approved drugs for FMS in concert with pharmaceutical industry marketing of these drugs . . . relative to IBS and CFS."[25] Walitt et al.[40,41] showed recently that most patients diagnosed with FMS in the US general population would probably not satisfy current FMS criteria. From malleable and unverifiable criteria in the community together with extensive "disease mongering" advertising, several persons with the diagnosis has been rising rather than falling, as might have been expected on the basis of historical models. Another success has been gaining at least partial acceptance of the diagnosis and its largely unverifiable symptoms and symptom severity by government and insurance agencies.

The intervention of pharmaceutical companies was a hugely important factor in the sustenance and growth of FMS. In support of the drug cyclobenzaprine, Merck began educational programs in the United States in 1985. The 1986 supplement publication of multiple research and concept articles in the then prestigious American Journal of Medicine—distributed freely to physicians, together with holidays and lecture programs at multiple resort sites provided major impetus to the growth of FMS that "would probably have remained on the fringe . . . if it were it not for [this] initiative."[22]

In 2007, Pfizer gained U.S. Food and Drug Administration (FDA) approval for using pregabalin for FMS treatment, and began extensive advertising, including daily pervasive direct-to-patient advertising. Pregabalin (and other putative FMS drugs) did not gain approval in Europe. Although at a much more limited level than in the United States and Japan, off-label use of "FMS drug" or a related diagnosis became common in Europe and other locations.[13,47] Although direct-to-patient advertising was not allowed in Europe and many other locations, access to patients was accomplished in "patient journals" and popular magazines.

Daily pervasive direct-to-patient advertising in the United States attracted those who might satisfy FMS criteria but are undiagnosed, but also those who are undiagnosed and would never satisfy FMS criteria—those identified in the Walitt et al.[40,41] studies. Extensive advertising in medical journals and grants to professional medical organizations and physicians inform and influence physicians to acknowledge and "understand" the diagnosis and to prescribe treatment for it. There is a conflicted relationship between pharmaceutical companies (Pfizer, in particular) and many FMS research physicians. Pfizer sponsors and helps with the writing and text for research and popular articles on FMS, often calling attention to the many "undiagnosed" patients.[2,10] "This concise review was developed by the FibroCollaborative, a diverse group of leading experts on FMS, to provide practical guidance regarding the current understanding of FMS pathophysiology and how it relates to FMS symptomatology, diagnosis, and management approaches."[10] Their financial and organizational sponsorship of the international "FibroCollaborative" led to the recruitment of physicians worldwide and initiated publications and advertising. Pmlive.com wrote, "Pfizer maintains lead in top CNS drug sales. Pfizer's number one spot is predominately from the blockbuster sales of its pain drug Lyrica (pregabalin), which saw $5.1 bn worth of revenue last year—a 12% jump on 2013." The influence of pharma on the growth and sustenance of FMS cannot be underestimated.

FMS, itself, has spawned a huge number of "research" and popular articles in a way that would not have been possible before the Internet era. Although many publications about FMS are of high quality, many are not. In recent years, there have been about 600 scientific publications annually that address FMS. Most compare patients with FMS with normal controls. However, comparing one end of the continuum with the other end ("normals" vs. FMS) almost always leads to statistically significant results. In fact, every feeling, symptom, physical finding, neuroscience measure, cost, and outcome will be worse in studies of this sort.[54] In addition, given FMS's position at the end of the spectrum, descriptive studies abound. Because such studies are so easy, publications proliferate and with them a drumbeat that suggests wide acceptance of FMS.

FMS today is sustained by pharmaceutical advertising and research physician advocates of FMS as a neurobiologic disease. There has been a recent tendency to further extend the definition of FMS. Some articles speak of subclinical, pre-FMS, or incomplete FMS,[9,29,55] and one major FMS research center wrote, "FMS is the current term for chronic widespread musculoskeletal pain for which no alternative cause can be identified."[38] These efforts vastly enlarge the diagnostic domain of FMS. It remains to be seen if this weakening of the FMS definition will swing the pendulum back somewhat from an organic disease to one based more on human complexity and a wide range of genetic, metabolic, behavioral, and environmental risk factors, perhaps leading to some patients leaving the diagnosis.

REFERENCES

1. Album D, Johannessen LE, Rasmussen EB. Stability and change in disease prestige: a comparative analysis of three surveys spanning a quarter of a century. *Soc Sci Med.* 2017;**180**:45–51.
2. Arnold LM, Clauw DJ, McCarberg BH; FibroCollaborative. Improving the recognition and diagnosis of fibromyalgia. *Mayo Clin Proc.* 2011;**86**(5):457–464.
3. Barker KK. Listening to Lyrica: contested illnesses and pharmaceutical determinism. *Soc Sci Med.* 2011;**73**(6):833–842.
4. Barker KK. Electronic support groups, patient-consumers, and medicalization: the case of contested illness. *J Health Soc Behav.* 2008;**49**(1):20–36.
5. Bolwijn PH, van Santen-Hoeufft MH, Baars HM, Kaplan CD, van der Linden S. The social network characteristics of fibromyalgia patients compared with healthy controls. *Arthritis Care Res.* 1996;**9**(1):18–26.
6. Boss LP. Epidemic hysteria: a review of the published literature. *Epidemiol Rev.* 1997;**19**(2):233–243.
7. Brown D, Mulvey M, Cordingley L, et al. The relationship between psychological distress and multiple tender points across the adult lifespan. *Arch Gerontol Geriatr.* 2016;**63**:102–107.
8. Brummett CM, Janda AM, Schueller CM, et al. Survey criteria for fibromyalgia independently predict increased postoperative opioid consumption after lower-extremity joint arthroplasty: a prospective, observational cohort study. *Anesthesiology.* 2013;**119**(6):1434–1443.
9. Brummett CM, Urquhart AG, Hassett AL, et al. Characteristics of fibromyalgia independently predict poorer long-term analgesic outcomes following total knee and hip arthroplasty. *Arthritis Rheumatol.* 2015;**67**(5):1386–1394.
10. Clauw DJ, Arnold LM, McCarberg BH; FibroCollaborative. The science of fibromyalgia. *Mayo Clin Proc.* 2011;**86**(9):907–911.
11. Cohen ML, Quintner JL. The derailment of railway spine: a timely lesson for post-traumatic fibromyalgia syndrome. *Pain Rev.* 1996;**3**:181–202.
12. Conrad P, Stults C. The internet and the experience of illness. *Handbook Med Sociol.* 2010;**6**:179–191.
13. Di Franco M, Iannuccelli C, Atzeni F, et al. Pharmacological treatment of fibromyalgia. *Clin Exp Rheumatol.* 2010;**28**(6 Suppl 63):S110–S116.
14. Dumit J. Illnesses you have to fight to get: facts as forces in uncertain, emergent illnesses. *Soc Sci Med.* 2006;**62**(3):577–590.
15. Edgar A. The dominance of big pharma: power. *Med Health Care Philos.* 2013;**16**(2):295–304.
16. Ehrlich GE. Pain is real; fibromyalgia isn't. *J Rheumatol.* 2003;**30**(8):1666–1667.
17. Ferrari R, Shorter E. From railway spine to whiplash—the recycling of nervous irritation. *Med Sci Monit.* 2003;**9**(11):HY27–HY37.
18. Ford CV. Somatization and fashionable diagnoses: illness as a way of life. *Scand J Work Environ Health.* 1997;**23(Suppl 3)**:7–16.
19. Grob GN. The rise of fibromyalgia in 20th-century America. *Perspect Biol Med.* 2011;**54**(4):417–437.
20. Groopman J. Sick but not sick. *New York Rev Books.* 2017;**64**(2). http://www.nybooks.com/articles/2017/02/09/sick-but-not-sick/. Accessed December 12, 2017.
21. Grue J, Johannessen LE, Rasmussen EF. Prestige rankings of chronic diseases and disabilities. A survey among professionals in the disability field. *Soc Sci Med.* 2015;**124**:180–186.

22. Hadler NM, Greenhalgh S. Labeling woefulness: the social construction of fibromyalgia. *Spine*. 2005;**30**(1):1–4.
23. Hazemeijer I, Rasker JJ. Fibromyalgia and the therapeutic domain. A philosophical study on the origins of fibromyalgia in a specific social setting. *Rheumatology*. 2003;**42**(4):507–515.
24. Janda AM, As-Sanie S, Rajala B, et al. Fibromyalgia survey criteria are associated with increased postoperative opioid consumption in women undergoing hysterectomy. *Anesthesiology*. 2015;**122**(5):1103–1111.
25. Jeffery DD, Bulathsinhala L, Kroc M, et al. Prevalence, health care utilization, and costs of fibromyalgia, irritable bowel, and chronic fatigue syndromes in the military health system, 2006–2010. *Mil Med*. 2014;**179**(9):1021–1029.
26. Josefsson U. Coping with illness online: the case of patients' online communities. *Informat Soc*. 2005;**21**(2):133–141.
27. Kendler KS, Zachar P, Craver C. What kinds of things are psychiatric disorders? *Psychol Med*. 2011;**41**(6):1143–1150.
28. Kirmayer LJ, Sartorius N. Cultural models and somatic syndromes. *Psychosom Med*. 2007;**69**(9):832–840.
29. Malin K, Littlejohn GO. Personality and fibromyalgia syndrome. *Open Rheumatol J*. 2012;**6**:273–285.
30. McBeth J, Silman AJ. The role of psychiatric disorders in fibromyalgia. *Curr Rheumatol Rep*. 2001;**3**(2):157–164.
31. McEvedy CP, Beard AW. Royal Free epidemic of 1955: a reconsideration. *Br Med J*. 1970;**1**(5687):7–11.
32. Murphree R. Are they crazy? *American Chiropractor*. 2007;**29**(5):44–46.
33. Perrot S. If fibromyalgia did not exist, we should have invented it. A short history of a controversial syndrome. *Reumatismo*. 2012;**64**(4):186–193.
34. Reed M, Herrmann M. The difficulties in developing and implementing fibromyalgia guidelines. In: *New Insights into Fibromyalgia*. INTECH Open Access Publisher; 2012. http://www.intechopen.com/books/new-insights-into-fibromyalgia. Accessed June 13, 2016.
35. Shorter E. Chronic fatigue in historical perspective. *Ciba Found Symp*. 1993;**173**:6–16; discussion 16.
36. Shorter E. *From the Mind Into the Body: The Cultural Origins of Psychosomatic Symptoms*. New York: Free Press; 1993;**250**.
37. Shorter E. *From Paralysis to Fatigue: A History of Psychosomatic Illness in the Modern Era*. New York: Free Press; 1993;**420**.
38. Sluka KA, Clauw DJ. Neurobiology of fibromyalgia and chronic widespread pain. *Neuroscience*. 2016;**338**:114–129.
39. Tikkinen KA, Leinonen JS, Guyatt GH, et al. What is a disease? Perspectives of the public, health professionals and legislators. *BMJ Open*. 2012;**2**(6):e001632.
40. Walitt B, Katz RS, Bergman MJ, et al. Three-quarters of persons in the US population reporting a clinical diagnosis of fibromyalgia do not satisfy fibromyalgia criteria: the 2012 National Health Interview Survey. *PLoS ONE*. 2016;**11**(6):e0157235.
41. Walitt B, Nahin RL, Katz RS, et al. The prevalence and characteristics of fibromyalgia in the 2012 National Health Interview Survey. *PLoS ONE*. 2015;**10**(9):e0138024.
42. Wallace DJ, Clauw DJ. *Fibromyalgia and Other Central Pain Syndromes*. Philadelphia, PA: Lippincott Williams & Wilkins; 2005.
43. Ware NC. Suffering and the social construction of illness: the delegitimation of illness experience in chronic fatigue syndrome. *Med Anthropol Q*. 1992;**6**(4):347–361.
44. Wessely S, Hotopf M. Is fibromyalgia a distinct clinical entity? Historical and epidemiological evidence. *Baillieres Best Pract Res Clin Rheumatol*. 1999;**13**(3):427–436.
45. Wessely S. Old wine in new bottles: neurasthenia and 'ME'. *Psychol Med*. 1990;**20**(1):35–53.
46. Wessely S. History of postviral fatigue syndrome. *Br Med Bull*. 1991;**47**(4):919–941.
47. Wettermark B, Brandt L, Kieler H, et al. Pregabalin is increasingly prescribed for neuropathic pain, generalised anxiety disorder and epilepsy but many patients discontinue treatment. *Int J Clin Pract*. 2014;**68**(1):104–110.

48. Wolfe F, Brähler E, Hinz A, Häuser W. Fibromyalgia prevalence, somatic symptom reporting, and the dimensionality of polysymptomatic distress: results from a survey of the general population. *Arthritis Care Res.* 2013;**65**(5):777–785.
49. Wolfe F, Clauw DJ, Fitzcharles MA, et al. Fibromyalgia criteria and severity scales for clinical and epidemiological studies: a modification of the ACR Preliminary Diagnostic Criteria for Fibromyalgia. *J Rheumatol.* 2011;**38**(6):1113–1122.
50. Wolfe F, Clauw DJ, Fitzcharles MA, et al. The American College of Rheumatology preliminary diagnostic criteria for fibromyalgia and measurement of symptom severity. *Arthritis Care Res.* 2010;**62**(5):600–610.
51. Wolfe F, Clauw DJ, Fitzcharles MA, et al. 2016 Revisions to the 2010/2011 fibromyalgia diagnostic criteria. *Semin Arthritis Rheum.* 2016;**46**(3):319–329.
52. Wolfe F, Smythe HA, Yunus MB, et al. The American College of Rheumatology 1990 Criteria for the classification of fibromyalgia. Report of the Multicenter Criteria Committee. *Arthritis Rheum.* 1990;**33**(2):160–172.
53. Wolfe F. Fibromyalgia and fibromyalgia criteria: problems in definition and validity. *Pain.* 2017; this issue.
54. Wolfe F. Criteria for fibromyalgia? What is fibromyalgia? Limitations to current concepts of fibromyalgia and fibromyalgia criteria. *Clin Exp Rheumatol.* 2017;**35 Suppl 105**(3):3–5.
55. Yunus MB, Aldag JC. The concept of incomplete fibromyalgia syndrome: comparison of incomplete fibromyalgia syndrome with fibromyalgia syndrome by 1990 ACR classification criteria and its implications for newer criteria and clinical practice. *J Clin Rheumatol.* 2012;**18**(2):71–75.

CHAPTER 3

Fibromyalgia Syndrome and Fibromyalgia Syndrome Criteria: Problems in Definition and Validity

Frederick Wolfe

Summary Points

- Fibromyalgia syndrome (FMS) is an arbitrarily and broadly defined disorder with widespread pain and multiple symptoms that is strongly influenced by culture, context, and social forces.
- Despite well-studied criteria, problems of validity and reliability remain. It is not clear when FMS starts or ends, or what to do with intermediate states.
- Criteria have changed over the years of FMS's existence.
- It is possible that despite criteria, most clinical patients are diagnosed by physicians based on the presence of pain and distressing symptoms rather than by criteria suggested by experts.

Fibromyalgia is, in part, a socially constructed disorder that is composed of symptoms that are common in populations. Its content and use are influenced by societal pressures and belief systems of physicians and patients.[4,18,31,32,40,47] From its onset, different sets of often incompatible criteria of varying degrees of validity and reliability have been used to define the disorder and its patients. The boundaries between FMS and similar disorders can be unclear,[12] and for many patients, it is uncertain when FMS starts or ends.[28] A patient going to a fatigue specialist, a rheumatologist, a psychiatrist, or a generalist may receive different diagnoses for the same set of symptoms, depending on the physician consulted.[1,41] In addition, disorders such as FMS can be shaped by the concepts and criteria we employ to define and classify them.[14] Furthermore, we review the development of criteria for FMS that began in the second half of the 20th century.

CRITERIA DEVELOPMENT AND ALTERATION: MANY CRITERIA SETS, MANY DIFFERENCES (TABLE 3.1)

From the 19th century through the early years of the 20th century, patients with what we now call FMS would probably have received a diagnosis of neurasthenia, as the multiplicity and content of symptoms associated with FMS fit within the concept of neurasthenia.[40] However, with the collapse and general abandonment of neurasthenia in the 1920s because it was perceived as being "psychiatric,"[42] what was to become modern FMS necessitated reinvention. By the end of World War II (WW2), and under the name "fibrositis,"[17] three overlapping concepts contended in the clinic: (a) local or regional musculoskeletal pain, (b) generalized musculoskeletal symptoms, and (c) what was called "psychogenic rheumatism." Freyberg,[16] perhaps the dominant US expert on nonarticular rheumatism and fibrositis, reflected ideas of the times when he wrote in 1951 that "psychogenic rheumatism" was a common form of nonarticular rheumatism. It was caused by "psychic trauma, fear, anxiety, apprehension or sorrow which led to arthralgia, muscle and tendon pain, stiffness and interference with joint motion resembling common forms of arthritis or fibrositis . . . It may be difficult to differentiate psychogenic rheumatism from fibrositis." Almost 60 years later, Kroenke,[23] writing on somatic symptom disorders, touched on the same issue: "the real divide . . . centers on the role of psychologic factors."

Fibrositis gradually gained prominence as the de facto generalized pain disorder largely because of the development of the new medical specialty of rheumatology—a specialty for which generalized fibrositis seemed designed. Clinicians could refer patients with generalized pain to rheumatology specialists, while those with local and regional musculoskeletal disorders were sent to orthopedic and physical medicine specialists. Ownership of FMS became more certain when rheumatologists renamed fibrositis as FMS in the 1970s and 1980s,[21] and in 1990 established the American College of Rheumatology (ACR) criteria for FMS.[50] The specter of psychogenic rheumatism was absorbed into FMS under the vigorously defended assertion that FMS was not a psychological disorder and that most psychological symptoms were secondary, not causative phenomena.[6] From the post-WW2 period through the 1970s, FMS was seen as a disorder of muscular ache and pain that was associated with multiple symptoms.[36] This conception of FMS would not change and was largely reformulated into the quantifiable Yunus criteria of 1981,[54] and further modified into the 2010/2011/2016 criteria of the 21st century.[47,45,46] Widespread (almost total body) pain was a common feature, but was not a necessary part of the definition. We can define this type of criteria broadly as substantial but not total body pain, together with many physical and psychological symptoms.

From the somewhat vague definition started in the 1950s, there were problems defining FMS and its boundaries. Many did not believe that FMS was a real (medical)

TABLE 3.1 Historical and current fibromyalgia syndrome criteria

Year	Reference	Widespread pain	Symptoms	Tender points	Items and new (N) items added by these criteria
19th to early 20th century	Neurasthenia[42]	Not required	Multiple	Not required	Many symptoms, including pain. Many would have satisfied fibromyalgia syndrome criteria
<1977	Freyberg, Traut[16,36]	Not required	Multiple	Not required	Ill-defined disorder of muscular aching and pain that was associated with multiple, various symptoms
1977	Smythe and Moldofsky[43]	Not required	Sleep + fatigue + morning stiffness	≥12 of 14	Simultaneous sleep disturbance, morning stiffness, and fatigue (N) Tender points (N)
1980–1989	Ad hoc modifications	Not required	Multiple	< "≥12 of 14"	Modification of Kroenke[23] to include symptoms and reduced tender point count
1981	Yunus[54]	Not required	Multiple	≥3	Multiple symptoms (N), trade-off of symptoms, and painful regions (N)
1990	ACR 1990[50]	Required	None	≥11 of 18	Tender points and widespread pain (N)
2010	ACR 2010[45]	Not required	Moderate-to-high symptom and painful site score	Not required	Multiple symptoms. PSD scale (N)
2011	Modified ACR 2011[46]	Not required	Moderate-to-high symptom and painful site score	Not required	Multiple symptoms. PSD scale, self-report version
2016	Modified ACR[47]	Required	Moderate-to-high symptom and painful site score	Not required	Multiple symptoms. PSD scale, self-report version, generalized pain (N)
2016	Clinical practice[37,38]	Not required	Yes	Unknown, probably not	National Health Interview Survey (NHIS) data compared to surrogate 2011 criteria. See text.

ACR, American College of Rheumatology; PSD, polysymptomatic distress scale.

disorder (a "condition for which individuals do not bear primary responsibility, afflictions of which the sufferer is at least to some extent a victim"),[36] a belief that still exists. Formal criteria that had scientific reliability were needed and appeared first with the 1977 publication of the semiquantitative criteria of Smythe and Moldofsky.[34] FMS diagnosis with these criteria required the presence of "widespread aching for longer than three months" and "disturbed sleep with morning fatigue and stiffness." However, none of these characteristics was defined in a measurable way, and their presence and severity through most of the history of FMS were, like beauty, in the eye of the beholder. Interestingly, sleep problems become a major defining characteristic of FMS from this time on (Moldofsky was a psychiatrist with a major interest in sleep), even though they were not mentioned by Freyberg[16] or were not an important symptom to neurasthenia physicians.[30] Smythe and Moldofsky provided one key quantitative measure that gave impetus to and was central to FMS, even to this day: tender points. Patients who "had" FMS were more sensitive (tender) to finger (digital) pressure than those without FMS; and a high count of tender points, which established this "decreased pain threshold" (or increased sensitivity to pain), became the central diagnostic criterion for FMS. To meet the Smythe and Moldofsky criteria, all four symptoms and the tender point criterion had to be satisfied. Soon thereafter, a clinical quantitative measure of pain threshold became available, the dolorimeter,[27] which confirmed decreased pain threshold in FMS. However, this more objective method, which removed the physician's opinion from the quantitation of pain threshold, never proved to be useful for diagnosis because it was insensitive and lacked discriminatory capabilities.[47,52] The malleable tender point count[27] that combined objectivity with physician and patient subjectivity was far superior in distinguishing those with from those without FMS and was clearly influenced by the patient–physician interview interaction performed before the tender point examination.[47] The Smythe and Moldofsky[34] 1977 paper was cited 424 times by the end of 2016, but the criteria it proposed were never used in clinical research, serving primarily an educational purpose that would stimulate further research.

Over the next decade, many researchers variously and arbitrarily modified the Smythe and Moldofsky FMS definition to require fewer tender points, as the original requirement (11 of 14 tender points) was too restrictive and failed to detect most cases of apparent FMS.[6] In 1990, the ACR published the influential "classification criteria" for FMS.[50] To have FMS, one needed to have at least 11 of 18 possible tender points *and* the presence of "widespread pain." Widespread pain, an ad hoc assessment of four-quadrant body pain, was added to the definition to make epidemiologic screening easier, but could have been eliminated with a less than 1% reduction in diagnostic accuracy. FMS was effectively established and characterized by tender points. Although alternative "preliminary" ACR criteria that did not use tender points were published 20 years later in 2010,[45] the 1990 criteria were not revoked by the ACR and remain "valid" and in force. The 1990 criteria were accepted by medical, regulatory, and educational authorities and had widespread influence. Thus, to get a diagnosis and medication, qualify for FMS-related disability benefits, prevail in lawsuits, and establish *bona fides* of being ill, one had to have 11 tender points. It was as simple and complex as that.

In contrast to the Smythe–Moldofsky 1977 paper in which all patients were required to have "disturbed sleep with morning fatigue and stiffness," the 1990 ACR paper noted the reality that each symptom was present in more than 75% of FMS patients, but, "only 56% of patients had all 3 symptoms, and 81% had 2 of the 3. . . . This 'consensus' definition differs from some previous definitions in that it recognizes that symptoms of sleep disturbance, fatigue, and stiffness may not all be present in patients with FMS." By the end of 2016, the ACR paper[50] had been cited more than 8,000 times.

Between the Smythe and Moldofsky 1977 criteria and the official ACR criteria of 1990, there was one other formal set of criteria, that of Yunus. From 1980 through 1990, when the ACR criteria were published, the Yunus criteria were very influential and were the de facto FMS criteria, being cited more than 1,000 times by the end of 2016.[54] These criteria presented a somewhat different idea of FMS. Following Traut,[16] Yunus required the "presence of generalized aches and pains or prominent stiffness involving 3 or more sites." There could be as few as three positive tender points. Yunus's "minor criteria" included "(A) modulation of symptoms by physical activity, (B) modulation of symptoms by weather factors, (C) aggravation of symptoms by anxiety or stress, (D) poor sleep, (E) general fatigue or tiredness, (F) anxiety, (G) chronic headache, (H) irritable bowel syndrome, (I) subjective swelling, and (J) numbness." Symptoms were balanced with tender points, and patients with few tender points required more symptoms. In comparison with the ACR 1990 criteria, the Yunus criteria could be characterized as having fewer tender points, more limited pain, and more symptoms. More importantly, the criteria admitted to the FMS diagnosis a nonhomogenous group of patients who varied in the number of tender points, the amount of pain, and the number and kind of symptoms—like the pre-1977 definition described earlier and the 2010 criteria that would follow.

In 2010, the ACR published "preliminary diagnostic criteria for FMS."[45] These criteria, based on an analysis of symptoms in FMS and non-FMS patients, included symptoms, but not tender points. The 2010 criteria required the physician to elicit and interpret the symptoms in order to make a diagnosis. "'Fibro fog', relabeled as cognitive difficulties, was [also] incorporated into the 2010 ACR FMS criteria. Prior to 1990, [however,] only one 'hit' [was] noted for fibro fog in a Google search, and the decade of the 1990s produced 104 hits. However, the next 10 years added 13,800 results."[51] The criteria required the physician to quantitate the degree of somatic symptom reporting, "Considering somatic symptoms in general, indicate whether the patient has (no) (few) (moderate) (a great deal) of symptoms." Although increased

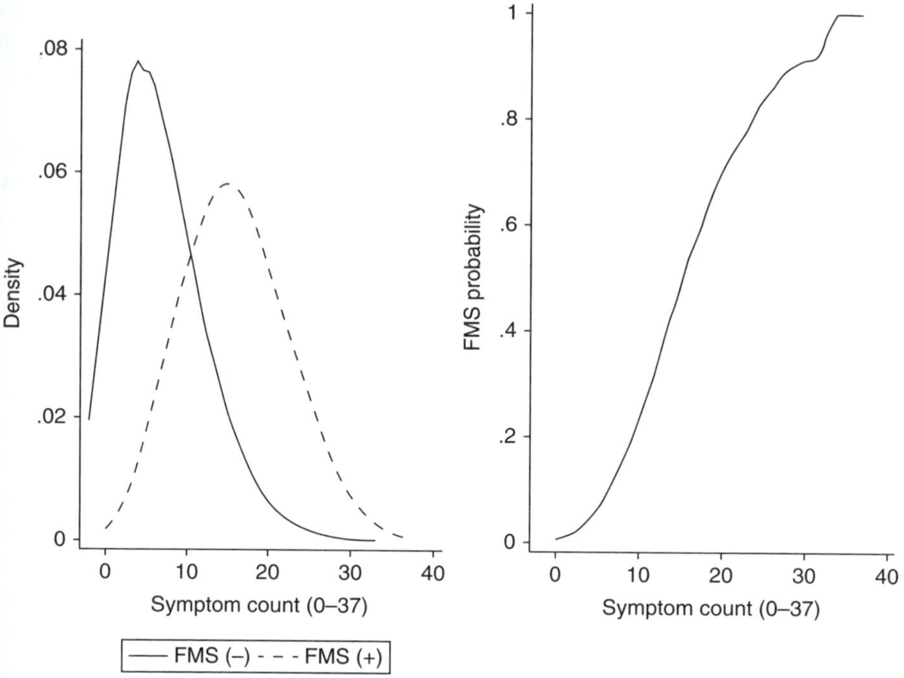

FIGURE 3.1 The distribution of the number of symptoms in 16,987 persons with mixed rheumatic disease who satisfy or do not satisfy 2016 FMS criteria (*left graph*) and predictive probability of FMS based on symptom count (*right graph*). FMS, fibromyalgia syndrome.

symptom reporting was always inherent in previous definitions of FMS, it had never been a specific part of a criteria set. Figure 3.1, using data from the National Data Bank for Rheumatic Diseases,[49] demonstrates the distribution and predictive value of a count of symptoms. It is likely that increased symptom reporting is a key identifying variable for primary care physicians. A self-report version of the 2010 criteria to be used for research was published in 2011,[46] and was further refined and modified in 2016.[47] By 2017, the 2010 criteria had been cited 1,642 times and the 2011 criteria 462 times.

The 2010/2011/2016 (2010+) criteria also included what has been called the polysymptomatic distress (PSD) scale, which was formed by summing the scores for self-reported painful regions (the *widespread pain index* [*WPI*]) and the self-reported symptom scores (*the symptom severity scale*). The PSD scale ranged from 0 to 31. A score ≥12 generally identified patients who satisfied FMS diagnostic criteria. The PSD functioned as a (the) latent continuous FMS variable (sometimes called fibromyalgianess).[10,53] Subsequent research with the PSD demonstrated that there was no distinct cutoff between FMS and "not FMS," and that FMS symptoms occur, in varying degrees, in all patients with pain. The idea that patients either have or do not have FMS is a convenient, but an incorrect understanding of the nature of the FMS and FMS symptoms. The 2016 criteria modification urged physicians to look at PSD scores as well as specific criteria.

In addition to the four criteria sets cited earlier, one study from the United States suggests that physicians may not use or use correctly any of the criteria cited previously. Using surrogate FMS criteria, Walitt et al.[37,38] analyzed the 2012 National Health Interview Survey (NHIS) and found that three-fourths of persons reporting a diagnosis of FMS did not satisfy the criteria. If these data are true generally, then FMS diagnosis extends haphazardly and in an ad hoc way, perhaps due to social pressure and extensive pharmaceutical company advertising,[4,22] to many persons with less symptomatic distress.

Although the ACR 1990 and the 2010+ criteria represent "official" criteria, by 2017, several other trends were noted. PSD scale data led to the acknowledgment that FMS symptoms represented a continuum.[51,44] In response, some articles began to speak of subclinical, pre-FMS, or incomplete FMS.[8,24,55] A major FMS research center wrote, "FMS is the current term for chronic widespread musculoskeletal pain for which no alternative cause can be identified."[33] These efforts vastly enlarge the diagnostic domain of FMS. Subclinical or pre-FMS is an incontestable, ipse dixit diagnosis, while conflating "chronic widespread pain" with FMS increases the overall prevalence of FMS from 2% to 4% to ≥11%.

In summary, the clinical definition of FMS based on criteria has changed repeatedly since its description as a generalized pain disorder in the mid-20th century, and symptoms and physical signs have been added and subtracted. Two general types of criteria are apparent. The first set relies on tender points that "[have] been largely responsible for defining a group of patients who display hyperalgesia and allodynia. These constructs have been extremely useful in attempting to elucidate the mechanisms operative in FMS."[27,7,29,56] The second set of criteria has been purely descriptive, relying on symptoms. The prototypes for this type of criteria are the Yunus et al.[54] and the 2010+ criteria.[47,45,46] These criteria have allowed low tender point counts and/or less than widespread pain, and have stressed patient symptoms.

New criteria items that have been introduced since the start of FMS include sleep disturbance, tender points, cognitive problems, and somatic symptom severity. Evidence suggests that community physicians do not use, or use correctly, published criteria, with the result that most patients receiving the diagnosis of FMS would not satisfy the criteria.[37,38] This trend may reflect extensive advertising and disease mongering by pharma,[4,3,9] as well as indicating that there is a separate community definition of FMS (pain and distress) that is widely used.[37,38] Current trends are strongly influenced by pharma, in its efforts to increase the number of persons adopting the FMS diagnosis.

PROBLEMS WITH FIBROMYALGIA SYNDROME AND FIBROMYALGIA SYNDROME DIAGNOSIS

There Is No Gold Standard for Fibromyalgia Syndrome

There have been two formal attempts at providing a gold standard for FMS that would allow a consistent, valid, and reliable definition. In the 1990 ACR criteria study, 16 physicians provided 135 cases of primary FMS and 135 control cases. The characteristics of these patients formed the basis of the de facto case definition of FMS. The physicians were deeply influenced by the Smythe–Moldofsky paper, and it should be no surprise that tender points were effective in diagnosing FMS because physicians referring cases to the study relied on tender points for their clinical diagnoses. But, the widely used (before 1990) 1981 Yunus criteria and the ACR 1990 criteria did not and could not identify the same cases.[54,50] It seems clear that the de facto definition of FMS (widespread pain and multiple tender points) that came out of the 1990 study could have been different, and other physicians/investigators with different patients might well have resulted in different criteria. Who is to say that the Yunus criteria did not identify FMS patients? If patients supplied to the 1990 criteria study had been referred using the Yunus criteria, it is certain that the 1990 criteria would have been very different. At a distance, the 1981 Yunus criteria that deemphasized tender points and emphasized symptoms have important resemblances to the ACR 2010 criteria.

The 2010 criteria attempted a definition of FMS that was based on the clinical features of serial patients from the practices of expert rheumatologists. To decide which symptoms worked best, the 1990 criteria were used as the gold standard. Thus, although the implicit definition of FMS of the 2010+ criteria was broader with respect to symptoms, it was still based on the arbitrary 1990 criteria.

The Walitt et al.[37] NHIS study of 2016, which showed that ~75% of persons with a physician diagnosis of FMS did not satisfy surrogate 2010+ criteria, can be interpreted in several ways. One interpretation is that community physicians do a poor job at diagnosis, but another interpretation is that the definition of FMS in the community is different from official expert diagnosis. "I don't know how to define FMS, but I know it when I see it," may be the default definition in the community.[a] "Pain, fatigue, and many complaints" may be a more accurate definition of FMS in the community than the nuanced criteria of specialist medicine.

Subsequent ad hoc attempts to broaden the definition of FMS by equating it to widespread pain, regional FMS, or subclinical FMS further underscore the problem of FMS definition.[8,24,33] Because criteria for disorders without a gold standard act to

---

[a] In the United States, the "I know it when I see it" standard derives from the famous statement about pornography made by the Supreme Court justice (*Jacobellis v. Ohio, 378 U.S. 184* (1964)).

define the disorder rather than to identify a defined disorder, the disorder content is always at the mercy of the criteria definers. The history of FMS indicates that criteria have been used in a nominalist way—"constructs that humans create to bring order to a disorderly world."[35] An essentialist-based approach to definition and criteria would consider FMS as a disease and seek evidence from neurobiologic investigation processes that might "cause" FMS. To date, there has been no criteria study meeting minimal scientific standards that has used this approach. Finally, criteria or not, many physicians do not believe that FMS is a legitimate disease. This concern has been approached uniquely by Tikkinen; the case against FMS has been detailed by others.[13,19,20]

The Validity and Reliability of Fibromyalgia Syndrome Criteria Items Are Questionable

The 1990 criteria were difficult to use, requiring training, practice, and interest that were usually absent from the nonspecialist medical evaluation. Even "expert" examinations had problems, as illustrated by the following exchange on an Internet chat group.

> "Ohanamama: Yes, you have to have the tender points. The key is finding a doctor who is good enough at finding them. I've seen 6-7 rheumatologists in my health career, and only one has been good enough at it to find just about all 18 of them . . . I'd leave other doctor's offices and they we're hard pressed to find four or five. So yes, you really do have to have them, and you'll find that a few of them are really obvious, but to get the diagnostic 11, you need a good doctor." In reply, "I agree with ohanamama, yes you have to have the tender points. Before being sent to my Rheumy by my internist, he tried to find the tender points and only found 6, but he told me that he wasn't trained to in doing them. The very first visit with my Rheumy, he found 16 of the 18 points."[26]

In addition to the difficulty in the performance of the tender point count, the validity and reliability of tender points are questionable. Measurement error, difficulty in the performance of the tender point examination, and subjective contribution of physicians and patients lead to reduced reliability and validity.[47] Available data show reliability coefficients of ≤0.71 for the tender point examination; and the examination is not objective and unbiased, as it almost always occurs after, and is influenced by, a patient interview. The 2010 criteria depend on physician interpretation, and the self-report 2010+ criteria can be problematic for use in the individual patient, while being useful for research investigations.[48] The measurement error inherent in the 2010+ criteria is such that they may not be able to reliably distinguish cases from controls near the diagnostic borderline.[48]

When Does Fibromyalgia Syndrome Begin and End?

FMS diagnostic criteria are based on reaching a sufficient level of symptom severity. However, persons with FMS may have many symptoms and multiple interactions with physicians for years before FMS is diagnosed.[28,39,43] If FMS is an entity, how should the patient's state before satisfying FMS criteria be defined? As a somatic symptom disorder?[23,5] Some have labeled it as subclinical, pre-FMS or incomplete FMS.[8,24,55] A similar conundrum exists if a patient with FMS "improves" or has fewer symptoms and, therefore, does not meet criteria anymore. Once FMS always FMS? Perhaps, if stressful states regularly lead to criteria-positive FMS, which may then remit. A number of studies have reported that one-third of patients diagnosed with FMS do not meet criteria on follow-up examinations, including the ACR 2010 criteria study.[46]

Fibromyalgia Syndrome Cannot Be Distinguished From Other Similar Disorders

Investigators coming from a background of somatic symptom disorders tend to see FMS as a non-separate somatic symptom disorder,[15] or at least a somatic symptom disorder in which musculoskeletal symptoms predominate in comparison with other somatic symptom disorders. FMS adherents more often consider FMS as primarily a pain disorder rather than being part of the somatoform family, and the model of neurobiologic causation fits better with the idea of amplified pain than it does with somatic symptoms.[10] However, (lifelong) multiple symptoms are one of the most distinguishing features of FMS. FMS is often similar to or indistinguishable from chronic fatigue (syndrome)[2,11,25] and overlaps with many other disorders.[57]

Fibromyalgia Syndrome May Not Be Diagnosed Even if Criteria Are Met

There are other issues. Ehrlich[13] wrote, "When one has tuberculosis, one has tuberculosis, whether or not it is diagnosed. The same is true for cancer, rheumatoid arthritis, hookworm infestation—really, of the gamut of diseases but not for FMS. No one has FMS until it is diagnosed." One of the implications of Ehrlich's statement is that the diagnosis of FMS is discretionary, and that patient-level psychosocial factors and external societal factors influence that discretion. Physicians may choose not to diagnose FMS, and use other terms to characterize FMS symptoms.[47,37]

Fibromyalgia Syndrome as a Continuum

It now seems clear that the diagnosis of FMS versus not FMS is often the result trying to dichotomize a continuous variable, and that a better way of looking at FMS is to use the PDS—a recommendation of the 2016 criteria.

REFERENCES

1. Aaron LA, Buchwald D. A review of the evidence for overlap among unexplained clinical conditions. *Ann Intern Med.* 2001;**134**(9 Pt 2):868–881.
2. Abbi B, Natelson B. Is chronic fatigue syndrome the same illness as fibromyalgia: evaluating the 'single syndrome' hypothesis. *QJM.* 2013;**106**(1):3–9.
3. Amber K, Brooks L, Ference T. Direct to consumer advertising's effect on medical students: the case of fibromyalgia. *Med Teach.* 2013;**35**(11):969–970.
4. Barker KK. Listening to Lyrica: contested illnesses and pharmaceutical determinism. *Soc Sci Med.* 2011;**73**(6):833–842.
5. Bass C, May S. Chronic multiple functional somatic symptoms. *BMJ.* 2002;**325**(7359):323–326.
6. Bennett RM. Fibrositis: misnomer for a common rheumatic disorder. *West J Med.* 1981;**134**:405–413.
7. Bennett RM. Emerging concepts in the neurobiology of chronic pain: evidence of abnormal sensory processing in fibromyalgia. *Mayo ClinProc.* 1999;**74**(4):385–398.
8. Brummett CM, Urquhart AG, Hassett AL, et al. Characteristics of fibromyalgia independently predict poorer long-term analgesic outcomes following total knee and hip arthroplasty. *Arthrit Rheumatol.* 2015;**67**(5):1386–1394.
9. Cetel JS. Disease-branding and drug-mongering: could pharmaceutical industry promotional practices result in tort liability. *Seton Hall L Rev.* 2012;**42**:643.
10. Clauw DJ. Fibromyalgia: a clinical review. *JAMA.* 2014;**311**(15):1547–1555.
11. Clayton EW. Beyond myalgic encephalomyelitis/chronic fatigue syndrome: an IOM report on redefining an illness. *JAMA.* 2015;**313**(11):1101–1102.
12. Dumit J. 7.Illnesses you have to fight to get: facts as forces in uncertain, emergent illnesses. *Soc Sci Med.* 2006;**62**(3):577–590.
13. Ehrlich GE. Pain is real; fibromyalgia isn't. *J Rheumatol.* 2003;**30**(8):1666–1667.
14. Eisenberg L. The social construction of mental illness. *Psychol Med.* 1988;**18**(01):1–9.
15. Fink P, Schroder A. One single diagnosis, bodily distress syndrome, succeeded to capture 10 diagnostic categories of functional somatic syndromes and somatoform disorders. *J Psychosom Res.* 2010;**68**(5):415–426.
16. Freyberg RH. Non-articular rheumatism. *Bull N Y Acad Med.* 1951;**27**(4):245–258.
17. Gowers WR. A lecture on lumbago: its lessons and analogues. *Br Med J.* 1904;**1**(2246):117–121.
18. Hadler NM, Greenhalgh S. Labeling woefulness: the social construction of fibromyalgia. *Spine.* 2005;**30**(1):1–4.
19. Hadler NM. "Fibromyalgia" and the medicalization of misery. *J Rheumatol.* 2003;**30**(8):1668–1670.
20. Hazemeijer I, Rasker JJ. Fibromyalgia and the therapeutic domain. A philosophical study on the origins of fibromyalgia in a specific social setting. *Rheumatology.* 2003;**42**(4):507–515.
21. Hench PK. Nonarticular rheumatism, 22nd rheumatism review: review of the American and English literature for the years 1973 and 1974. *Arthritis Rheum.* 1976;**19**(Suppl):1081–1089.
22. Jeffery DD, Bulathsinhala L, Kroc M, Dorris J. Prevalence, health care utilization, and costs of fibromyalgia, irritable bowel, and chronic fatigue syndromes in the military health system, 2006–2010. *Mil Med.* 2014;**179**(9):1021–1029.
23. Kroenke K. Somatoform disorders and recent diagnostic controversies. *Psychiatr Clin North Am.* 2007;**30**(4):593–619.
24. Malin K, Littlejohn GO. Personality and fibromyalgia syndrome. *Open Rheumatol J.* 2012;**6**(1):273–285.
25. Meeus M, Ickmans K, Struyf F, et al. What is in a name? Comparing diagnostic criteria for chronic fatigue syndrome with or without fibromyalgia. *Clin Rheumatol.* 2016;**35**(1):191–203.
26. Ohanamoma. Fibromyalgia tender points. 2009. http://www.medhelp.org/posts/Fibromyalgia/Fibro-w-out-tender-points/show/931836.
27. Petzke F, Gracely RH, Park KM, Ambrose K, Clauw DJ. What do tender points measure? Influence of distress on 4 measures of tenderness. *J Rheumatol.* 2003;**30**(3):567–574.

28. Rief W, Rojas G. Stability of somatoform symptoms—implications for classification. *Psychosom Med.* 2007;**69**(9):864–869.
29. Russell I. Neurochemical pathogenesis of fibromyalgia. *Z Rheumatol.* 1998;**57**(2):S63–S66.
30. Sharpley A, Clements A, Hawton K, Sharpe M. Do patients with "pure" chronic fatigue syndrome (neurasthenia) have abnormal sleep? *Psychosom Med.* 1997;**59**(6):592–596.
31. Shorter E. *From the Mind Into the Body: The Cultural Origins of Psychosomatic Symptoms.* New York, NY: Free Press; 1994.
32. Shorter E. *From Paralysis to Fatigue: A History of Psychosomatic Illness in the Modern Era.* New York, NY: Simon and Schuster; 2008.
33. Sluka KA, Clauw DJ. Neurobiology of fibromyalgia and chronic widespread pain. *Neuroscience.* 2016:**338**:114–129.
34. Smythe HA, Moldofsky H. Two contributions to understanding of the "fibrositis" syndrome. *Bull Rheum Dis.* 1977;**28**:928–931.
35. Tikkinen KA, Leinonen JS, Guyatt GH, Ebrahim S, Järvinen T. What is a disease? Perspectives of the public, health professionals and legislators. *BMJ Open.* 2012;**2**(6):e001632.
36. Traut EF. Fibrositis. *J Am Geriatr Soc.* 1968;**16**:531–538.
37. Walitt B, Katz RS, Bergman MJ, Wolfe F. Three-quarters of persons in the US population reporting a clinical diagnosis of fibromyalgia do not satisfy fibromyalgia criteria: the 2012 National Health Interview Survey. *PLoS One.* 2016;**11**(6):e0157235.
38. Walitt B, Nahin RL, Katz RS, Bergman MJ, Wolfe F. The prevalence and characteristics of fibromyalgia in the 2012 National Health Interview Survey. *PLoS One.* 2015;**10**(9):e0138024.
39. Wallace DJ. What constitutes a fibromyalgia expert? *Arthrit Care Res.* 1999;**12**(2):82–84.
40. Wessely S, Hotopf M. Is fibromyalgia a distinct clinical entity? Historical and epidemiological evidence. *Baillieres Best Pract Res Clin Rheumatol.* 1999;**13**(3):427–436.
41. Wessely S, White PD. There is only one functional somatic syndrome. *Br J Psychiat.* 2004;**185**(2): 95–96.
42. Wessely S. Old wine in new bottles: neurasthenia and "M.E.002001D; *Psychol Med.* 1990;**20**:35–53.
43. Wolfe F, Anderson J, Harkness D, et al. A prospective, longitudinal, multicenter study of service utilization and costs in fibromyalgia. *Arthritis Rheum.* 1997;**40**(9):1560–1570.
44. Wolfe F, Brähler E, Hinz A, Häuser W. Fibromyalgia prevalence, somatic symptom reporting, and the dimensionality of polysymptomatic distress: results from a survey of the general population. *Arthitis Care Res.* 2013;**65**(5):777–785.
45. Wolfe F, Clauw D, Fitzcharles MA, et al. The American College of Rheumatology preliminary diagnostic criteria for fibromyalgia and measurement of symptom severity. *Arthritis Care Res.* 2010;**62**(5):600–610.
46. Wolfe F, Clauw D, Fitzcharles MA, et al. Fibromyalgia criteria and severity scales for clinical and epidemiological studies: a modification of the ACR preliminary diagnostic criteria for fibromyalgia. *J Rheumatol.* 2011;**38**:1113–1122.
47. Wolfe F, Clauw DJ, Fitzcharles M-A, et al. 2016 Revisions to the 2010/2011 Fibromyalgia Diagnostic Criteria. *Semin Arthritis Rheum.* 2016;**46**:319–329.
48. Wolfe F, Fitzcharles MA, Goldenberg D, et al. Comparison of physician-based and patient-based criteria for the diagnosis of fibromyalgia. *Arthritis Care Res.* 2016;**68**:652–659.
49. Wolfe F, Michaud K. The National Data Bank for rheumatic diseases: a multi-registry rheumatic disease data bank. *Rheumatology.* 2011;**50**(1):16–24.
50. Wolfe F, Smythe HA, Yunus MB, et al. The American College of Rheumatology 1990 criteria for the classification of fibromyalgia. Report of the Multicenter Criteria Committee. *Arthritis Rheum.* 1990;**33**(2):160–172.
51. Wolfe F, Walitt B. Culture, science and the changing nature of fibromyalgia. *Nat Rev Rheumatol.* 2013;9:751–755.

52. Wolfe F. The relation between tender points and fibromyalgia symptom variables: evidence that fibromyalgia is not a discrete disorder in the clinic. *Ann Rheum Dis*. 1997;**56**(4):268–271.
53. Wolfe F. Fibromyalgianess. *Arthritis Rheum*. 2009;**61**(6):715–716.
54. Yunus M, Masi AT, Calabro JJ, Miller KA, Feigenbaum S. Primary fibromyalgia (fibrositis): clinical study of 50 patients with matched normal controls. *Semin Arthritis Rheum*. 1981;**11**(1):151–171.
55. Yunus MB, Aldag JC. The concept of incomplete fibromyalgia syndrome: comparison of incomplete fibromyalgia syndrome with fibromyalgia syndrome by 1990 ACR classification criteria and its implications for newer criteria and clinical practice. *J Clin Rheumatol*. 2012;**18**(2):71–75.
56. Yunus MB. Towards a model of pathophysiology of fibromyalgia: aberrant central pain mechanisms with peripheral modulation. *J Rheumatol*. 1992;**19**(6):846–850.
57. Yunus MB. Central sensitivity syndromes: a new paradigm and group nosology for fibromyalgia and overlapping conditions, and the related issue of disease versus illness. *Semin Arthritis Rheum*. 2008;**37**(6):339–352.

CHAPTER 4

Chronic Widespread Pain and Fibromyalgia Syndrome—A Difference?

Winfried Häuser and Serge Perrot

Summary Points

- Different definitions of chronic widespread pain (CWP) are used in studies and clinical practice.
- Recent diagnostic criteria of fibromyalgia syndrome (FMS) do not use anymore the American College of Rheumatology 1990 definition of CWP, but criteria of widespreadness or multisite pain.
- There is a continuum of pain sites, somatic and psychological symptoms in the general population.
- FMS can be regarded to be the end of a continuum of somatic and psychological symptom burden (distress).
- People with FMS demonstrate abnormal pain processing: Increased allodynia and evoked pain with a global decrease of pain thresholds related to central sensitization, increased temporal summation, and impaired pain controls.
- In clinical care, the assessment of the amount of somatic and psychological symptom burden in patient with chronic pain is more important than the use of categorical diagnostic categories (CWP with or without FMS).

WHAT IS WIDESPREAD PAIN?

A simple classification of chronic pain is based on several pain sites or pain areas into local pain (one pain site), regional pain (some pain sites in one body area, e.g., right shoulder and right arm), and widespread pain. Interestingly, the question how to define CWP is not definitely answered and different criteria for CWP are used in research and clinical practice.

By the American College of Rheumatology 1990 (ACR 1990) definition, CWP became the fundamental feature of FMS and is defined as pain lasting 3 months or longer, located axially (cervical spine, thoracic spine, anterior chest, or low back), above and below the waist, and on the left and right sides of the body. In this definition, shoulder and buttock pain is considered as pain for each involved side. "Low back" pain is considered as lower segment pain. The 1990 definition, however, is inexact because it does not state which body areas should be included in the body pain assessment. In addition, rare patients who otherwise met the 1990 criteria could satisfy the ACR widespread pain definition with pain in only a few areas. For example, in the axial pain, low back pain and pain in the right hand and left foot would qualify as widespread pain. This occurs because pain in a single site can be expanded to include more than one region, as when right-hand pain is scored for right side and for upper extremity.[19,18]

Another measure of CWP that was frequently used in epidemiology studies, the London Fibromyalgia Epidemiological Study Screening Questionnaire (LFESSQ), defined CWP by pain in four areas: right and left shoulders, arms, or hands, and right and left legs or feet.[13]

Recent diagnostic criteria of FMS avoided the term "CWP." The ACR 2010 preliminary diagnostic criteria[15] and the modified 2011 criteria[16] used the term "widespread pain," which was defined by at least 5 of 19 pain sites in the widespread pain index. The 2016 criteria revision used the term "generalized pain," which requires pain in at least four of five regions. Jaw, chest, and abdominal pain are not included in generalized pain definition.[17] Most recently, the term "multisite pain" defined as the pain in ≥8/≥10 body sites (adults/children) indicated on four-view body manikins was created.[2]

In clinical practice, CWP can be easily identified by pain in all four body quadrants, the neck and back in a pain drawing of the patient.[12]

Prevalence of Chronic Widespread Pain

A systematic review on the prevalence of CWP found that estimates for CWP prevalence ranged from 0% to 24%, with most estimates between 10% and 15%. When only studies at low risk of bias were considered pooled, prevalence increased to 11.8% (95% confidence interval 10.3 to 13.3), with reduced but still high heterogeneity. Prevalence was higher in women and in those aged 40 years and older.[8]

Chronic Widespread Pain or Fibromyalgia Syndrome—Does It Matter?

The prevalence of FMS is lower than the one of CWP. A review reported a global prevalence of FMS as 2.7%. FMS was more prevalent in women, in patients older than 50 years of age, in subjects with low education level, with low socioeconomic status, living in rural areas, and possibly in obese women.[10] In epidemiology studies in the general population, persons with CWP meeting FMS criteria reported more somatic and psychological symptoms and more disability than persons with CWP without meeting FMS criteria. These findings were independent of which criteria for CWP and FMS were used.[2,1,14,6]

In samples of the general population, the number of pain sites is highly associated with the number of somatic and psychological symptoms. Multiple pain sites are associated with higher pain intensity, longer pain duration, and greater disability.[6,7] The clinical distinction of local, regional, and widespread pain with and without FMS was confirmed by a cluster analysis of the number of pain sites, somatic and psychological symptoms in a general population sample.[6]

Based on these findings, CWP with and without FMS can be regarded as separate clinical entities with FMS to be the end of a continuum of somatic and psychological symptom burden (distress).[6] The findings in the general population support that ACR 2010 criteria[15] dispensed with tender point examination and instead used a measure of the widespreadness of pain and a measure of the number of somatic symptoms experienced, such as fatigue and cognitive impairment for the clinical diagnosis of FMS. The new criteria place FMS at one extreme on a spectrum of polysymptomatic distress (PSD) that includes CWP.

Chronic Widespread Pain and Fibromyalgia Syndrome: Differences in Spontaneous and Evoked Pain

Hyperalgesia, tenderness, allodynia, and evoked pain are important symptoms to test in CWP and FMS. FMS is characterized by abnormal pain modulation, whereas CWP mainly refers to diffuse spontaneous pain, but not to specific pain hypersensitivity or dysfunction.

Individuals with FMS present with diffuse hyperalgesia (increased pain to normally painful stimuli) and/or allodynia (pain to normally non-painful stimuli, also called tenderness). The ACR 1990 classification criteria[15] included tender point examination, to test allodynia in specific sites. In the recent criteria, allodynia is no longer required because diffuse tenderness is variable, not limited to the tender points and related to physician training.[17] However, tender point count and tender point sensitivity are important to consider for pathophysiological mechanisms, especially in the distinction between CWP and FMS. Allodynia and evoked pain reflect that there are impaired pain and sensory processing in FMS, probably more specific to FMS.

Contrary to allodynia and tenderness, hyperalgesia can be found in CWP and FMS and is mainly related to peripheral mechanisms and explained by increased pain sensitivity of nociceptors located in deep tissue (peripheral sensitization) or by increased responses from dorsal horn neurons (central sensitization).[5]

Because diffuse tenderness is a defining feature of FMS, more sophisticated methods have been used to investigate pain sensitivity in FMS, especially Quantitative Sensory Testing (QST). These studies show the following:

1. FMS patients are more sensitive to pressure anywhere in their body.[11]
2. Spontaneous pain intensity is predicted by mechanical and heat hyperalgesia in FMS.[3]

3. FMS patients also display a decreased threshold to other noxious stimuli, heat, cold, and electrical stimuli.[4]
4. FMS patients are more sensitive to other sensory stimuli such as sound.[14]

Thus, pain testing suggests that FMS might represent a specific CWP with diffuse allodynia and increased evoked pain, related to amplification of all sensory stimuli gains, in the center and perhaps also the periphery, together with impaired pain modulation, for example, decreased pain inhibition.

Comorbid Fibromyalgia Syndrome and Chronic Widespread Pain in Rheumatic Disorders

The recent concept of comorbid FMS emphasizes the previous concept of the continuum between CWP and FMS. Several authors have demonstrated that FMS may be present in up to 20% to 30% of chronic inflammatory painful rheumatisms.[9] Comorbid FMS could be related to impaired pain mechanisms induced by chronic inflammation, and represent a distinct clinical entity, which should be treated, independent of the underlying rheumatic disorder.

Consequences of Clinical Practice

The medical system requires to use categorical diagnosis, for example, a person meets any of the FMS criteria or does not. However, in patients with chronic pain, it is more useful to take into consideration the continuous spectrum of pain sites and somatic and psychological symptoms. The Fibromyalgia Survey/Symptom Questionnaire (also called PSD scale)[16] allows one to see and follow the extent of PSD (fibromyalgianess) without having to make sometimes categorical diagnosis. High scores on the PSD indicate that a patient with chronic pain will probably not benefit from monodisciplinary treatment, but most probably needs a multicomponent approach.

REFERENCES

1. Cöster L, Kendall S, Gerdle B, Henriksson C, Henriksson KG, Bengtsson A. Chronic widespread musculoskeletal pain—a comparison of those who meet criteria for fibromyalgia and those who do not. *Eur J Pain*. 2008;**12**:600–610.
2. Dean LE, Arnold L, Crofford L, et al. The impact of moving from a widespread to multi-site pain definition on other fibromyalgia symptoms. *Arthritis Care Res*. 2017;**69**:1878–1886.
3. Desmeules JA, Cedraschi C, Rapiti E, et al. Neurophysiologic evidence for a central sensitization in patients with fibromyalgia. *Arthritis Rheumatol*. 2003;**48**(5):1420–1429.
4. Geisser ME, Casey KL, Brucksch CB, Ribbens CM, Appleton BB, Crofford LJ. Perception of noxious and innocuous heat stimulation among healthy women and women with fibromyalgia: association with mood, somatic focus, and catastrophizing. *Pain*. 2003;**102**:243–250.
5. Graven-Nielsen T, Arendt-Nielsen L. Assessment of mechanisms in localized and widespread musculoskeletal pain. *Nat Rev Rheumatol*. 2010;**6**(10):599–606.

6. Häuser W, Schmutzer G, Brähler E, Glaesmer H. A cluster within the continuum of biopsychosocial distress can be labeled "fibromyalgia syndrome"0020014;evidence from a representative German population survey. *J Rheumatol.* 2009;**36**:2806–2812.
7. Kamaleri Y, Natvig B, Ihlebaek CM, et al. Number of pain sites is associated with demographic, lifestyle and health-related factors in the general population. *Eur J Pain.* 2008;**12**:742–748.
8. Mansfield KE, Sim J, Jordan JL, Jordan KP. A systematic review and meta-analysis of the prevalence of chronic widespread pain in the general population. *Pain.* 2016;**157**:55–64.
9. Perrot S, Peixoto M, Dieudé P, et al. Patient phenotypes in fibromyalgia comorbid with systemic sclerosis or rheumatoid arthritis: influence of diagnostic and screening tests. Screening with the FiRST questionnaire, diagnosis with the ACR 1990 and revised ACR 2010 criteria. *Clin Exp Rheumatol.* 2017;**105**(3):35–42.
10. Queiroz LP. Worldwide epidemiology of fibromyalgia. *Curr Pain Headache Rep.* 2013;**17**:356.
11. Staud R, Weyl EE, Price DD, Robinson ME. Mechanical and heat hyperalgesia highly predict clinical pain intensity in patients with chronic musculoskeletal pain syndromes. *J Pain.* 2012;**13**(8):725–735.
12. Staud R. Chronic widespread pain and fibromyalgia: two sides of the same coin? *Curr Rheumatol Rep.* 2009;**11**:433–436.
13. White KP, Harth M, Speechley M, Ostbye T. Testing an instrument to screen for fibromyalgia syndrome in general population studies: the London Fibromyalgia Epidemiology Study Screening Questionnaire. *J Rheumatol.* 1999;**26**:880–884.
14. White KP, Nielson WR, Harth M, Ostbye T, Speechley M. Chronic widespread musculoskeletal pain with or without fibromyalgia: psychological distress in a representative community adult sample. *J Rheumatol.* 2002;**29**:588–594.
15. Wolfe F, Clauw D, Fitzcharles MA, Goldenberg D, Katz RS, Mease P. The American College of Rheumatology Preliminary Diagnostic Criteria for fibromyalgia and measurement of symptom severity. *Arthritis Care Res.* 2010;**62**:600–610.
16. Wolfe F, Clauw DJ, Fitzcharles MA, et al. Fibromyalgia criteria and severity scales for clinical and epidemiological studies: a modification of the ACR preliminary diagnostic criteria for fibromyalgia. *J Rheumatol.* 2011:**38**:1113–1122.
17. Wolfe F, Clauw DJ, Fitzcharles M-A, Goldenberg DL, Häuser W, Katz RL. 2016 Revisions to the 2010/2011 Fibromyalgia Diagnostic Criteria. *Semin Arthritis Rheumatol.* 2016;**46**:319–329.
18. Wolfe F, Egloff N, Häuser W. Widespread pain and low widespread pain index scores among fibromyalgia positive cases assessed with 2010/2011 fibromyalgia criteria. *J Rheumatol.* 2016;**43**:1743–1748.
19. Wolfe F, Smythe HA, Yunus MB, Bennett RM, Bombardier C, Goldenberg DL. The American College of Rheumatology 1990 Criteria, for the classification of fibromyalgia. Report of the Multicenter Criteria Committee. *Arthritis Rheumat.* 1990;**33**:1863–1864.

CHAPTER 5

Classification

Winfried Häuser

Summary Points

- There is an ongoing debate on the classification of fibromyalgia syndrome (FMS): Rheumatic disease, neurology disease, pain disorder, functional somatic syndrome, central sensitivity syndrome, overlapping pain condition, somatoform disorder, depressive spectrum disorder, and somatic symptom disorder.
- All classification systems available only capture some parts of this poly-symptomatic condition.
- The debate on the classification of FMS is linked with the debate as to which specialty should treat FMS patients and which treatment options should be preferred.

BACKGROUND

FMS is a controversial condition.[24] One of the "FMS wars" are fought on the classification of FMS. The discussion on the classification is linked with the debate on the presumed pathophysiology and on the "ownership" of FMS: Which specialty should treat patients with FMS and which treatments should be preferred?[16]

FIBROMYALGIA SYNDROME

Syndrome, Disease, or Disorder?

The answer to this question depends on the definition of syndrome, disease or disorder used.[7] A satisfactory definition of disease is surprisingly difficult. What counts as a disease also changes over historical time, partly due to the changes in diagnostic ability, but mostly for a mixture of social and economic reasons. One example is osteoporosis, which after being officially recognized as a disease by the World Health Organization (WHO) in 1994 switched from being an unavoidable part of normal ageing to a pathology. This has consequences for the patients for their ability to get the treatment reimbursed by health service providers.[15] If the official recognition by the WHO is required as condition for a disease, FMS is a disease. In 1994, the 10th revision of the *International Classification of Diseases* (*ICD-10*) listed FMS under "diseases of the musculoskeletal system and connective tissue."[25]

If defined etiology and pathophysiology are required for the definition of a disease, FMS is not a disease.[6] Therefore, the term "fibromyalgia syndrome" is frequently used in the literature. However, the term "syndrome" is not consistently used in the medical literature. A syndrome can be defined by the aggregation of symptoms, which by themselves are not characteristic of the disease, to form a characteristic disease pattern. The German guideline classified FMS as a first-order syndrome or a symptom complex with unknown or unclear etiology, heterogeneous pathogenesis, and a defined phenotype.[6] Second-order syndromes are defined by unknown etiologies, homogeneous pathogenesis, and defined phenotypes (e.g., Cushing's syndrome). Third-order syndromes are defined by homogeneous etiologies, unknown pathogenesis, and defined phenotypes (e.g., Down syndrome and Marfan syndrome).[13] The WHO uses the term "disorder" throughout the classification of mental disorders, so as to avoid even greater problems inherent in the use of terms such as "disease" and "illness." "Disorder" is not an exact term, but it is used here to imply the existence of a clinically recognizable set of symptoms or behavior associated in most cases with distress and with interference with personal functions.[25]

A Rheumatology Disorder?

The fact that FMS is listed under "diseases of the musculoskeletal system and connective tissue"[5] suggests a rheumatology disease. The first official definition of FMS by the 1990 American College of Rheumatology Criteria with specific tender points in the muscle[23] have suggested that FMS was a rheumatologic condition. However, no consistent and broadly recognized structural changes in the musculoskeletal system and connective tissue have been demonstrated until now.[20]

A Pain Disorder?

The International Association for the Study of Pain (IASP) established a Task Force for the classification of chronic pain for the upcoming 11th revision of the *ICD* (*ICD-11*).[18] The goal is to create a classification system that is applicable in primary care and clinical settings for specialized pain management. One category is chronic primary pain which is defined as pain in one or more anatomic regions that persists or recurs for longer than 3 months and is associated with significant emotional distress or functional disability (interference with activities of daily life and participation in social roles) and that cannot be better explained by another chronic pain condition. This is a new phenomenologic definition, created because the etiology is unknown for many forms of chronic pain. The term "primary pain" was chosen in close liaison with the *ICD-11* revision committee, who felt that this was the most widely acceptable term, in particular, from a nonspecialist perspective.[18] Dysfunction in pain modulation, demonstrated by allodynia and spontaneous pain, suggest that FMS could be a disease of pain by an increase of pain sensitivity and a decrease of pain inhibitory controls.[4]

However, whether FMS is a pain disorder is contested. In 1989, Turk and Flor[19] stated that FMS is more than a chronic widespread pain and tender points. The new diagnostic criteria of FMS give unrefreshed sleep and fatigue a nearly equal weight for diagnosis and even include depression as a minor symptom.[21,22]

A Neurology Disease?

Because of small fiber pathology findings in FMS–patients, some authors claimed that FMS is a neurology disease (small fiber neuropathy).[14] However, small fiber pathology findings cannot be detected in every patient meeting established FMS criteria. In addition, some small pathology findings such as decreased intraepidermal nerve fiber density (IENFD) have been noted in most chronic pain conditions where this has been examined, and in many conditions not normally associated with pain, such as postural tachycardia syndrome and amyotrophic lateral sclerosis.[20,5] Finally, the clinical picture of patients with small fiber neuropathy differs from that of FMS patients.[20]

A Mental Disorder?

Patients with FMS symptoms receive other diagnostic labels by mental health care specialists. For some psychiatrists FMS is a "masked" depression or a affective spectrum disorder.[11] However, not every patient with FMS is depressed and not every patient with depressive disorder reports chronic widespread pain.[6,8]

The absence of a defined pathology and the association of FMS symptoms with psychosocial stress prompted some specialists in psychosomatic medicine, to use the diagnostic label "persistent somatoform pain disorder" (ICD-10 F45.4). However, only 60% to 80% of FMS patients meet the diagnostic criterion of the onset or aggravation of FMS symptoms together with psychosocial stress and emotional conflicts.[10]

Recently, the American Psychiatric Association (APA) substituted the category "pain disorder" by "somatic symptom disorder (SSD)" for the 5th version of the *Diagnostic and Statistical Manual of Psychiatric Diseases*.[1] The diagnosis of SSD may be made when there are persistent (i.e., typically longer than 6 months) somatic symptoms that are distressing and/or significantly disrupt daily life (criteria A and C) that are accompanied by excessive and disproportionate symptom-related thoughts, feelings, and behaviors regarding these symptoms (criteria B). The first papers have been published that classify FMS to be an SSD.[17,12] However, in one study only 26% of

FMS patients met the criteria of a SSD. The construct validity and the clinical utility of the diagnostic label SSD was limited in one study.[9]

Besides these approaches that try to classify FMS into established classification systems (WHO, APA), FMS is classified to belong to categories that were defined by specialties but are not officially recognized.

Fibromyalgia Syndrome and Functional Somatic Syndromes

The term "functional somatic syndrome" is mainly used in general internal medicine. Functional somatic syndromes are defined by a clinical complex of physical symptoms, a defined time period and the absence of the causative somatic disease factors that explain the symptoms (e.g., structural tissue damage, biochemical disorder, or specific laboratory findings).[2] The German guideline classifies FMS as a functional somatic syndrome. Examples for other functional somatic syndromes are irritable bowel syndrome (IBS) or tension headache.[6]

Fibromyalgia Syndrome and Central Sensitivity Syndromes

Dr. Yunus, a rheumatologist, created the term "central sensitivity syndromes (CSS)" to point out the overlap of FMS with other pain disorders such as IBS and tension headache, chronic fatigue, and multiple chemical syndrome and posttraumatic stress disorder. He rejects some assumptions of the categories "functional somatic syndrome" and "somatoform disorder." To his opinion, CSS can be medically explained and psychological processes such as somatization are not relevant.[26]

Fibromyalgia Syndrome and Chronic Overlapping Pain Conditions

Recently, a group of U.S. researches coined the term "chronic overlapping pain conditions" to capture the overlap of vulvodynia, temporomandibular disorders, myalgic encephalomyelitis/chronic fatigue syndrome, IBS, interstitial cystitis/painful bladder syndrome, FMS, endometriosis, chronic tension-type headache, chronic migraine headache, and chronic low back pain.[3]

CONCLUSION

The debate on the classification of FMS continues. FMS is a polysymptomatic disease/syndrome situated between general internal medicine, neurology, pain medicine, psychiatry, psychosomatic medicine, and rheumatology. The classification systems of these specialties only capture some parts of a complex and heterogeneous disorder.

REFERENCES

1. American Psychiatric Association. *Diagnostic and statistical manual of mental disorders*. 5th ed. Arlington, VA: American Psychiatric Publishing; 2013.
2. Barsky AJ, Borus JF. Functional somatic syndromes. *Ann Intern Med.* 1999;**130**:910–921.
3. Chronic Pain Research Alliance. Impact of chronic overlapping pain conditions on public health and urgent need for safe and effective treatments. http://www.chronicpainresearch.org/public/CPRA_WhitePaper_2015-FINAL-Digital.pdf Accessed October 20, 2016.
4. Clauw DJ. Fibromyalgia: a clinical review. *JAMA*. 2014;**311**:1547–1555.
5. Clauw DJ. What is the meaning of small fiber neuropathy in fibromyalgia? *Pain*. 2015; **156**:2115–2116.
6. Eich W, Bär KJ, Bernateck M, et al. Definition, classification, clinical diagnosis and prognosis of fibromyalgia syndrome: updated guidelines 2017 and overview of systematic review articles. *Schmerz*. 2017;**31**:231–238.
7. Emson HE. Health, disease and illness: matters for definition. *Can Med Assoc J.* 1987;**136**:811–814.
8. Gracely RH, Ceko M, Bushnell MC. Fibromyalgia and depression. *Pain Res Treat.* 2012; **2012**:486590.
9. Häuser W, Bialas P, Welsch K, Wolfe F. Construct validity and clinical utility of current research criteria of DSM-5 somatic symptom disorder diagnosis in patients with fibromyalgia syndrome. *J Psychosom Res.* 2015; **78**:546–552.
10. Häuser W, Henningsen P. Fibromyalgia syndrome: a somatoform disorder? *Eur J Pain.* 2014; **18**:1052–1059.
11. Hudson JI, Pope HG. The concept of affective spectrum disorder: relationship to fibromyalgia and other syndromes of chronic fatigue and chronic muscle pain. *Baillieres Clin Rheumatol.* 1994;**8**:839–856.
12. Klaus K, Fischer S, Doerr JM, Nater UM, Mewes R. Classifying fibromyalgia syndrome as a mental disorder?-an ambulatory assessment study. *Int J Behav Med.* 2017;**24**:230–238.
13. Leiber B. *Die klinischen Syndrome (Clinical syndromes)*. Stuttgart: Urban & Schwarzenberg; 1990
14. Oaklander AL, Herzog ZD, Downs HM, Klein MM. Objective evidence that small-fiber polyneuropathy underlies some illnesses currently labeled as fibromyalgia. *Pain*. 2013;**154**:2310–2316.
15. Scully JL. What is a disease? *EMBO Rep*. 2004;**5**:650–653.
16. Shir Y, Fitzcharles MA. Should rheumatologists retain ownership of fibromyalgia? *J Rheumatol.* 2009;**36**:667–670.
17. Tavel ME. Somatic symptom disorders without known physical causes: one disease with many names? *Am J Med.* 2015;**128**:1054–1058.
18. Treede RD, Rief W, Barke A, et al. A classification of chronic pain for ICD-11. *Pain.* 2015;**156**(6):1003–1007.
19. Turk DC, Flor H. Primary fibromyalgia is greater than tender points: toward a multiaxial taxonomy. *J Rheumatol Suppl.* 1989;**19**:80–86.
20. Üçeyler N, Burgmer M, Friedel E, et al. Etiology and pathophysiology of fibromyalgia syndrome: updated guidelines 2017, overview of systematic review articles and overview of studies on small fiber neuropathy in FMS subgroups. *Schmerz.* 2017;**31**:239–245.
21. Wolfe F, Clauw DJ, Fitzcharles MA, et al. The American College of Rheumatology preliminary diagnostic criteria for fibromyalgia and measurement of symptom severity. *Arthritis Rheum.* 2010;**62**:(6):600–610.
22. Wolfe F, Clauw DJ, Fitzcharles MA, et al. Fibromyalgia criteria and severity scales for clinical and epidemiological studies: a modification of the ACR Preliminary Diagnostic Criteria for Fibromyalgia. *J Rheumatol.* 2011;**38**:(6):1113–1122.
23. Wolfe F, Smythe HA, Yunus MB, et al. The American College of Rheumatology 1990 Criteria for the Classification of Fibromyalgia. Report of the Multicenter Criteria Committee. *Arthritis Rheum.* 1990;**33**:160–172.
24. Wolfe F. Fibromyalgia wars. *J Rheumatol.* 2009;**36**:671–678.
25. World Health Organization. International Classification of Diseases (ICD). *WHO* [online], http://www.who.int/ classifications/icd/en (2015). Accessed January 2, 2016.
26. Yunus MB. Fibromyalgia and overlapping disorders: the unifying concept of central sensitivity syndromes. *Semin Arthritis Rheum.* 2007;**36**:335–356.

SECTION 2

Clinical Features of Fibromyalgia Syndrome

CHAPTER 6

Clinical Features of Fibromyalgia Syndrome

Fabiola Atzeni, Ignazio Francesco Masala, and Piercarlo Sarzi-Puttini

Summary Points

- Pain, fatigue, and sleep disturbances are the hallmark symptoms of fibromyalgia syndrome (FMS).
- Patients typically suffer from hyperalgesia or allodynia, thus suggesting that the original problem is distorted pain or sensory processing.
- Poor sleep quality can correlate with worsening symptoms of FMS.
- Treating the pain, fatigue, and sleep disturbances associated with FMS and related conditions is a great challenge.
- Multidisciplinary approach is essential and physicians need to bear in mind all of the potential comorbidities and overlapping conditions to avoid treatment failures.

Pain is the hallmark symptom of FMS and is associated with fatigue and sleep disturbances.[6] The pain of FMS is quite different from that of other rheumatic diseases and, unlike arthritis, osteoarthritis, or other painful soft tissue conditions, it cannot be adequately explained on the basis of the degree of peripheral tissue inflammation or damage.[6] Patients typically suffer from hyperalgesia (increased pain induced by normally painful stimuli) or allodynia (pain induced by normally non-painful stimuli), thus suggesting that the original problem is distorted pain or sensory processing rather than a local or regional abnormality.

CHARACTERISTICS OF PAIN

Pain is usually present in all four limbs, as well as the upper or lower back; many patients state that they "hurt all over," and this is often a discriminant when evaluating patient complaints. It may be regional or generalized and "non-anatomically" distributed, and perceived as originating in muscles or deep in bones[17] and, rarely, articular[29]; no structural or nerve root distribution can be detected. Hyperalgesia and allodynia, persistent pain, summation effects, skin hyperpathia, and tenderness on examination are the most common characteristics, and patients describe their pain as sharp, burning, searing, tingling, shooting or stabbing, and deeply aching, or say they feel bruised all over.[17] Its intensity is aggravated by cold or humid weather, anxiety or stress, overuse or inactivity, poor sleep,[39,5] and noise.[27]

Tenderness is a unique and typical sign, but is not limited to the canonic tender points.[21] The pain and other symptoms of FMS are invisible and, although they are always present in the majority of patients, they are also quite variable: That is, their intensity changes from day to day, and during the day.[2,40,3,4] The unpredictability of these symptoms, together with the difficulty of family, friends, and physicians to accept their reality, are further sources of stress and distress, but other factors that strongly influence pain perception are coping styles (particularly catastrophizing) and having an external locus of control, which positively correlate with pain and other symptoms, whereas self-efficacy is associated with reduced pain perception.[4,15,33,36]

Sleeping With Fibromyalgia Syndrome Pain

Most patients with FMS complain that the quality of their sleep is poor.[35,32,1] They take longer to fall asleep, wake up during the night more frequently, sleep fewer hours, and wake up unrefreshed significantly more often than healthy controls and patients with other rheumatic diseases or pain disorders.[11,10] Polysomnography partly confirms the poor quality of sleep: The most consistent findings are decreased sleep efficiency (total sleep time/time in bed), a higher proportion of sleeping time in light sleep, and more time of wakefulness before the onset of sleep.[30] In 1975, Moldofsky et al.[25] observed that patients with FMS had more frequent alpha rhythms during non–rapid eye movement (NREM) sleep than healthy controls and, as alpha electroencephalographic frequencies are usually associated with wakefulness, they hypothesized that this was responsible for nonrestorative sleep pattern in FMS patients. Several studies have also observed that in comparison with healthy controls, the occurrence of alpha electroencephalographic frequencies during deep NREM delta-wave sleep is also increased in patients with FMS.[25,22]

However, it should be noted that alpha-wave intrusions into NREM sleep are not specific to FMS, but are also seen in patients with other pain syndromes as well as healthy controls, and may actually indicate good quality sleep rather than sleep disturbance. This means that the cyclic alternating pattern (CAP), a measure of sleep stability/instability that has been found to be more frequent in patients with FMS than in healthy controls may be a better marker of sleep quality as it correlates negatively with sleep efficiency and positively with the tender point index.[30]

Sleep disorders such as obstructive sleep apnea and restless legs syndrome seem to be more common in (particularly male) patients with FMS than in the general population, and their presence is associated not only with worse perceived sleep quality, but also with pain, fatigue, and greater symptom severity.[35]

Effects of Loss of Sleep on Fibromyalgia Syndrome Pain

Several prospective studies have found correlations between poor sleep quality and worsening symptoms of FMS.[19,13] Sleep deprivation in healthy individuals can cause symptoms of FMS, including myalgia, tenderness, and fatigue, suggesting that sleep dysfunction might be not only a consequence of pain, but also pathogenic.[9] However, there is some disagreement regarding the direction of these associations: One model shows the path going from disturbed sleep via pain and an ineffective coping style to distress and functional limitations[13]; the other shows the path to start with pain and go via sleep quality and self-efficacy to distress and daily functioning.

A path analysis found that a night of disturbed sleep was associated with increased pain, worsened physical functioning, and subsequent mood disturbances.[38] The ability to recover from stressful days, and the effects of several nights of inadequate sleep are cumulative[22] and sleep disturbances and pain are both associated with symptoms of depression and anxiety and functional limitations. Some studies suggest that a bidirectional relationship exists between sleep disturbance on the one hand, and anxiety and depression on the other. Data from a large population-based study in Norway suggest that poor sleep quality predisposes adolescents to mental illnesses.[34]

Finally, clinical trials of pharmacologic and nonpharmacologic therapies have shown that improving sleep quality can reduce pain and fatigue, supporting the hypothesis that sleep dysfunction is a pathogenic stimulus of FMS.[9]

At least 75% of FMS patients report fatigue,[14,31] the levels of which are perceived as being significantly higher than those reported by healthy controls and patients with other rheumatic diseases.[31] However, despite the obvious importance of this symptom, it remains somewhat unclear because, although, major initiatives for defining relevant outcome measures for FMS such as Outcome Measures in Rheumatology (OMERACT) or the Patient-Reported Outcomes Measurement Information System (PROMIS) identify it as important, they fail to define it.[23,24,7] The descriptors used by patients indicate that fatigue is a complex multisystem concept that has physical, emotional and mental/cognitive dimensions, but the only assessment instrument that includes all of these dimensions is the Multidimensional Fatigue Inventory, and in observational studies, FMS patients have simply been asked to rate the severity of their fatigue on a visual analogue or numerical rating scale, which completely ignores this complexity. A wide range of negative factors have been found to be associated with fatigue,[37] including pain, stiffness, sleep disturbances, anxiety and depression; furthermore, positive events have been associated with decreased fatigue.[26]

Treatment

Treating the pain, fatigue, and sleep disturbances associated with FMS and related conditions is a great challenge, and clinicians are well aware of the fact that pain and its associated symptoms are graded and prioritized. Patients most frequently complain of pain and, fortunately, various drugs and nondrug therapies have proved to have positive effects on at least some symptoms and, more generally, chronic pain.[20] Since the past few decades, our increasing understanding of the pathophysiology of FMS, our improved knowledge of central system mechanisms, and our ability to define symptom domains more precisely have allowed substantial advances in particularly pharmacologic and non-pharmacologic treatment. A recent meta-analysis comparing the efficacy profile on six FMS core symptoms—pain, sleep disturbance, fatigue, affective symptoms (depression/anxiety), functional deficit, and cognitive impairment—of pharmacologic and non-pharmacologic treatment showed that only amitriptyline exhibited a significant effect on the three symptom domains: pain, sleep disturbance and fatigue, but it exhibited many adverse effects, whereas growth hormone exhibited significant effect on pain and function. None of the other pharmacologic treatments showed a large effect on sleep disturbances.[28] Among non-pharmacologic interventions, pain was the symptom that was most frequently relieved: Balneotherapy and repetitive transcranial magnetic stimulation (rTMS) demonstrated large effects on pain. Pool/water exercise, cognitive behavior therapy (CBT), homeopathy, and massage all showed medium effect sizes on pain. Pool/water exercise showed consistent medium-to-large effects on all six domains.[28] Systematic reviews of CBTs, aerobic exercise, and drugs showed that only aerobic exercise and CBT,[18] have a clinically relevant effect on fatigue. In contrast, some drugs (amitriptylin and pregabalin) have a clinically relevant effect on sleep problems, but none of the non-pharmacologic treatment options.[16] Moreover, fatigue and sleep problems may need different approaches as suggested by the new European League against Rheumatism (EULAR) recommendations because centrally acting drugs can worsen fatigue[20] and induce somnolence and dizziness leading to discontinuation of therapy.

CONCLUSION

In conclusion, experts have pointed that a multidisciplinary approach is essential as physicians need to bear in mind all of the potential comorbidities and overlapping conditions to avoid treatment failures and ensure that the most active problem is confronted in a timely and effective manner.[8,12]

REFERENCES

1. Bigatti SM, Hernandez AM, Cronan TA, Rand KL. Sleep disturbances in fibromyalgia syndrome: relationship to pain and depression. *Arthritis Rheum.* 2008;**59**:961–967.
2. Borchers AT, Gershwin ME. Fibromyalgia: a critical and comprehensive review. *Clin Rev Allergy Immunol.* 2015;**49**:100–151.
3. Bossema ER, vanMiddendorp H, Jacobs JW, Bijlsma JW, Geenen R. Influence of weather on daily symptoms of pain and fatigue in female patients with fibromyalgia: a multilevel regression analysis. *Arthritis Care Res.* 2013;**65**:1019–1025.

4. Burckhardt CS, Clark SR, O'Reilly CA, Bennett RA. Paincoping strategies of women with fibromyalgia: relationship to pain, fatigue, and quality of life. *J Musculoskel Pain*. 1997;**5**(3):5–21.
5. Campbell SM, Clark S, Tindall EA, Forehand ME, Bennett RM. Clinical characteristics of fibrositis. I. A "blinded,002001D; controlled study of symptoms and tender points. *Arthritis Rheum*. 1983;**26**:817–824.
6. Cassisi G, Sarzi-Puttini P, Casale R, et al. Pain in fibromyalgia and related conditions. *Reumatismo*. 2014;**66**:72–86.
7. Cella D, Yount S, Rothrock N, et al. The patient-reported outcomes measurement information system (PROMIS): progress of an NIH roadmap cooperative group during its first two years. *Med Care*. 2007;**45**(5 Suppl 1):S3–S11.
8. Chinn S, Caldwell W, Gritsenko K. Fibromyalgia pathogenesis and treatment options update. *Curr Pain Headache Rep*. 2016;**20**:25.
9. Choy EH. The role of sleep in pain and fibromyalgia. *Nat Rev Rheumatol*. 2015;**11**:513–520.
10. Cöster L, Kendall S, Gerdle B, Henriksson C, Henriksson KG, Bengtsson A. Chronic widespread musculoskeletal pain-a comparison of those who meet criteria for fibromyalgia and those who do not. *Eur J Pain*. 2008;**12**:600–610.
11. Diaz-Piedra C, Di Stasi LL, Baldwin CM, Buela-Casal G, Catena A. Sleep disturbances of adult women suffering from fibromyalgia: a systematic review of observational studies. *Sleep Med Rev*. 2015;**21**:86–99.
12. Gerardi MC, Batticciotto A, Talotta R, Di Franco M, Atzeni F, Sarzi-Puttini P. Novel pharmaceutical options for treating fibromyalgia. *Expert Rev Clin Pharmacol*. 2016 Feb;**16**:1–7.
13. Hamilton NA, Affleck G, Tennen H, Karlson C, Luxton D, Preacher KJ. Fibromyalgia: the role of sleep in affect and in negative event reactivity and recovery. *Health Psychol*. 2008;**27**:490–497.
14. Hamilton NA, Pressman M, Lillis T, Atchley R, Karlson C, Stevens N. Evaluating evidence for the role of sleep in fibromyalgia: a test of the Sleep and Pain Diathesis Model. *Cogn Ther Res*. 2012;**36**:806–814.
15. Hassett AL, Cone JD, Patella SJ, Sigal LH. The role of catastrophizing in the pain and depression of women with fibromyalgia syndrome. *Arthritis Rheum*. **200**;43:2493–2500.
16. Häuser W, Walitt B, Fitzcharles MA, Sommer C. Review of pharmacological therapies in fibromyalgia syndrome. *Arthritis Res Ther*. 2014;**16**(1):201.
17. Jain KA, Carruthers M, Van De Sande MI, Barron R, Donaldson S, Dunne JV. Fibromyalgia syndrome: Canadian clinical working case definition, diagnostic and treatment protocols – a consensus document. *J Musculoskel Pain*. 2003;**11**:3–107.
18. Langhorst J, Häuser W, Lauche R, et al. Complementary and alternative medicine for the treatment of fibromyalgia. *Evid Based Complement Alternat Med*. 2014;**2014**:408–436.
19. Lentz, MJ, Landis CA, Rothermel J, Shaver JL. Effects of selective slow wave sleep disruption on musculoskeletal pain and fatigue in middle aged women. *J. Rheumatol*. 1999;**26**:1586–1592.
20. Macfarlane GJ, Kronisch C, Dean LE, et al. EULAR revised recommendations for the management of fibromyalgia. *Ann Rheum Dis*. 2017;**76**:318–328.
21. Macfarlane GJ. Generalized pain, fibromyalgia and regional pain: an epidemiological view. *Best Pract Res Clin Rheumatol*. 1999;**13**:403–414.
22. Mahowald ML, Mahowald MW. Nighttime sleep and daytime functioning (sleepiness and fatigue) in less well-defined chronic rheumatic diseases with particular reference to the 'alpha-delta NREM sleep anomaly'. *Sleep Med*. 2000;**1**:195–207.
23. Mease PJ, Arnold LM, Crofford LJ, et al. Identifying the clinical domains of fibromyalgia: contributions from clinician and patient Delphi exercises. *Arthritis Rheum*. 2008;**59**:952–960.
24. Mease PJ, Clauw DJ, Christensen R, et al. Toward development of a fibromyalgia responder index and disease activity score: OMERACT module update. *J Rheumatol*. 2011;**38**:1487–1495.
25. Moldofsky H, Scarisbrick P, England R, Smythe H. Musculosketal symptoms and non-REM sleep disturbance in patients with "fibrositis syndrome" and healthy subjects. *Psychosom Med*. 1975;**37**:341–51.

26. Parrish BP, Zautra AJ, Davis MC. The role of positive and negative interpersonal events on daily fatigue in women with fibromyalgia, rheumatoid arthritis, and osteoarthritis. *HealthPsychol.* 2008; **27**:694–702.
27. Pellegrino MJ. Atypical chest pain as an initial presentation of primary fibromyalgia. *Arch Phys Med Rehabil.* 1990;**71**:526–528
28. Perrot S, Russell IJ. More ubiquitous effects from non-pharmacologic than from pharmacologic treatments for fibromyalgia syndrome: a meta-analysis examining six core symptoms. *Eur J Pain.* 2014;**18**:1067–1080.
29. Reilly PA, Littlejohn GO. Peripheral arthralgic presentation of fibrositis/fibromyalgia syndrome. *J Rheumatol.* 1992;**19**:281–283.
30. Rizzi M, Sarzi-Puttini P, Atzeni F, et al. Cyclic alternating pattern: a new marker of sleep alteration in patients with fibromyalgia? *J Rheumatol.* 2004;**31**(6):1193–1199.
31. Roehrs T, Diederichs C, Gillis M, et al. Nocturnal sleep, daytime sleepiness and fatigue in fibromyalgia patients compared to rheumatoid arthritis patients and healthy controls: a preliminary study. *Sleep Med.* 2013;**14**:109–115.
32. Roizenblatt S, Moldofsky H, Benedito-Silva AA, Tufik S. Alpha sleep characteristics in fibromyalgia. *Arthritis Rheum.* 2001;**44**:222–230.
33. Sánchez AI, Martínez MP, Miró E, Medina A. Predictors of the pain perception and self-efficacy for pain control in patients with fibromyalgia. *Span J Psychol.* 2011;**14**:366–373.
34. Sivertsen B, Harvey AG, Pallesen S, Hysing M. Mental health problems in adolescents with delayed sleep phase: results from a large population-based study in Norway. *J. Sleep Res.* 2014;**24**:11–18.
35. Spaeth M, Rizzi M, Sarzi-Puttini P. Fibromyalgia and sleep. *Best Pract Res Clin Rheumatol.* 2011;**25**:227–239.
36. Van Liew C, Brown KC, Cronan TA, Bigatti SM, Kothari DJ. Predictors of pain and functioning over time in fibromyalgia syndrome: an autoregressive path analysis. *Arthritis Care Res.* 2013;**65**(2):251–256.
37. Vincent A, Benzo RP, Whipple MO, McAllister SJ, Erwin PJ, Saligan LN. Beyond pain in fibromyalgia: insights into the symptom of fatigue. *Arthritis Res Ther.* 2013;**15**:221.
38. Yunus MB, Ahles TA, Aldag JC, Masi AT. Relationship of clinical features with psychological status in primary fibromyalgia. *Arthritis Rheum.* 1991;**34**:15–21.
39. Yunus MB, Masi AT, Aldag JC. A controlled study of primary fibromyalgia syndrome: clinical features and association with other functional syndromes. *J Rheumatol Suppl.* 1989;**19**:62–71.
40. Zautra AJ, Fasman R, Parish BP, Davis MC. Daily fatigue in women with osteoarthritis, rheumatoid arthritis, and fibromyalgia. *Pain.* 2007;**128**:128–135.

CHAPTER 7

Fibrofog: The Experience and Science of Cognitive Symptoms of Fibromyalgia Syndrome

Benjamin Coleman, Traian Popa, Joseph Snow, and Brian Walitt

Summary Points

- "Fibrofog" is the subjective experience of impaired thinking seen in fibromyalgia syndrome (FMS) patients.
- Evidence from the current literature demonstrates that subjective cognitive complaints substantially interferes with the activities of daily living for FMS patients.
- There is no evidence to support that fibrofog has been measured or can be measurable using standard objective cognitive tests.
- No clear relationship exists between subjective cognitive impairment and objective cognitive performance as measured by current neuropsychologic tests in FMS patients.
- Progress in the field will require a reconsideration of the scientific methods brought to bear on this frustrating clinical problem.

Dyscognition, the complaint that one's ability to perform thinking tasks is impaired, has become a common refrain in FMS. Patients often refer to this problem as "fibrofog" and report that it impairs proper thinking and substantially interferes with their occupational and domestic capabilities. Increases in physician appreciation of cognitive symptoms in FMS have led to the recognition of dyscognition as an important domain of symptom assessment[29] and as a criterion for diagnosis.[51] For many patients, the alterations in their cognitive experiences are very concerning, raising for them the specter of severe dementing disorders such as Alzheimer's disease, as well as the possibility that FMS is a dementing illness of its own.

Despite the ubiquity of dyscognitive complaints in FMS patients, the state of knowledge regarding the complaint is very limited. There is no clear definition or consensus of what constitutes FMS dyscognition. Several score of small research studies have attempted to document neurocognitive alterations in FMS patients, but only a handful have attempted to explore the relationship between subjective dyscognition and objective cognitive performance. There have also been a few attempts to describe the neuro-correlates of dyscognition using functional imaging techniques. Review of the literature suggests that there are systematic problems with the current direction of scientific inquiry. This chapter critically reviews the topic, with the goal to orient clinicians and scientists to what is known and unknown about the dyscognition of FMS.

A BRIEF HISTORY OF THE TERM "FIBROFOG"

The initial description of FMS, and its antecedent disorder fibrositis, was mainly concerned with pain and tenderness. There is no description of dyscognition in the historic fibrositis literature (1900 to 1988). Case descriptions from the time do not feature problems with concentration, memory, or thinking clearly. The closest a description from the period's literature comes to dyscognition is that of "ponderous thinking, [and] indecisiveness" in fibrositis patients.[5]

Around the time of the 1988 to 1990 transition from the fibrositis to FMS nomenclature, it was appreciated by the medical community that FMS patients frequently experienced a wide range of symptoms, including anxiety, fatigue, poor sleep, depression, subjective swelling, paresthesias, headaches, irritable bowel syndrome, and dysmenorrhea.[55] Descriptions of other, more specific cognitive symptoms were conspicuously absent from the literature. Cognitive complaints were not considered in the studies that led to the 1990 American College of Rheumatology FMS diagnostic criteria.[52] Dyscognition also was not part of the Fibromyalgia Impact Questionnaire (FIQ) (1991), the first validated questionnaire specifically intended to measure the spectrum and severity of FMS symptoms.[4] The FMS of 1990 was primarily a disorder of painful tenderness and unrefreshing sleep, with some appreciation of concomitant fatigue, mood alteration, and gastric and menstrual complaint.

The striking absence of cognitive complaint from the descriptions of fibrositis and FMS may be, in part, due to physicians of the time viewing cognitive complaints as features of a depression diagnosis[19] rather than its own specific medical problem. Historically, cognitive symptoms have been often considered part of the content of psychiatric syndromes. One example of this is "pseudodementia," a diagnosis that was loosely used in the 1960s to 1970s to describe the cognitive deficits of depression, especially in older adults.[25,22] Prevailing ideas about the "psychiatry of symptoms" often influence how physicians describe clinical disorders.

Over the next two decades, the 1990-style FMS became regarded by many physicians and scientists to be the "archetypical" central pain disorder.[54] The guiding principle, that of central sensitization, cast FMS as a disorder of amplification of peripheral stimulation, a disorder analogous to "the volume control setting being turned up too high."[9] This powerful analogy greatly influenced how FMS was subsequently discussed, described, and inquired about by patients and doctors alike. Cognitive complaints were not initially part of this discussion.

The absence of cognitive complaint from the 1990 FMS narrative was not due to the absence of the concept of dyscognition. Descriptions of acedia[38] and neurasthenia[2] ("brain fag") from centuries ago resemble modern descriptions of dyscognition. Physicians recognized "chemobrain" as dyscognition that could complicate recovery from chemotherapy and recognized "brain fog" as a defining characteristic of several modern medical syndromes, including Gulf War illness, myalgic encephalomyelitis/chronic fatigue syndrome (ME/CFS), and post-Lyme disease syndrome. The cognitive symptoms of these disorders are typically described as memory, executive function, speech, and language deficits.[22,32,34,14] However, such symptoms are poorly defined when compared to the cognitive defects seen and measured in certain neurologic and psychiatric syndromes.

In fact, it was the investigators familiar with the "brain fog" of ME/CFS and Lyme disease who first suggested that there is a cognitive aspect to FMS. The 1987 article entitled "The Chronic Fatigue Syndrome: Definition, Current Studies, and Lessons for Fibromyalgia Research" is the first to mention this aspect.[53] The first objective measurements of cognitive function in FMS were conducted as part of a 1992 study of Lyme disease, in which FMS patients were selected as a control group because the "symptoms in the[se] illness[es] may be similar."[23]

Following this initial publication, multiple investigative teams started to measure subjective and objective alterations in cognitive functioning in FMS patients. Pincus was the first to characterize cognitive symptoms in a 1996 abstract using the Cognitive Symptoms Inventory. FMS patients were shown to have an increased frequency of cognitive complaints compared to other rheumatic diseases.[37] By the late 1990s, the first studies seeking to measure objective cognitive performance in FMS were performed. Grace notes in 1998 that cognitive complaints were "not as commonly documented in the literature," and justifies performing cognitive testing in FMS based on "anecdotal reports from both healthcare professionals and patients suggest[ing] possible deficits in attention, concentration, and memory."[20] The first mention of the term "fibrofog" in the medical literature was by Katz et al. in 2004:

> Co-occurring disturbances in memory and mental clarity are popularly referred to as fibrofog, a label prominent in the electronic media and largely established by anecdote. It connotes fog-like feelings, also referred to as brain fog. The syndrome is unified by a wide range of difficulties, including forgetfulness, blurring of mental activities, sensory overload, and diminished ability to think, process information, or follow conversations.[24]

As Katz suggests, the term fibrofog and its description emerged from the advocacy community rather than from the physicians and scientists studying FMS. One of the earliest descriptions of fibrofog was by patient advocate and author Devin Starlanyl in 1998:

> Cognitive deficits is the technical term for what many of us call "fibrofog" when we are communicating with each other over the Internet. To be in fibrofog means that you feel as if your brain isn't fully engaged. In fibrofog, it is as if your body was a large electrical system, and some of the circuit breakers have shut down and many of the fuses have blown. Your brain may feel clouded or stuffed with cotton. It's extremely difficult to function. You forget the names of nouns, especially, and your use of the word "thing" rises exponentially. Sentences like "it's not the thing itself, but it's the thingie on the thingie-do that causes the thing" don't convey a whole lot of meaning to most people. For those of us with fibromyalgia syndrome, however, we understand them all too well. We've been there. You begin "tongue-tripping"—having difficulty pronouncing simple everyday words. Sometime, you say a word that begins with the same letter of the word you wanted to say, but it will be entirely inappropriate. These are just some of the "cognitive deficits" that can turn your life into an obstacle course.[43]

It does not appear that Starlanyl's description captures the full content of the FMS dyscognition. Searches on the internet for descriptions of fibrofog provide a wide various descriptions. One website dated April 2016 (themighty.com/2016/04/what-fibro-fog-feels-like/) provides 21 different descriptions, including feeling like "living your life underwater while trying to do your daily tasks," "having to solve complicated math in your head before you can think of an answer," "like a turtle trying to run in peanut butter," "wading through quicksand," and "getting startled awake in the middle of the night to find you're on stage with a live audience and you have to recite a song with duct tape on your mouth." Such anecdotal descriptions also provide a sense that fibrofog is more of a variable "state" that comes and goes than a constant "trait" experience. Fibrofog is used by patients and clinicians to refer to a wide range of problems, from difficulty in intellectual engagement, absentmindedness, general slowness, a sense of knowing something without being able to communicate it, being able to remember something well enough to know that you cannot remember it, an inability to multitask, and a sense of anxiety regarding having to think in public and in time-sensitive situations.

Once recognized, the incorporation of dyscognition into the FMS diagnosis was quick. By 2008, Mease et al. used the Delphi method to have patients rank the importance of the clinical domains of FMS from 0 to 10, with 10 being "extremely important." Using predefined questions, the authors found that FMS patients report difficulty concentrating (7.57 of 10), difficulty thinking or "fibrofog" (7.04 of 10), difficulty remembering things (7.15 of 10), memory loss (6.13 of 10), difficulty answering a question quickly (5.9 of 10), and difficulty expressing "yourself"

(4.79 of 10).[30] Self-reported cognitive complaints were also measured during the process of creating the 2010 FMS criteria. During the process of developing the criteria, substantial correlation between cognitive complaint and tender point count ($r = 0.58$) and widespread pain index ($r = 0.59$) was noted.[51] The severity of cognitive symptoms ("trouble thinking or remembering") is now part of the diagnostic criteria for FMS, although the criteria are not explicit about what exactly "trouble thinking or remembering" means.

A full accounting of what fibrofog represents has not been formulated yet. Questionnaires filled by FMS patients report subjective alterations in memory,[20] attention, concentration, and language abilities.[48,45] It is unclear whether these static cognitive "traits" capture the dynamic "state" nature of fibrofog. It is also an open question whether self-perception and recollection of one's cognitive state are constant or variable over time. As of 2017, there is still an absence of qualitative research designed to capture the content of the cognitive complaints of FMS in an unbiased fashion.

The absence of clear definitions of the concepts of dyscognition and fibrofog inevitably complicates the scientific study of the cognitive function of FMS patients.

THE SCIENTIFIC STUDY OF DYSCOGNITION AND COGNITIVE FUNCTION IN FIBROMYALGIA SYNDROME PATIENTS

The first focused study of the cognitive aspects of FMS dates to Sletvold et al.'s work in 1995.[42] Since this initial work, a total of 28 studies have been published (Table 7.1). Nearly all the studies (26) use the same exploratory cross-sectional group comparison design based on the hypothesis that objective cognitive performance is altered in FMS.

The design is simple. First, FMS patients and comparators volunteers are recruited. Comparator groups are typically healthy volunteers (27) but also have included depression (2), older adults (2), rheumatoid arthritis (1), musculoskeletal disorders (2), and other chronic pain disorders (2). Second, researchers administered a battery of neurocognitive tests and symptom questionnaires at a single point in time. Mean group differences are then calculated, with the statistical significance typically determined with *t*-tests or chi-square methods. This research strategy can determine if there are differences between the groups being studied.

It is important to be mindful of statistical and clinical issues when interpreting results of cross-sectional comparative studies. As has been said in many different contexts, "not all differences are created equal." Of central importance, the results of cross-sectional comparative studies are heavily influenced by the sample sizes of the populations being studied.

TABLE 7.1 **Description of studies attempting to characterize objective cognitive impairment in patients with fibromyalgia syndrome**

Year	Author	Groups (*N*)	Objective cognitive measures	Positive results	Negative results	Comments
1992	Kaplan et al.[23]	Lyme (20) FMS (11) MD (11)	WMS, CVLT, RCFT	CVLT: FMS > Lyme in final learning trial and 20-min recall ($\bar{x}_{diff} = 2.3$ points, $p \leq 0.01$)	FMS not lower than other groups	No healthy comparators
1995	Sletvold et al.[42]	FMS (25) MD (22) HC (18)	DST, TMT-A, TMT-B, PASAT, APT-RT	• DST: FMS lower ($\bar{x}_{diff} = 3.0$ points, $p < 0.05$; 0.9 standard deviation (*SD*) below HC) • PASAT: FMS lower ($\bar{x}_{diff} = 24$ points, $p < 0.05$; 1.5 *SD* below HC) • Left-hand reaction time: FMS > HC ($\bar{x}_{diff} = 90$ ms, $p < 0.05$; 2.4 *SD* above HC)	• TMT-A and B • Right-hand reaction time • FMS + MD: no difference	Subgroup analysis showed effects are attenuated in nondepressed FMS
1997	Cote and Moldofsky[11]	FMS (10) HC (9)	SO, PAB, SW	SW: FMS lower ($\bar{x}_{diff} = 206$ points, $p < 0.001$; 1.6 *SD* below HC)	• PAB • SO	Military measures are difficult to apply to daily civilian life
1997	Landro et al.[27]	FMS (25) MD (22) HC (18)	DS-F, DS-B, RMT, CMT, FAS, KRRFT	• RMT: FMS lower ($\bar{x}_{diff} = 1.4$ points, $p < 0.05$; 2 *SD* below HC) • CMT: FMS lower ($\bar{x}_{diff} = 28$ points, $p < 0.05$; 1.3 *SD* below HC) • FAS: FMS lower ($\bar{x}_{diff} = 11$ points, $p < 0.05$; 1 *SD* below HC)	• DS-F and B • KRRFT • FMS + MD: no difference	Nondepressed FMS subgroup too small to find differences in performance (*N* = 14)

1999	Grace et al.[20]	FMS (30) HC (30)	WMS, RAVLT, PASAT, SDMT	• WMS: FMS lower in general memory ($\bar{x}_{diff}$ = 9.7 points, $p = 0.01$), verbal memory ($\bar{x}_{diff}$ = 8.4 points, $p = 0.01$), and delayed recall ($\bar{x}_{diff}$ = 8.5 points, $p = 0.03$) • PASAT: FMS lower ($\bar{x}_{diff}$ = 14 points, $p = 0.01$)	• RAVLT • SDMT	Minimal clinical significance (all differences < 1 *SD*)
2001	Park et al.[35]	FMS (23) HC (23) OA (22)	Nonstandard tests: processing speed, working and recognition memory, free recall, verbal knowledge	• FMS lower in working memory, free recall, recognition memory, and verbal knowledge • FMS + OA no difference except in verbal knowledge	Processing speed	Statistical analyses used were one-tailed *t*-tests
2002	Dick et al.[12]	FMS (20) RA (20) MSK (20) HC (20)	TEA	TEA: FMS lower in overall score ($\bar{x}_{diff}$ = 1.8 points, $p < 0.005$; 1.3 *SD* below HC), selective attention ($\bar{x}_{diff}$ = 8.2 points, $p < 0.005$; 1 *SD* below HC), and working memory ($\bar{x}_{diff}$ = 4.3 points, $p < 0.005$; 1 *SD* below HC)	TEA: sustained attention and attention switching subscales	FMS had same performance as RA and MSK

(*Continued*)

TABLE 7.1 **Description of studies attempting to characterize objective cognitive impairment in patients with fibromyalgia syndrome** ***(Continued)***

Year	Author	Groups (N)	Objective cognitive measures	Positive results	Negative results	Comments
2002	Grisart et al.[21]	CP (17) FMS (16) HC (20)	Nonstandard word list learning task	FMS slightly lower performance	—	—
2003	Suhr[44]	FMS (23) CP (22) HC (21)	WCST, SCWT, RAVLT, RCFT, PASAT, AS-WAIS, DS-F, DS-B, LNS, DST, SST, FAS, TMT-A, TMT-B	—	No differences in test performance	• Test administration issues • Study not designed to capture negative results
2005	Glass et al.[39]	FMS (23) HC (23) OA (22)	Nonstandard word list learning	FMS lower compared to HC ($\bar{x}_{diff}$ = 8%, p = 0.005)	FMS + OA: No difference	One-tailed t-test was used in analyses
2006	Leavitt and Katz[28]	FMS (35) HC (35)	WMS—logical memory and paired associates, LNS, ACT, DS-F, DS-B, PASAT	• PASAT: FMS lower (1 SD below norm, p = 0.01) • LNS: FMS lower (0.6 SD below norm, p = 0.05) • ACT: FMS lower in all trials (2.2 SD below norm, p = 0.001)	• WMS • DS-F and B	• HC performed below normative mean • No raw scores • Technical issues

2008	Dick et al.[13]	FMS (30) HC (30)	TEA, ACT, RST	• TEA: FMS lower in overall score ($\bar{x}_{diff}$ = 11 points, $p = 0.002$) and auditory verbal working memory ($\bar{x}_{diff}$ = 3.3 points, $p = 0.006$) • RST: FMS lower in working memory ($\bar{x}_{diff}$ = 14 points, $p = 0.001$) and grammatical judgment ($\bar{x}_{diff}$ = 1.1 points, $p = 0.01$) • ACT: FMS lower in 36-s delay trial ($\bar{x}_{diff}$ = 2.9 points, $p = 0.005$)	• TEA: selective attention and sustained attention • ACT: all other trials	• Minimal clinical significance (all differences < 1 *SD*) • Opioid medicated FMS (*N* = 9) + non-opioid medicated FMS (*N* = 21): no difference
2008	Munguia-Izquierdo et al.[33]	FMS (81) HC (35)	DS-F, DS-B, TMT-A, TMT-B, PASAT, RAVLT, FAS	• DS-F and DS-B: FMS lower ($\bar{x}_{diff}$ = 2.2 points, $p < 0.001$; 1.4 *SD* below HC) • TMT-A: FMS lower ($\bar{x}_{diff}$ = 30 s, $p < 0.001$; 1.3 *SD* below HC) • TMT-B: FMS lower ($\bar{x}_{diff}$ = 74 s, $p < 0.001$; 2.2 *SD* below HC) • PASAT: FMS lower ($\bar{x}_{diff}$ = 15.8 points, $p < 0.001$; 1.4 *SD* below HC) • RAVLT: FMS lower all subscales ($p < 0.001$) • FAS: FMS lower ($\bar{x}_{diff}$ = 10.6 points, $p < 0.001$; 0.9 *SD* below HC)	—	Issues with TMT administration

(*Continued*)

TABLE 7.1 Description of studies attempting to characterize objective cognitive impairment in patients with fibromyalgia syndrome (*Continued*)

Year	Author	Groups (*N*)	Objective cognitive measures	Positive results	Negative results	Comments
2008	Walitt et al.[49]	FMS (27) MSK (18) HC (27)	ANAM, TMT-A, TMT-B, SCWT	• ANAM: FMS better in math processing ($\bar{x}_{diff} = 0.7$ points, $p < 0.05$) after adjusting for premorbid IQ and depression • SCWT: FMS + MSK better ($\bar{x}_{diff} = 4.1$ points, $p < 0.05$) after adjusting	FMS not lower in any test	—
2009	Canovas et al.[6]	FMS (15) HC (15)	DS-B, CBTT, DS-F, 10/36, VR-BR, VR-MWM	VR-BR and VR-MWM: • FMS more errors ($\bar{x}_{diff} = 3$ errors and 1.5 errors at final trial, $p < 0.05$) • No difference in distance or time	• DS-F and B • CBTT • 10/36	VR tasks adapted from standard test for animal models
2009	Verdejo-Garcia et al.[47]	FMS (36) HC (36)	WCST, IGT	• IGT: FMS lower in block 3 ($\bar{x}_{diff} = 3$ in score, $p < 0.05$) • WCST: FMS more non-perseverative errors ($\bar{x}_{diff} = 6$ in score, $p = 0.04$; 0.6 *SD* above HC) and lower number of categories ($\bar{x}_{diff} = 1.3$ cat., $p = 0.007$; 1.8 *SD* below HC)	• IGT: no difference for other blocks • WCST: No difference in perseverative errors	No learning curve in IGT for either group

2011	Glass et al.[18]	FMS (18) HC (14)	Nonstandard response inhibition task	—	No differences in performance	—
2011	Miro et al.[31]	FMS (33) HC (28)	ANT-I	Reaction time: FMS > HC	No differences in performance	—
2011	Walteros et al.[50]	FMS (15) HC (15)	SCWT, WAIS-III, CALT, IGT	• CALT: FMS more perseveration errors in verbal trials ($\bar{x}_{diff}$ = 3 errors in final block, $p = 0.05$) • IGT: FMS significantly impaired in blocks 3 and 5 ($\bar{x}_{diff}$ = 7 in score in final block, $p < 0.05$)	• WAIS-III • SCWT	Unclear clinical significance
2012	Kim et al.[26]	FMS (23) HC (24)	DS-F, DS-B, RAVLT, RCFT, CPT, WCST	• RAVLT: FMS lower in delayed recall ($\bar{x}_{diff}$ = 1.7 points, $p = 0.011$; 1.1 *SD* below HC) • RCFT: FMS lower ($\bar{x}_{diff}$ = 8 points, $p = 0.01$; 1.4 *SD* below HC)	• DS-F and B • CPT • WCST	Significance disappears in RAVLT after controlling for depression
2012	Veldhuijzen et al.[46]	FMS (35) HC (35)	SCWT, MSIT	Reaction time (both tests): FMS > HC ($\bar{x}_{diff}$ = 200 ms, $p < 0.01$; 1.3 *SD* below HC)	No differences in performance	—

(*Continued*)

TABLE 7.1 **Description of studies attempting to characterize objective cognitive impairment in patients with fibromyalgia syndrome** ***(Continued)***

Year	Author	Groups (*N*)	Objective cognitive measures	Positive results	Negative results	Comments
2014	Cherry et al.[8]	FMS (43) HC (44)	ADWL, SCWT, DS-F, DS-B, TMT-A, TMT-B, AN, DST, EPT	• DST: FMS lower ($\bar{x}_{diff}$ = 11 points, $p < 0.005$; 1 *SD* below HC) • SCWT: FMS lower ($\bar{x}_{diff}$ = 17.5 s, $p < 0.05$; 0.7 *SD* below HC)	• ADWL • DS-F and B • TMT-A and B • AN • DST • EPT	—
2014	Seo et al.[40]	FMS (19) HC (22)	0-back, 2-back	• FMS greater reaction time ($\bar{x}_{diff}$ = 100 ms, $p < 0.05$) • FMS lower accuracy in 2-back ($\bar{x}_{diff}$ = 8%, $p < 0.05$)	No difference 0-back accuracy	Minimal clinical significance
2014	Shmygalev et al.[41]	FMS (43) HC (129)	GDA	Non-inferiority for FMS in every test except motor coordination ($\bar{x}_{diff}$ = 1.7 points)	—	Non-inferiority analysis
2015	Ceko et al.[7]	FMS (28) HC (23)	0-back, 1-back, 2-back, 3-back	No differences	—	—
2015	Tesio et al.[48]	FMS (30) HC (30)	RAVLT, 1-back, TOL, TMT-A, TMT-B, DS-F, DS-B, FAS	• DS-B: FMS lower ($\bar{x}_{diff}$ = 0.6 points, $p = 0.031$) • RAVLT: FMS lower in delayed recall ($\bar{x}_{diff}$ = 1.8 points, $p = 0.033$) • TMT-B: FMS lower ($\bar{x}_{diff}$ = 21.6 s, $p = 0.020$) • 1-back: FMS longer reaction time ($\bar{x}_{diff}$ = 170 ms, $p < 0.0001$)	• TMT-A • DS-F • 1-back accuracy • FAS	• No adjustments for multiple comparisons • Minimal clinical significance (all differences < 0.8 *SD*) • Technical issues

2016	Gelonch et al.[15]	FMS (82) HC (42)	FAS, PASAT, 2-back, 3-back, TMT-A, TMT-B, SCWT, WCST	SCWT: FMS lower ($\bar{x}_{diff} = 0.5\ SD$, $p = 0.03$)	• FAS • PASAT • 2 and 3-back • TMT-A and B • WCST	Minimal clinical significance for SCWT
2016	Walitt et al.[48]	FMS (16) HC (13)	0-back, 2-back	—	No differences	—

Patient Groups:

CP, chronic pain; FMS, fibromyalgia syndrome; HC, healthy controls; MD, major depression patients; MSK, musculoskeletal pain; OA, older adults; RA, rheumatoid arthritis.

Memory Cognitive Tests:

ACT, Auditory Consonant Trigram; CALT, Conditional Associative Learning Task; CMT, Code Memory Test; CVLT, California Verbal Learning Test; KRRFT, Kimura Recurring Recognition Figures Test; RAVLT, Rey Auditory Verbal Learning Test; RMT, Randt Memory Test; WMS, Wechsler Memory Scale.

Visuospatial Processing Tests:

CBTT, Corsi Block Tapping Test; RCFT, Rey– Osterrieth Complex Figure Test; 10/ 36, 10/ 36 Spatial Recall Test.

Attention/Concentration Tests:

DS-F, Digit Span-Forward; DS-B, Digit Span-Backward; LNS, Letter Number Sequencing; PASAT, Paced Auditory Serial Addition Task; SDMT, Symbol Digit Modalities Test; TEA, Test of Everyday Attention; TMT-A, Trail-Making Test-A; TMT-B, Trail-Making Test-B.

Executive Function Tests:

IGT, Iowa Gambling Task; SCWT, Stroop Color and Word Test; WCST, Wisconsin Card Sorting Test.

Language Tests:

ADWL, Consortium to Establish a Registry for Alzheimer's Disease 10-item word list; AN, Animal Naming; FAS, Verbal Fluency Test; RST, Reading Span Test.

Other Tests:

ANAM, Automated Neuropsychological Assessment Metrics; ANT-I, Attentional Network Test—Interactions; APT-RT, Automated Psychological Test—Reaction Time; AS-WAIS, Arithmetic Scale from the Wechsler Adult Intelligence Scale-III; CPT, Continuous Performance Test; DST, Digit Symbol Test; EPT, Everyday Problems Test; GDA, German national recommendations for tests to determine driving ability; MSIT, Multisource Interference Test; PAB, Walter Reed Performance Assessment Battery; SO, Sustained Operations; SST, Symbol Search Test; SW, Synthetic Work; TOL, Tower of London test for inhibition; VR-BR, Virtual Reality Boxes room; VR-MWM, Virtual Reality Morris Water Maze; WAIS-III, Wechsler Adult Intelligence Scale-III.

In brief, cross-sectional comparative studies rely on the predictability of normal probability (bell curve) distributions. This allows data collected by researchers to be "fit" to standard curves and then to compare the curves to each other. The predictability of normal distributions makes it possible to determine the probability that two groups are not the same. By convention, a difference is considered statistically significant when it is 95% likely the groups are different. How well collected data fit these normal probability models is determined by the number of unique measurements made and the precision of the measurements.

Sample size is very important in understanding cross-sectional comparative studies. Large, obvious differences between groups can be demonstrated with relatively small sample sizes. Small, subtle differences between groups require large sample sizes to detect. Small sample sizes tend to overestimate effect sizes. This tendency is responsible for the Proteus effect, the high frequency of initially promising findings from small studies that cannot be reproduced in follow-up work.[5] In research fields comprised entirely of studies of small sample size, it can be expected that many studies would demonstrate some promising finding, but that the promising findings in all of the studies would not be the same.

Sample size also impacts the efficiency of cross-sectional comparative research. When designing clinical research experiments, it is efficient to make multiple different measurements simultaneously. However, as increasing numbers of measurements are performed, the probability of erroneous inference increases. It becomes increasingly likely with each additional simultaneous measurement that at least one difference noted is due to random sample error alone. The more simultaneous measurements compared, the harder it becomes to demonstrate that any differences noted are not sampling error. This is the problem of multiple comparisons. To mathematically address the problem, it is typical to use statistical adjustments, such as the Bonferroni correction, that consider the possibility of random sampling errors in determining group differences. These statistical adjustments increase the probability of what is considered statistically significant to be substantially higher than 95% likely that the groups are different.

Studies making multiple comparisons have a higher bar for demonstrating statistical significance than those making single comparisons. If a study of objective cognitive function made 10 simultaneous measurements, a Bonferroni's correction would require any individual measure to be 99.5% likely to be different to be considered statistically significant. In this way, sample size is at the heart of the problem of multiple comparisons. Large sample sizes, such as those used in population studies, ensure that there are enough unique measurements to account for the possibility of random sample errors.

Studies with large numbers of simultaneous measurements and small sample sizes often find it difficult to demonstrate any group differences after adjusting for multiple comparisons. Rather than adjusting for comparisons, some studies will describe themselves as "exploratory" or "hypothesis generating." It is important to consider these studies as such, as they increase the likelihood of reporting a sample error as a relevant group difference.

A final consideration required for interpreting the literature is a sense of what a "clinically meaningful" difference between groups is. Not all differences that can be measured have clinical relevance. It is important to set a threshold for what magnitude of difference is clinically impactful. For the purposes of this review, we have selected performance that is 1.5 standard deviations (*SDs*) below the mean test score of the healthy comparator group to serve as a guidepost for clinical significance. Our selected standard threshold has been applied to studies of mild cognitive impairment, early Parkinson's disease, and cognitive impairment in systemic lupus erythematosus, and has been demonstrated to have clinical relevance.[39,1,36]

MEASUREMENT OF SUBJECTIVE DYSCOGNITION IN FIBROMYALGIA SYNDROME PATIENTS

Of the 27 studies of objective cognition performance in FMS, only 9 concomitantly measured subjective cognitive complaint (Table 7.2). These studies use questionnaires to characterize cognitive symptoms. Three studies used questionnaires that only measure subjective memory complaints,[20,35,17] one used an executive function complaint questionnaire, and four used questionnaires that assess subjective complaints in all cognitive domains. All questionnaire responses result in a score that describes the severity or frequency of dyscognition, allowing FMS patients' cognitive complaints to be quantified and compared to control groups.

As outlined in Table 7.2, these studies found robust statistical and clinically meaningful differences between FMS patients and comparator groups in their subjective cognitive complaint questionnaire scores. Except for one study, all that have assessed subjective cognitive complaints in FMS report at least 1.5 *SD*s greater subjective cognitive complaint scores in FMS than the mean complaint scores of comparator groups (Table 7.2). This 1.5 standard difference indicates that FMS patients appraise their cognitive abilities to be at or below the seventh percentile of what is seen in healthy volunteers, a powerful demonstration of the clinical importance of the complaint. These measured differences are of such a large magnitude that they are robust despite small sample sizes, remaining statistically significant after post-hoc adjustments for multiple comparisons.

Although studies have demonstrated that FMS patients report clinically significant dyscognition, it remains unclear what the exact nature of these cognitive complaints are. To date, four studies have tried to better describe the dyscognition of FMS using questionnaire subscores. However, the information that can be gleaned from this literature is limited. The full experience of FMS dyscognition is not likely captured by current questionnaires. These questionnaires also seek to quantify experiences over weeks to months, limiting their usefulness in understanding day-to-day or moment-to-moment variability of fibrofog. It appears exceedingly important

TABLE 7.2 **Description of studies characterizing subjective cognitive impairment in patients with fibromyalgia syndrome**

Year	Author	Groups (*N*)	Subjective cognitive measures	Objective cognitive measures	Subjective results	Correlations between subjective complaints and objective measures	Comments
1997	Cote and Moldofsky[11]	FMS (10) HC (9)	VAS	SO, PAB, SW	• Perception of accuracy: FMS lower ($\bar{x}_{diff}$ = "13%"; $F = 12.73$, $p < 0.01$) • Perception of reaction time: No difference	None performed	Military measures are difficult to apply to daily civilian life
1999	Grace et al.[20]	FMS (30) HC (30)	MOQ	WMS, RAVLT, PASAT, SDMT	FMS more memory complaints ($\bar{x}_{diff} = 22.3$ points, 2.17 *SD* diff, $p = 0.0001$)	No statistically significant correlations for either group	Correlations were found for all group pooled data
2001	Park et al.[35]	FMS (23) HC (23) OA (22)	PCSI	Nonstandard tests: processing speed, working and recognition memory, free recall, verbal knowledge	FMS more cognitive complaints than HC ($F = 38.99$, $p < 0.0001$) and OA ($F = 25.447$, $p < 0.0001$)	In FMS: • Processing speed: $r = -0.507$, $p = 0.005$ • Working memory: $r = -0.406$, $p = 0.049$ • Free recall: $r = -0.448$, $p = 0.028$ • Correlations for other tests not significant	• Nonstandard tests used • No adjustments for multiple comparisons

2003	Suhr[44]	FMS (23) CP (22) HC (21)	MMQ—Memory effort subscale	WCST, SCWT, RAVLT, RCFT, PASAT, AS-WAIS, DS-F, DS-B, LNS, DST, SST, TMT-A, TMT-B	FMS more memory complaints than HC ($\bar{x}_{diff}$ = 23.6 points, 1.1 *SD*) and CP ($\bar{x}_{diff}$ = 26.5 points, 1.5 *SD*) $F = 12.61$, $p < 0.001$ (post hoc tests not included)	No statistically significant correlations	• Correlations were constructed based on all group data
2005	Glass et al.[17]	FMS (23) HC (23) OA (22)	MIA	Nonstandard word list learning	FMS have more complaints than HC in memory: • Capacity ($\bar{x}_{diff}$ = 13.9 points, 1.3 *SD*; $F = 20.22$, $p < 0.001$) • Stability ($\bar{x}_{diff}$ = 13 points, 1.1 *SD*; $F = 15.77$, $p < 0.001$) Effect remains, albeit attenuated, for OA comparison ($p < 0.05$)	• In FMS, correlation between memory capacity and free recall task ($r = 0.467$, $p < 0.01$) • No statistically significant correlations for other groups	• Nonstandard test used • No adjustment for multiple comparisons
2011	Glass et al.[18]	FMS (18) HC (14)	MASQ	Nonstandard response inhibition task	FMS more cognitive complaints ($\bar{x}_{diff}$ = 29.9 points, 2.1 *SD*; *t*-test $p < 0.001$)	None	Nonstandard test used

(*Continued*)

TABLE 7.2 **Description of studies characterizing subjective cognitive impairment in patients with fibromyalgia syndrome *(Continued)***

Year	Author	Groups (N)	Subjective cognitive measures	Objective cognitive measures	Subjective results	Correlations between subjective complaints and objective measures	Comments
2015	Tesio et al.[45]	FMS (30) HC (30)	FACT-CS	RAVLT, 1-back, TOL, TMT-A, TMT-B, DS-F, DS-B, FAS	FMS more cognitive complaints ($\bar{x}_{diff}$ = 0.7 points, 1.8 *SD*; *t*-test $p < 0.0001$)	• DS-B and verbal fluency complaint score ($r = 0.395$, $p < 0.05$) • TMT-B and verbal fluency complaint score ($r = -0.361$, $p < 0.05$) • Reaction time and quality of life ($r = -0.377$, $p < 0.05$) • Other correlations not significant (including total FACT-CS score)	• No adjustments for multiple comparisons • Correlations not reported for HC
2016	Gelonch et al.[15]	FMS (82) HC (42)	BRIEF-A	FAS, PASAT, 2-back, 3-back, TMT-A, TMT-B, SCWT, WCST	• FMS more global executive function complaints ($\bar{x}_{diff}$ = 18.5 points, 2.1 *SD*; MANOVA $p = 0.03$) and working memory complaints ($\bar{x}_{diff}$ = 21.6 points, 1.9 *SD*; MANOVA $p = 0.002$) controlling for anxiety and depression	• 3-Back performance and working memory complaints subscale ($r = -0.295$, $p < 0.001$), among other BRIEF-A subscales • WCST performance and working memory complaints subscale ($r = -0.245$, $p < 0.05$)	—

					• No differences in other executive function subscale	• Other correlations not significant	
2016	Walitt et al.[48]	FMS (16) HC (13)	MASQ	0-back, 2-back	—	Performance and MASQ in HC ($r = -0.66$, $p = 0.02$), but not FMS	—

Patient Groups:
CP, chronic pain; FMS, fibromyalgia syndrome; HC, healthy controls; OA, older adults.
Subjective Cognitive Complaint Scales:
BRIEF-A, Behavior Rating Inventory of Executive Function—Adult Version; FACT-CS, Functional Assessment of Cancer Therapy Cognition Scale; MASQ, Multiple Abilities Self-Report Questionnaire; MIA, Metamemory in Adulthood Questionnaire; MMQ, Metamemory Questionnaire; MOQ, Memory Observation Questionnaire; PCSI, Pincus Cognitive Symptoms Inventory; VAS, perception of performance—Speed and Accuracy Visual Analog Scale.
Memory Cognitive Tests:
RAVLT, Rey Auditory Verbal Learning Test; WMS, Wechsler Memory Scale.
Visuospatial Processing Tests:
RCFT, Rey–Osterrieth Complex Figure Test.
Attention/Concentration Tests:
DS-B, Digit Span–Backward; DS-F, Digit Span–Forward; DST, Digit Symbol Test; LNS, Letter Number Sequencing; PASAT, Paced Auditory Serial Addition Task; SDMT, Symbol Digit Modalities Test; SST, Symbol Search Test; TMT-A, Trail-Making Test-A; TMT-B, Trail-Making Test-B.
Executive Function Tests:
SCWT, Stroop Color and Word Test; WCST, Wisconsin Card Sorting Test.
Language Tests:
FAS, Verbal Fluency Test.
Other Tests:
AS-WAIS, Arithmetic Scale from the Wechsler Adult Intelligence Scale-III; PAB, Walter Reed Performance Assessment Battery; SO, sustained operations; SW, synthetic work; TOL, Tower of London test for inhibition.

to study fibrofog with qualitative tools to best understand the content and variability of fibrofog. Common sense suggests that a clear understanding of the qualities of fibrofog is essential for designing studies that have a chance to successfully capture differences in objective cognitive performance.

MEASUREMENT OF OBJECTIVE COGNITIVE PERFORMANCE IN FIBROMYALGIA SYNDROME PATIENTS

To date, there have been 28 studies that have sought to measure objective cognitive performance in FMS patients. Each of these studies' test battery, design, results, and potential problems are detailed in Table 7.1. Collectively, these studies utilized 40 different standardized neurocognitive tests. Learning and memory were assessed in 18 studies, complex attention was assessed in 15 studies, language was assessed in 5 studies, and 4 studies evaluated the cognitive domain of visuospatial processing. Four studies used tests or a testing battery that was not standard, making it difficult to accurately localize what cognitive domain was being tested.[35,21,18,17] Of note, no study has evaluated social cognition in FMS.

Attention

Attention is the most studied cognitive domain in FMS. Overall, the results are inconsistent.

Seven controlled studies used the *Trail Making A/B* tests. Five of them found no differences in performance between groups.[42,44,49,8,15] One found a clinically irrelevant decrease in performance in the Trail Making B test only (t-test: <0.8 SD differences, $p = 0.020$).[45] Munguia-Izquierdo et al. ($N = 81/35$) reported differences in Trail Making A (1.3 SD difference, $p < 0.001$) and B (2.2 SD difference, $p < 0.001$).[33] However, 37% of FMS patients and 8% of the healthy volunteers did not perform the Trail Making B test correctly, raising concerns about its administration.

Eight controlled studies used the *Digit Span Forward and Backwards* tests as part of their battery. Six of them reported no statistical differences between groups.[27,44,28,26,8] Two found statistically but not clinically significant differences between groups (<1.5 SD in magnitude).[33]

The *Paced Auditory Serial Addition Task* has been the most consistent among all chosen tests of attention in identifying relevant differences. Four studies found FMS patients had statistically lower scores in this task, while two found no differences.[20,42,44,28,33,15] However, only two of the four statistically significant studies reported clinically relevant differences (around 1.5 SD in magnitude).[42,33]

Overall, the literature does not demonstrate a clinically substantial impairment in concentration in FMS patients when compared to healthy volunteers.

Memory

Memory function has been extensively studied in FMS. Five studies utilized *Rey Auditory Verbal Learning Test*, three of which found statistically significant group differences in performance.[45,33,26] However, results of one these studies disappear after adjusting for depression scores (analysis of covariance [ANCOVA]: $p = 0.857$),[26] and the difference reported in another is not clinically relevant (<0.8 *SD* difference).[45] Two studies utilized the *Wechsler Memory Scale*.[20,28] One of them found a clinically irrelevant decrease in performance on the General Memory and Verbal Memory subscales (t-test: <1 *SD* difference, $p = 0.01$), while the other found no differences.[28]

Overall, the literature does not demonstrate a clinically substantial impairment in memory in FMS patients when compared to healthy volunteers.

Executive Function

Executive function has been studied using various tests in FMS, typically with the *Stroop Color Word* tests. Clinically irrelevant differences on the Stroop Color Word Test were reported by two studies (<0.7 *SD* differences).[8,15] Four studies found no diminished performance in the Stroop Color Word Test.[44,49,50,46]

No substantial differences have been demonstrated in the four studies utilizing the *Wisconsin Card Sort Test*. Three found no differences in performance, the fourth found no differences in perseverative errors (t-test: $p = 0.54$).[44,47,26,15] No substantial differences have been shown in the two studies using the *Iowa Gambling Test*.[47,50]

Overall, the literature does not demonstrate a clinically substantial impairment in executive function in FMS patients when compared to healthy volunteers.

Language

Language has not been studied extensively in FMS. Four studies reported no differences in performance between patients and healthy controls in the *verbal fluency task*.[45,27,44,15]

Overall, the literature does not demonstrate a clinically substantial impairment in language in FMS patients when compared to healthy volunteers.

Visuospatial Processing

Visuospatial processing has not been studied extensively in FMS. Two studies using the *Rey Complex Figure Test* provide contrasting results. Only one reported differences that approached but did not reach clinical relevance after controlling for depression (ANCOVA: 1.4 *SD* difference, $p = 0.01$).[26]

Overall, the literature does not demonstrate a clinically substantial impairment in visuospatial processing in FMS patients when compared to healthy volunteers.

Functional Imaging

Table 7.3 reviews the four studies that address the cognitive aspects of FMS using functional magnetic resonance imaging (fMRI). One study used the Go/No-Go response inhibition task,[18] where no difference in performance between patients and comparators was expected. Three studies used the N-Back to measure cognitive performance.[48,40,7] One study found FMS patients to have lower accuracy than healthy controls in 2-back (8% difference, *t*-test: $p < 0.05$),[16] while the other two found no differences for the 0- or 2-back.[48,40,7] No fMRI study demonstrated a clinically relevant difference in cognitive performance. All of the fMRI studies demonstrated a difference in the pattern blood oxygen level dependent (BOLD) imaging during task performance. A consistent pattern of BOLD activation was not seen between the four studies. The observed BOLD differences in all these studies cannot be attributed to differences in objective cognitive performance. One study suggests that group differences in the pattern of BOLD activity are correlated with subjective appraisal of symptoms.[48]

Overall, the literature does not support that fibrofog is related to a specific alteration of BOLD activation as measured by fMRI.

Test-Taking Effort

As noted previously, a clinically relevant alteration in objective cognitive performance has not been consistently demonstrated in FMS. If a large effect on objective cognitive testing had been found in fibrofog, it would be reasonable to attempt to study whether differential test-taking effort or invalid performance profiles rather than true cognitive deficits account for differences in performance. That is, perhaps any differences seen in studies of objective cognitive performance are related to group differences in test-taking effort.

To date, only one study by Gervais et al. tried to determine if performance validity measures, which can serve as an index of differential test-taking effort, have a relevant role in the cognitive performance of FMS patients.[16] Their study was focused on the impact of having a disability claim on cognitive performance. FMS patients were split into two groups, one comprised of patients who had or were applying for disability benefits ($N = 46$) and one with patients without disability claims ($N = 50$). To examine test-taking effort, they used the Word Memory Test and the Computerized Assessment of Response Bias, tasks designed for participants to perceive as difficult but are in fact very easy. They found that FMS patients with disability claims performed statistically (ANOVA: $p < 0.001$) and clinically (> 1.5 *SD* differences) worse than FMS patients without disability claims, rheumatoid arthritis patients, traumatic brain injury patients, and healthy controls in both tests. FMS patients without disability claims did not perform statistically or clinically worse than healthy controls on these tests. These results suggest that disability claims may have a clinically relevant impact on the effort put forth in cognitive testing, but differential test-taking effort

TABLE 7.3 **Neuroimaging of cognitive dysfunction/fibrofog**

Refs.	Groups (*N*)	Age/gender	Imaging modality ROI	Statistical corrections	Cognitive test/ measurement	fMRI findings	Conclusions	Biases and limitations
Glass et al.[18]	FMS (18) HC (14)	43.6 ± 9.8, all *F* 41.1 ± 11.9, all *F*	Task—fMRI; functional connectivity Whole brain; seed in the right inferior temporal gyrus/ fusiform gyrus	Cluster correction for multiple comparisons ($p < 0.05$, derived from an uncorrected $p < 0.005$ on the voxel level, with a cluster extent of 92 contiguous voxels estimated with AFNI AlphaSim)	Response inhibition: Go/No-Go task (not cued)	No difference in task performance Hypo-activation in FMS bilaterally in PMC, SMA, MCC, putamen, right IPL, left MFC, and, after controlling for anxiety, in the right IC Hyper-activation in FMS the right inferior temporal gyrus/fusiform gyrus Mental fatigue scores in FMS correlated positively with the BOLD response in left IC and putamen, and negatively with the right temporal gyrus and orbitofrontal cortex, and left anterior cerebellum	–Inhibition and pain perception rely on partially overlapping networks (with an intersection in the posterior ACC/MCC/ SMA), which might divert resources from the inhibition task to pain processing in FMS. This might trigger additional resource allocation from other related areas. –Longitudinal studies of FMS subjects with pain improving over time might clarify this hypothesis	–Multiple correlations outside the main question of the study –Post hoc connectivity analyses –Small cohort sizes

(*Continued*)

TABLE 7.3 **Neuroimaging of cognitive dysfunction/fibrofog (*Continued*)**

Refs.	Groups (*N*)	Age/gender	Imaging modality ROI	Statistical corrections	Cognitive test/ measurement	fMRI findings	Conclusions	Biases and shortcomings
Seo et al.[40]	FMS (19) HC (22)	38.7 ±7.7, all *F* 38.3±8.5, all *F*	Task—fMRI Whole brain	$P < 0.01$, FDR corrected for multiple comparisons across the whole brain	Working memory: 0-back vs. 2-back Pain sensitivity: pressure on the left thumbnail of 1–6 kg/m^2 in 0.5 increments	Lower pain threshold, lower task accuracy, and higher response time in FMS vs. HC Hypo-activation in FMS bilaterally in DLPFC, VMPFC, and SMA, and right IPL for the 2-back task Depression and anxiety scores correlated %BOLD change in DLPFC, VLPFC, and IPL. If depression and anxiety are included in the fMRI analysis, the differences between FMS and HC disappear bilaterally for the DLPFC and for the right VLPFC.	–Working memory deficit, if any, found in FMS patients may be attributable to differences in neural activation of the frontoparietal memory network and may result from both pain itself or from depression and anxiety associated with pain	–Small cohort sizes –Medication might be a possible confounder (there was no controlling for antidepressants)
Ceko et al.[7]	FMS (28) HC (23)	48.7 ± 7.8, all *F* 48.8 ± 7.7, all *F*	Task—fMRI mask around DMN	Cluster-correction for multiple comparisons ($p < 0.05$) with Monte Carlo simulation (AFNI 3dClustSim) across independently defined masks external and internal to DMN	Working memory: multilevel N-back (0-back vs. 1 . . . 3-back, easy to hard)	DMN is more deactivated (negative fMRI response) with increased task difficulty in HC DMN is very low or not deactivated with increasing task difficulty in FMS No difference in task performance No differences in extra DMN activations involved in the task	–A responsive DMN might not be needed for successful –No structures appeared to compensate for DMN lack of modulation in patients	–Use of medications such as anticonvulsants could have in several patients contributed to decreased recruitment and possibly also decreased responsiveness of brain regions during the cognitive task

Walitt et al.[48]	FMS (15) HC (12)	44.9 ± 10.2, all *F* 44.2 ± 11.2, all *F*	Task—fMRI Whole brain	–Uncorrected voxel-wise threshold of $p < 0.01$ –Cluster corrected for multiple comparisons ($p < 0.05$) using random-field theory	Working memory: 0-back vs. 2-back	No difference in task performance No significant differences between groups in the 2back > 0back BOLD contrast, but similar activations in DLPFC, VLPFC, SPL, IPL, SMA, ACC, IC, precuneus, and cerebellum Positive correlation in HC between 2-back task accuracy and BOLD response in right IC, putamen, frontal operculum, PMC, DLPFC and left caudate, and putamen No correlation in FMS between 2-back task accuracy and BOLD response FMS lack the negative correlation between cognitive appraisal and BOLD response in the anterior IC and putamen observed in HC	–Lack of relationship between subjective experience and objective performance as a key property of "fibrofog" –"Fibrofog" does not appear to interfere with proper activation of task-related brain networks –Lack of activation in the putamen and IC during cognitive appraisal might contribute to "fibrofog" –"Fibrofog" is better characterized by subjective rather than objective cognitive impairment	–Small cohort size –Difficulty in separating different cognitive abilities from psychiatric comorbidities (e.g., anxiety or depression)

ACC, anterior cingulate cortex; AFNI, Analysis of Functional NeuroImages; BOLD, blood oxygen level dependent; DLPFC, dorsolateral prefrontal cortex; DMN, default-mode network; FDR, false discovery rate; FMS, fibromyalgia syndrome; fMRI, functional magnetic resonance imaging; HC, healthy controls; IC, insular cortex; IFG, inferior frontal gyrus; IPL, inferior parietal lobule; ITC, inferior temporal cortex; MCC, mid-cingulate cortex; MFC, middle frontal cortex; PMC, premotor cortex; ROI, region of interest; SMA, supplementary motor area; SPL, superior parietal lobule; STG, superior temporal gyrus; VLPFC, ventrolateral prefrontal cortex; VMPFC, ventromedial prefrontal cortex.

does not appear to have a clinically important impact on objective cognitive testing in FMS.

CORRELATION BETWEEN SUBJECTIVE COMPLAINT AND OBJECTIVE PERFORMANCE

The relationship between the subjective dyscognition and objective cognitive performance is essential to determine if the current psychometric approaches are capable of being accurate surrogates of fibrofog. A successful objective measurement of fibrofog should approximate the severity of dyscognitive symptoms reported.

To date, seven studies examined the relationship between subjective cognitive complaints and objective cognitive performance in FMS (Table 7.2). Three studies did not find any significant correlations.[20,48,44] Interestingly, Walitt et al. ($N = 16$) found a strong correlation between subjective cognitive difficulty and task accuracy on the 2-back task in healthy controls ($r = -0.66$, $p = 0.02$) that was not seen in FMS patients ($r = 0.18$, $p = 0.52$). Rather than correlating with objective performance, subjective cognitive complaint in FMS patients was found to correlate ($r = 0.65$, $p = 0.005$) with overall FMS symptom severity as determined by the FIQ.[48] In a separate, small ($n = 8$) longitudinal study, Walitt et al. also noted that substantial clinical improvement after 8 weeks of multimodal therapy (median change in FIQ score 33.9 [0 to 100 scale], $p = 0.002$) had no impact on neuropsychological performance.[49]

The other four of the seven studies found at least one correlation between subjective cognitive symptom severity and objective cognitive testing performance in FMS. However, two of those studies can be considered as negative, given that they did not adjust for multiple comparisons when 37 and 100 correlations were reported.[45,15] The other studies do not demonstrate a clear, consistent relation between specific subjective complaints and objective test performance in the domain of the subjective complaint.[35,17]

No clear relationship exists between the reporting of subjective cognitive impairment and objective cognitive performance as measured by current neuropsychological tests. This is a striking finding. Valid objective measures of fibrofog require tight correlation with the subjective experience. It seems clear that current methods of psychometric assessment fail to approximate the experience of fibrofog.

SYSTEMATIC METHODOLOGIC ISSUES IN THE STUDY OF SUBJECTIVE DYSCOGNITION AND OBJECTIVE COGNITIVE FUNCTION IN FIBROMYALGIA SYNDROME

The cross-sectional comparison method has now been applied to the study of subjective dyscognition and objective cognitive function for nearly two decades. Of published studies, 22 state in the conclusions that FMS patients are "cognitively impaired" in at least one way. The view evolved from the initial suggestion of Grace in 1999 that the "primary problems with attention/concentration are another characteristic of FMS which can be added to the list of ancillary features" to the Tesio 2015 statement that "our results confirmed the impairments of attention, long-term memory, and shifting and updating executive functions in FMS patient compared to healthy controls." Many contemporary scientists, clinicians, patients, and their advocates believe that a definitive cognitive impairment has been clearly demonstrated. Some have suggested that the mechanisms underlying this cognitive impairment are responsible for the experience of fibrofog.[10]

Our review of the literature demonstrates that FMS patients report clinically substantial and easily reproducible differences in subjective dyscognition compared to healthy comparators. On the other hand, objective testing of cognitive function has failed to demonstrate equivalent findings. These studies have reported small, inconsistent, and clinically irrelevant differences in objective neurocognitive testing. Finally, the literature fails to demonstrate a meaningful, reproducible relationship between the subjective complaint and objective test performance. It appears that standard neurocognitive testing has been unable to capture the essence of fibrofog.

Currently, there is a systematic scientific bias that impacts the entire neurocognitive literature of FMS. This bias is not the result of any single investigative group, but rather the consequence of many investigative groups working independently with small sample sizes and the same exploratory study design. Assuming no overlap of participants between studies, the entire literature to date encompasses only 804 FMS patients. Only four studies have more than 40 participants. Most studies have small patient cohorts of 10 to 30 subjects per group and are comprised exclusively of women (90% to 100%). These sample sizes predispose to false positive findings from sampling error, to overestimating effect sizes, and cannot be generalized to the population at large. The predisposition of small sample size studies to report false positives as true differences was markedly increased by the use of liberal statistical methods. Most authors considered their individual studies to be "exploratory" and did not select conservative statistical approaches. It is important for clinicians and scientists to be mindful that exploratory studies frequently suggest promise, but never provide definitive answers.

In addition, only 2 of 27 studies adjusted for multiple comparisons despite administering, on average, four tests (range 1 to 14). A noteworthy example can be seen in Tesio 2015, where none of the reported results would meet statistical significance after basic Bonferroni correction ($p = 0.005$ for 10 comparisons). All major statistical analysis packages include some form of multiple comparisons correction. Because controlling for false positives is widely available and straightforward, it seems to be the case that investigators do not want to jeopardize their results through the application of more stringent conditions.

Also, only 4 of 27 studies included a chronic pain patient comparator group, while most other studies used healthy controls as their sole comparator group. The absence of a positive control group may confound results, as we cannot determine whether to attribute any differences observed to FMS specifically or chronic pain in general. Moreover, only 2 of 27 studies controlled for centrally acting agents (such as opioids) in their analyses, and 10 of 27 studies controlled for depression, both of which may affect cognitive function. These potential confounders would serve to increase the magnitude of the objective cognitive deficit. However, the lack of a substantial and reproducible objective cognitive deficit in the literature suggests that these factors are of negligible importance.

ADVANCING THE STUDY OF FIBROFOG

The current state of science provides no insight into the mechanistic nature of fibrofog. As no objective cognitive test is a reliable correlate of subjective dyscognition, it appears that science has so far failed to measure fibrofog. However, the inability of medical science to adequately measure fibrofog does not make the problem disappear or make it less "real" for those who are inconvenienced and disabled by it. The need for an effective scientific approach to its measurement remains.

A renewed scientific approach to fibrofog should begin with its detailed qualitative assessment. Broad collection of qualitative symptom narratives from patients to identify common themes would be valuable in developing working definitions of fibrofog. Qualitative interviews can also provide insight into questions about the static, dynamic, and recalled content of fibrofog. This information can be used to develop new methods of measuring the subjective symptom content and severity of fibrofog over various temporal horizons. There are currently no qualitative tools able to provide meaningful and reliable point estimates of fibrofog.

Once developed, new insights into the subjective nature of fibrofog should be considered when choosing objective methods for measurement. The data reviewed above suggest that standard neurocognitive tests fail to adequately measure fibrofog. Future objective cognitive tests should be carefully chosen to best estimate the thematic elements of fibrofog. Aspects of fibrofog that seem important to patients such as Starlanyl's "tongue-tripping" will likely require the development of novel tests to objectively capture. Designing objective tests based on careful subjective description is likely to be the essential successful measurement of fibrofog. It is doubtful that continued use of standard testing will provide new, meaningful insight.

Study designs should also be considered with more care. Rather than using single time-point cross-sectional designs, study participants should be measured on multiple occasions. This will enable a better understanding of day-to-day fluctuations in symptoms, performance, and their relationship. Such a design will also address problems that are associated with memory and symptom recall. It will also better elucidate the clinical relevance of fibrofog symptoms and what amount of change is meaningful to patients.

Studies should also elaborate specific hypotheses and ensure that they have large enough sample sizes to analyze their data with statistical rigor. Statistical methods should be chosen that address the problem of multiple comparisons. Alternative ways of considering the data beyond means and *SD* are also needed. Presenting data in terms of medians and percentiles can smooth out the effects of outliers on results. Exploratory studies in this field have already shown their predisposition to mislead and should be avoided. The point of future studies should be to prove a well-considered idea, not running experiments in order to "just publish something."

A successful approach to objectively measure fibrofog will become obviously apparent. Any meaningful objective measure should strongly correlate with subjective symptom reporting, should change in proportion to changes in subjective symptom reporting, and should be reproducible in multiple studies. Objective tests that fail to correlate meaningfully with subjective symptoms should be categorically rejected.

The hope is that a reconsidered scientific approach to fibrofog will provide an objective method to quantify the subjective experience. With such a scientific tool in hand, it becomes possible to begin looking at the biologic underpinnings of the fibrofog experience.

ACKNOWLEDGMENTS

This chapter was supported (in part) by the Intramural Research program of the NIH, National Institute of Nursing Research, National Institute of Neurological Diseases and Stroke, and National Institute of Mental Health.

REFERENCES

1. Antonchak MA, Saoudian M, Khan AR, Brunner HI, Luggen ME. Cognitive dysfunction in patients with systemic lupus erythematosus: a controlled study. *J Rheumatol.* 2011;**38**(6):1020–1025.
2. Beard G. Neurasthenia, or nervous exhaustion. *Boston Med Surg J.* 1869;**80**(13):217–221.
3. Bennett RM. Fibrositis: misnomer for a common rheumatic disorder. *West J Med.* 1981;**134**(5):405–413.
4. Burckhardt CS, Clark SR, Bennett RM. The fibromyalgia impact questionnaire: development and validation. *J Rheumatol.* 1991;**18**(5):728–733.
5. Button KS, Ioannidis JP, Mokrysz C, et al. Power failure: why small sample size undermines the reliability of neuroscience. *Nat Rev Neurosci.* 2013;**14**(5):365–376.
6. Canovas R, Leon I, Roldan MD, Astur R, Cimadevilla JM. Virtual reality tasks disclose spatial memory alterations in fibromyalgia. *Rheumatology.* 2009;**48**(10):1273–1278.
7. Ceko M, Gracely JL, Fitzcharles MA, Seminowicz DA, Schweinhardt P, Bushnell MC. Is a responsive default mode network required for successful working memory task performance? *J Neurosci.* 2015;**35**(33):11595–11605.

8. Cherry BJ, Zettel-Watson L, Shimizu R, Roberson I, Rutledge DN, Jones CJ. Cognitive performance in women aged 50 years and older with and without fibromyalgia. *J Gerontol B Psychol Sci Soc Sci.* 2014;**69**(2):199–208.
9. Clauw DJ, Arnold LM, McCarberg BH. FibroCollaborative. The science of fibromyalgia. *Mayo Clin Proc.* 2011;**86**(9):907–911.
10. Coppieters I, Ickmans K, Cagnie B, et al. Cognitive performance is related to central sensitization and health-related quality of life in patients with chronic Whiplash-associated disorders and fibromyalgia. *Pain Physician.* 2015;**18**(3):E389–E401.
11. Cote KA, Moldofsky H. Sleep, daytime symptoms, and cognitive performance in patients with fibromyalgia. *J Rheumatol.* 1997;**24**(10):2014–2023.
12. Dick B, Eccleston C, Crombez G. Attentional functioning in fibromyalgia, rheumatoid arthritis, and musculoskeletal pain patients. *Arthritis Rheum.* 2002;**47**(6):639–644.
13. Dick BD, Verrier MJ, Harker KT, Rashiq S. Disruption of cognitive function in fibromyalgia syndrome. *Pain.* 2008;**139**(3):610–616.
14. Gaudino EA, Coyle PK, Krupp LB. Post-Lyme syndrome and chronic fatigue syndrome. Neuropsychiatric similarities and differences. *Arch Neurol.* 1997;**54**(11):1372–1376.
15. Gelonch O, Garolera M, Valls J, Rossello L, Pifarre J. Executive function in fibromyalgia: comparing subjective and objective measures. *Compr Psychiatry.* 2016;**66**:113–122.
16. Gervais RO, Russell AS, Green P, Allen LM, 3rd, Ferrari R, Pieschl SD. Effort testing in patients with fibromyalgia and disability incentives. *J Rheumatol.* 2001;**28**(8):1892–1899.
17. Glass JM, Park DC, Minear M, Crofford LJ. Memory beliefs and function in fibromyalgia patients. *J Psychosom Res.* 2005;**58**(3):263–269.
18. Glass JM, Williams DA, Fernandez-Sanchez ML, et al. Executive function in chronic pain patients and healthy controls: different cortical activation during response inhibition in fibromyalgia. *J Pain.* 2011;**12**(12):1219–1229.
19. Goldenberg DL. Psychological symptoms and psychiatric diagnosis in patients with fibromyalgia. *J Rheumatol Suppl.* 1989;**19**:127–130.
20. Grace GM, Nielson WR, Hopkins M, Berg MA. Concentration and memory deficits in patients with fibromyalgia syndrome. *J Clin Exp Neuropsychol.* 1999;**21**(4):477–487.
21. Grisart J, Van der Linden M, Masquelier E. Controlled processes and automaticity in memory functioning in fibromyalgia patients: relation with emotional distress and hypervigilance. *J Clin Exp Neuropsychol.* 2002;**24**(8):994–1009.
22. Kang H, Zhao F, You L, et al. Pseudo-dementia: a neuropsychological review. *Ann Ind Acad Neurol.* 2014;**17**(2):147–154.
23. Kaplan RF, Meadows ME, Vincent LC, Logigian EL, Steere AC. Memory impairment and depression in patients with Lyme encephalopathy: comparison with fibromyalgia and nonpsychotically depressed patients. *Neurology.* 1992;**42**(7):1263–1267.
24. Katz RS, Heard AR, Mills M, Leavitt F. The prevalence and clinical impact of reported cognitive difficulties (fibrofog) in patients with rheumatic disease with and without fibromyalgia. *J Clin Rheumatol.* 2004;**10**(2):53–58.
25. Kiloh LG. Pseudo-dementia. *Acta psychiatrica Scandinavica.* 1961;**37**:336–351.
26. Kim SH, Kim SH, Kim SK, Nam EJ, Han SW, Lee SJ. Spatial versus verbal memory impairments in patients with fibromyalgia. *Rheumatol Int.* 2012;**32**(5):1135–1142.
27. Landro NI, Stiles TC, Sletvold H. Memory functioning in patients with primary fibromyalgia and major depression and healthy controls. *J Psychosom Res.* 1997;**42**(3):297–306.
28. Leavitt F, Katz RS. Distraction as a key determinant of impaired memory in patients with fibromyalgia. *J Rheumatol.* 2006;**33**(1):127–132.
29. Mease P, Arnold LM, Choy EH, et al. Fibromyalgia syndrome module at OMERACT 9: domain construct. *J Rheumatol.* 2009;**36**(10):2318–2329.

30. Mease PJ, Arnold LM, Crofford LJ, et al. Identifying the clinical domains of fibromyalgia: contributions from clinician and patient Delphi exercises. *Arthritis Rheum.* 2008;**59**(7):952–960.
31. Miró E, Lupiáñez J, Hita E, Martínez MP, Sánchez AI, Buela-Casal G. Attentional deficits in fibromyalgia and its relationships with pain, emotional distress and sleep dysfunction complaints. *Psychol Health.* 2011;26(6):765–780.
32. Mitchell T, Turton P. 'Chemobrain': concentration and memory effects in people receiving chemotherapy—a descriptive phenomenological study. *Eur J Canc Care.* 2011;**20**(4):539–548.
33. Munguia-Izquierdo D, Legaz-Arrese A, Moliner-Urdiales D, Reverter-Masia J. Neuropsychological performance in patients with fibromyalgia syndrome: relation to pain and anxiety. *Psicothema.* 2008;**20**(3):427–431.
34. Ocon AJ. Caught in the thickness of brain fog: exploring the cognitive symptoms of Chronic Fatigue Syndrome. *Front Physiol.* 2013;**4**:63.
35. Park DC, Glass JM, Minear M, Crofford LJ. Cognitive function in fibromyalgia patients. *Arthritis Rheum.* 2001;**44**(9):2125–2133.
36. Pedersen KF, Larsen JP, Tysnes OB, Alves G. Natural course of mild cognitive impairment in Parkinson disease: a 5-year population-based study. *Neurology.* 2017;**88**(8):767–774.
37. Pincus T, Swearingen C, Callahan LF. A self-report cognitive symptoms inventory to assess patients with rheumatic diseases: results in eosinophilia-myalgia syndrome, fibromyalgia, rheumatoid arthritis, and other rheumatic diseases. *Arthritis Rheum.* 1996;**39:** S261.
38. Rabinbach A. *The Human Motor: Energy, Fatigue, and the Origins of Modernity.* Berkeley and Los Angeles, CA: University of California Press; 1992.
39. Schinka JA, Loewenstein DA, Raj A, et al. Defining mild cognitive impairment: impact of varying decision criteria on neuropsychological diagnostic frequencies and correlates. *Am J Geriatr Psychiatry.* 2010;**18**(8):684–691.
40. Seo J, Kim SH, Kim YT, et al. Working memory impairment in fibromyalgia patients associated with altered frontoparietal memory network. *PloS One.* 2012;**7**(6):e37808.
41. Shmygalev S, Dagtekin O, Gerbershagen HJ, Marcus H, Jübner M, Sabatowski R, et al. Assessing cognitive and psychomotor performance in patients with fibromyalgia syndrome. *Pain Ther.* 2014;3(2):85–101.
42. Sletvold H, Stiles TC, Landro NI. Information processing in primary fibromyalgia, major depression and healthy controls. *J Rheumatol.* 1995;**22**(1):137–142.
43. Starlanyl DJ. *The Fibromyalgia Advocate: Getting the Support You Need to Cope With Fibromyalgia and Myofascial Pain Syndrome.* Oakland, CA: New Harbinger Publications; 1998.
44. Suhr JA. Neuropsychological impairment in fibromyalgia: relation to depression, fatigue, and pain. *J Psychosom Res.* 2003;**55**(4):321–329.
45. Tesio V, Torta DM, Colonna F, et al. Are fibromyalgia patients cognitively impaired? Objective and subjective neuropsychological evidence. *Arthritis Care Res.* 2015;**67**(1):143–150.
46. Veldhuijzen DS, Sondaal SF, Oosterman JM. Intact cognitive inhibition in patients with fibromyalgia but evidence of declined processing speed. *J Pain.* 2012;**13**(5):507–515.
47. Verdejo-Garcia A, Lopez-Torrecillas F, Calandre EP, Delgado-Rodriguez A, Bechara A. Executive function and decision-making in women with fibromyalgia. *Arch Clin Neuropsychol.* 2009;**24**(1): 113–122.
48. Walitt B, Ceko M, Khatiwada M, et al. Characterizing "fibrofog": subjective appraisal, objective performance, and task-related brain activity during a working memory task. *NeuroImage Clin.* 2016;**11**:173–180.
49. Walitt B, Roebuck-Spencer T, Bleiberg J, Foster G, Weinstein A. Automated neuropsychiatric measurements of information processing in fibromyalgia. *Rheumatol Int.* 2008;**28**(6):561–566.
50. Walteros C, Sanchez-Navarro JP, Munoz MA, Martinez-Selva JM, Chialvo D, Montoya P. Altered associative learning and emotional decision making in fibromyalgia. *J Psychosom Res.* 2011;**70**(3):294–301.

51. Wolfe F, Clauw DJ, Fitzcharles MA, et al. The American College of Rheumatology preliminary diagnostic criteria for fibromyalgia and measurement of symptom severity. *Arthritis Care Res.* 2010;**62**(5): 600–610.
52. Wolfe F, Smythe HA, Yunus MB, et al. The American College of Rheumatology 1990 criteria for the classification of fibromyalgia. Report of the Multicenter Criteria Committee. *Arthritis Rheum.* 1990;**33**(2):160–172.
53. Wolfe F. The design of a fibromyalgia criteria study. *J Rheumatol Suppl.* 1989;**19**:180–184.
54. Woolf CJ. Central sensitization: implications for the diagnosis and treatment of pain. *Pain.* 2011;**152**(3 Suppl):S2–S15.
55. Yunus MB, Masi AT, Aldag JC. A controlled study of primary fibromyalgia syndrome: clinical features and association with other functional syndromes. *J Rheumatol Suppl.* 1989;**19**:62–71.

CHAPTER 8

Chronic Overlapping Pain Conditions

Christin Veasley

Summary Points

- Fibromyalgia syndrome (FMS) often exists in combination with a number of other chronic pain disorders, particularly those that solely or predominantly affect women. The clinical state of overlap of a subset of these disorders is termed chronic overlapping pain conditions (COPCs).
- Delays in the accurate diagnosis and effective treatment commonly experienced by individuals with COPCs can have serious consequences, including worsening of both site-specific and body-wide symptoms, which in turn make COPCs more difficult to treat effectively; a vicious cycle ensues, leading to poorer health outcomes, diminished quality of life, and increased disability and financial burden.
- Mounting evidence demonstrates that COPCs share common underlying disease mechanisms, mainly in the immune, neural, and endocrine systems.
- Systematic reviews summarize the current poor state of evidence for most of the treatments used to manage individual COPCs. In theory, those with multiple conditions are thought to have more "centralized" pain and are therefore treated with medications that target the CNS, although no studies have been conducted comparing the efficacy of a specific treatment in those with multiple COPCs versus in those with one COPC. In general, treatment is shifting toward a biopsychosocial, multimodal, personalized model that in addition to pain identifies non-pain domains that may be affected, for example, sleep, mood, and fatigue, and develops a treatment plan that is personalized to each individual.
- Research trends have shifted from studying each COPC in isolation to studying multiple conditions simultaneously in well-designed, multisite, prospective studies. This approach is more holistic, cost-effective, and patient-centric and is beginning to parse out both commonalities and uniqueness among COPC subgroups.

Fibromyalgia syndrome (FMS) frequently coexists with other chronic pain disorders, particularly those that solely or predominantly affect women. Although various terms have been used to describe the clinical state of overlap among a subset of these conditions (e.g., functional pain syndromes, central sensitivity syndromes, complex persistent pain conditions, dysfunctional pain), in 2012, the National Institutes of Health (NIH) termed them *COPCs* (Fig. 8.1).[113] In addition to FMS, they include vulvodynia, temporomandibular disorders (TMDs), myalgic encephalomyelitis/chronic fatigue syndrome (ME/CFS), irritable bowel syndrome (IBS), interstitial cystitis/painful bladder syndrome (IC/PBS), endometriosis, chronic migraine headache (cMigraine), chronic tension-type headache (cTTH), and chronic low back pain (cLBP) (see Table 8.1 for disorder summaries). FMS has also been reported to overlap with various other conditions, including but not limited to rheumatoid arthritis, osteoarthritis, diabetes mellitus, inflammatory bowel disease, lupus, and hypothyroidism.[182]

Most studies conducted to date have examined COPC comorbidity rates within a specific index condition, that is, prevalence rates of IBS and CFS in a population of patients with FMS, or prevalence rates of IC and vulvodynia in a population of patients with IBS. Furthermore, most of these studies have been cross-sectional and include only patients from specialized tertiary clinics. The reported prevalence rates

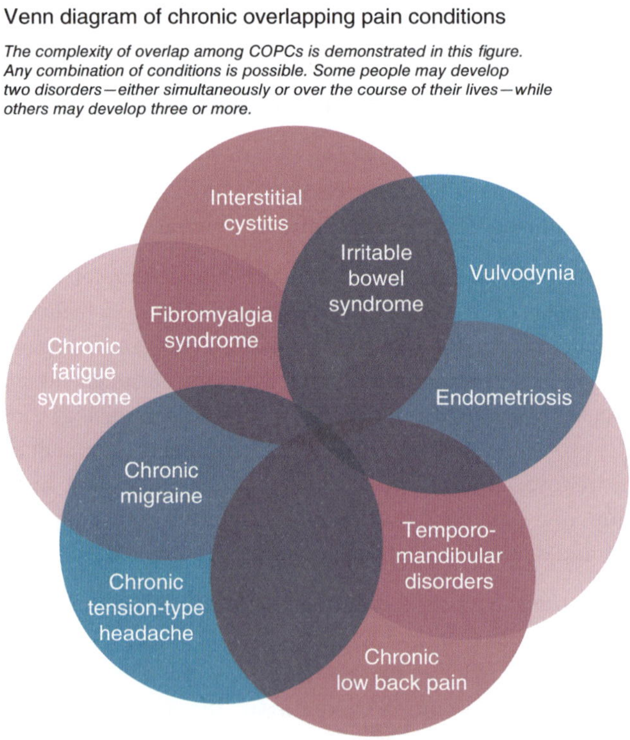

FIGURE 8.1 Venn diagram of chronic overlapping pain conditions.

TABLE 8.1 **COPC descriptions and rates of co-occurrence in FMS**

Condition	Disorder description and symptoms	% of Prevalence (range) of FMS
Vulvodynia	Chronic pain of the vulva—the area surrounding the vaginal opening—without an identifiable cause. The most common symptom is burning.	16–31[182]
Temporomandibular disorders (TMD)	Pain in the jaw joint and surrounding muscle and tissues, along with limitations in jaw movement. One or both joints may be involved, affecting one's ability to speak, chew, swallow, make facial expressions, and even breathe.	13–52[182]
Myalgic encephalomyelitis/ chronic fatigue syndrome (ME/ CFS)	Profound fatigue lasting for 6 or more consecutive months that is not improved by bed rest and that may be worsened by physical or mental activity. The nature and severity of symptoms vary, and include severe muscle and joint pain, cognitive impairment, unrefreshing sleep and a worsening of symptoms with mental or physical exertion.	16–80[182]
Irritable bowel syndrome (IBS)	Pain or discomfort in the abdomen, along with changes in bowel movement patterns. Four subtypes exist: with diarrhea, with constipation, mixed, and unknown.	20–65[182]
Interstitial cystitis/ painful bladder syndrome (IC/PBS)	Pain, pressure, or discomfort of the bladder in the absence of infection or other pathology, typically accompanied by urinary frequency and urgency	12–22[182]
Endometriosis	Chronic neuro-endocrine-immune system disease, in which the endometrial tissue is found outside of the uterus, causing pain, infertility, and other problems. The most common symptoms are pain before/during menstruation and/or sexual activity, pain with bowel movements and during urination, fatigue, infertility, and heavy bleeding.	2–56[49,144,149]
Chronic migraine headache (cMigraine)	Primary headache disorder that affects one-half of the head is pulsating in nature, lasts from 2 to 72 hours, and is generally made worse with physical activity. Associated autonomic symptoms include nausea; vomiting; and sensitivity to light, sound, or smell. Up to one-third of those with migraine perceive an aura—a transient visual, sensory, language, or motor disturbance.	10–22[182]

(*Continued*)

TABLE 8.1 **COPC descriptions and rates of co-occurrence in FMS (*Continued*)**

Condition	Disorder description and symptoms	% of Prevalence (range) of FMS
Chronic tension type headache (cTTH)	Primary headache disorder characterized by pain (pressure, tightening, or feeling like the head is being squeezed with a vice), frequently on both the left and right sides of the head. The pain can radiate from the lower back of the head, neck, eyes, or other muscle groups. Individuals also report sensitivity to light and sound and may experience nausea.	23–36[182]
Chronic low back pain (cLBP)	Low back pain that occurs at least half of the days in the past 6 months. Symptoms include dull aching, sharp pain, tingling or burning sensations, and/or weakness in the legs or feet, among others, in the low back, defined as the lumbar region of the back between the posterior margin of the rib cage and the horizontal gluteal fold.	19–67[182,170]

COPC, chronic overlapping pain conditions; FMS, fibromyalgia syndrome.

also differ for the same two disorders in the other condition, that is, studies report different prevalence rates of FMS in patients with vulvodynia, compared with rates of vulvodynia in FMS patients. For these and other reasons, the reported rates of co-occurrence vary substantially. Table 8.1 summarizes the estimated prevalence rates of FMS in other COPCs, which ranges from 2% to 80%. Efforts are under way at the NIH to develop a clinical research tool that will enable investigation of these conditions in any population, thereby eliminating the need for an index study condition. This will help us to elucidate the true rates of co-occurrence within virtually any study population. Furthermore, specialized phenotyping studies are beginning to yield rigorous epidemiologic data on rates of co-occurrence and relative risk, as well as the temporal relationship among COPCs (see the section Promising National Studies).

DISEASE BURDEN

Cumulatively, evidence demonstrates that COPC patients are at increased risk of developing a new and different COPC as the number of COPCs they have increases.[146,111,168,2,181,9,14,88,148,177,18] Furthermore, research suggests that the delay in accurate diagnosis and effective treatment commonly experienced by individuals with COPCs can have serious consequences, including worsening of both

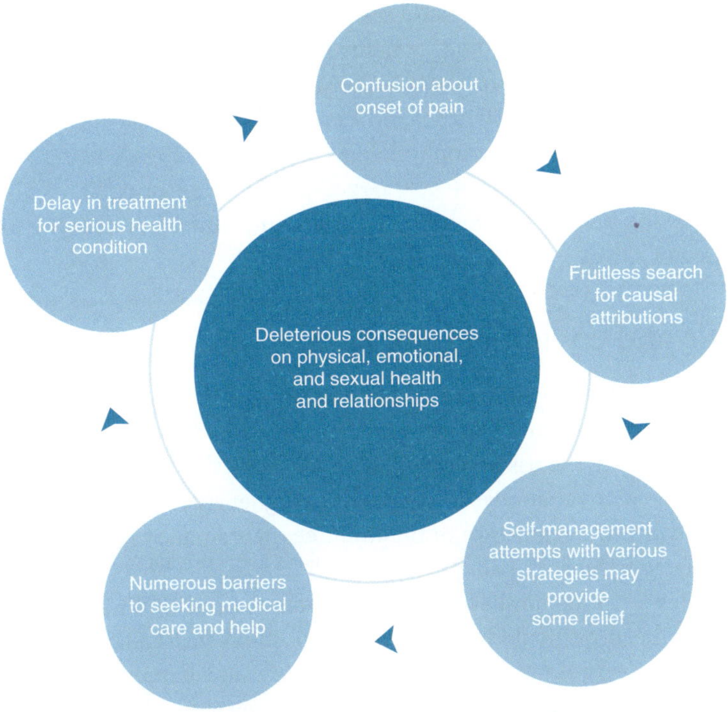

FIGURE 8.2 Profound quality-of-life impact experienced by COPC patients. This figure depicts a typical pattern experienced by individuals with COPCs. Because our health system is fragmented by medical specialties, this cycle is further complicated as the affected individual develops additional conditions; seeks care from different medical specialists (e.g., urologist for bladder pain, rheumatologist for fibromyalgia syndrome, and gynecologist for vulvodynia); receives multiple treatment recommendations; deals with disagreement among providers; lacks a primary clinician to coordinate medical care; and experiences further stigma and invalidation, poorer health and quality-of-life outcomes, and increased levels of disability. COPCs, chronic overlapping pain conditions.

site-specific and body-wide symptoms, which in turn increases treatment recalcitrance; a vicious cycle ensues, leading to poorer health and quality-of-life outcomes, as well as increased costs and disability rates.[88,85,90,12,167,150,118,169,136,45,32,1,91] Numerous studies elucidate the profound impact that these stigmatizing disorders have on all aspects of health and quality of life, even putting patients at increased risk of suicide (see Fig. 8.2).[146,111,85,12,118,91,42,115,27,106,69,154]

COMMON UNDERLYING DISEASE MECHANISMS

Mounting evidence further substantiates that these conditions share common underlying disease mechanisms, mainly in the immune, neural, and endocrine systems.

Those affected with any one of these conditions are more likely to be female, exhibit similar symptom profiles, and benefit from similar treatments. Furthermore, studies increasingly support the idea that COPCs are heterogeneous and that patient populations—both within and across disorders—cluster into phenotypic subgroups with common pathophysiologic mechanisms, each being responsive to treatment modalities that specifically target those mechanisms.[12,80,176] The following summarizes the findings of emerging research on common underlying mechanisms of disease in COPCs.

Genetic and Environmental Factors

Pain genetics research demonstrates that there are likely numerous genetic variations that determine the sensitivity of an individual's nervous system to pain and other sensory input, as well as the risk of developing chronic pain.[178,116,147] Studies have identified a number of genetic variations associated with a higher risk of developing COPCs, most of which involve the regulation of the immune, neural, and endocrine systems, specifically related to sensory/pain processing.[67,164,46,40,96,161,119,101,128,131] Likewise, research demonstrates a strong familial component to developing COPCs.[161,38,39,11,5,75,10] Twin studies have been particularly helpful in establishing that COPCs co-aggregate, are strongly genetic, and are separable from anxiety and depression.[103,162,76,117,122,159,73] Gene expression studies in this area are also beginning to yield insights into the molecular pathways implicated in symptom expression and treatment response.[95,28,35,107] As with most illnesses that may have a genetic underpinning, environmental factors, such as infection, trauma, surgery, and injury, may play a prominent role in triggering the onset of COPCs.[101,62,13,165,37,50,83,173] Genome-wide epigenetic studies have not yet been conducted to assess the molecular basis of various environmental factors in the etiology of these disorders. Once COPCs are triggered, the factors and mechanisms responsible for ongoing symptom expression are complex and multifactorial.

Abnormal Pain and Sensory Processing

Once COPCs develop, the abnormalities most consistently detected are pain and sensory processing dysfunction. Compared with healthy individuals, those with COPCs report enhanced pain perception—both increased pain intensity and lower sensory and pain thresholds—with the application of a variety of sensory stimuli (e.g., pressure, thermal, vibratory, electrical). These sensitivities are found not only at the body site where a person experiences chronic pain, but also at distal locations, such as the thumb, shin, and arm.[67,108,84,59,55,89,17,33,137,15] Recent studies, including those utilizing functional magnetic resonance imagine (MRI), also provide evidence that other sensory input, such as light, sound, and odor, are biologically amplified in patients with COPCs.[33,52,6,139,175,19] The insula—the brain region that plays a critical role in sensory integration—most consistently shows hyperactivity.

Using experimental pain testing, two pathogenic mechanisms have been found to contribute to enhanced pain perception and low sensory thresholds in individuals with COPCs.

Attenuated Diffuse Noxious Inhibitory Control (DNIC)/Conditioned Pain Modulation (CPM)

In healthy people and lab animals, application of an intense painful stimulus for 2 to 5 minutes produces generalized whole-body analgesia, that is, "pain inhibits pain." This analgesic effect has been consistently observed to be attenuated or absent in many, but not all, individuals with COPCs.[84,71,114,81,109,121,126]

Increased Wind-Up/Temporal Summation

Studies also suggest that some individuals with COPCs exhibit evidence of "wind-up" or temporal summation, in which repeated painful stimuli cause increased pain perception, indicative of sensitization of the central nervous system.[59,17,71,82,171,22,184]

Autonomic Nervous System Abnormalities

Increased sympathetic-to-parasympathetic balance has been demonstrated in some subgroups of individuals with COPCs, raising the possibility that dysfunction of the autonomic nervous system could be one of the common clustering pathophysiologic mechanisms.

Neuroimaging Abnormalities

A growing body of evidence shows that individuals with COPCs are more likely to exhibit changes in gray and white matter volume and cortical thickness in various brain regions. These findings closely align with what is increasingly reported in the general pain research literature—that chronic pain may be a neurodegenerative disorder.[8,102,74,179,141,135,127,70] These subtle changes in size and shape of cortical and subcortical areas in chronic pain states are improving our knowledge of "neuroplasticity," a term that is probably much more accurate than "neurodegeneration," because studies have found reversal of imaging findings following treatment.[142,64]

Neural functional magnetic resonance imaging (fMRI) provides a visual picture of how the brain processes the sensory experience of pain. Studies of people with COPCs indicate that in response to painful stimuli, similar brain regions show increased activity or are "activated," including those that integrate and process sensory information, cognition, and affect.[80,139,110,61,97,166,29,77,78] A more recent advancement in the use of fMRI is to look at patterns of connectivity among different brain regions, either while a person is at rest or while he or she is performing a specific task.[123] A resting-state analysis enables one to evaluate brain changes associated with chronic spontaneous pain, as well as examine how chronic pain may disrupt non–pain-related functions, such as cognition. Functional connectivity studies of individuals with COPCs show altered connectivity among several regions of the brain, such as the default mode, executive attention, and pain modulatory and sensory-motor networks.[77,68,94,180,140,79] This technique holds considerable promise in identifying potential biomarkers for pain intensity and/or mechanism.

Central Nervous System Versus Peripheral Nervous System Contribution

Several hypotheses have been proposed regarding the relative contribution of the peripheral nervous system (PNS) and the central nervous system (CNS) in the development and maintenance of COPCs. One theory is that they both exert influence on a continuum. In individuals with mild to moderate symptoms, there may be a greater contribution from the PNS (e.g., upregulation of afferent pathways), which is influenced by environmental factors, such as an infection or injury. In those with moderate to severe symptoms, the CNS is proposed to have a greater contribution, resulting in disinhibition of CNS pain processing, which then leads to a lack of pain inhibition in the PNS. Furthermore, with increasing severity and number of pain conditions/symptoms, contributory factors, such as life stressors, poor coping, and mood alterations, become more prevalent.[80] What is unclear at this time is whether the CNS dysfunction can be the sole source of pathogenesis, as some studies demonstrate that persistent nociceptive input from the PNS is needed to maintain CNS abnormalities.[151,125,16,183]

Female Predominance and Role of Ovarian Hormones

COPCs have a female predominance, proposed to result from multiple factors. Basic science studies suggest that ovarian hormones have distinct effects on inflammation, affective states, stress response, modulatory pain systems, and afferent sensory systems that increase or decrease pain reactivity.[132,104] Clinical studies demonstrate alterations in pain severity, thresholds, and tolerance during different phases of the menstrual cycle, and recent neural imaging studies have even indicated important sex differences in the connectivity between brain regions that process emotion and cognition.[132,158,65,3,31] Advanced knowledge of the mechanisms by which ovarian hormones modulate pain is necessary and will aid in understanding why pain tends to be more frequent, severe, and disabling in women.[87]

Neuroendocrine and Neuroimmune Abnormalities

Chronic pain research establishes that there is a complex interplay among immune cells, glia, and neurons—through the release of inflammatory mediators and interactions with neurotransmitters and their receptors—that affects immune response and modulates pain pathways and sensitivity in both the PNS and the CNS.[47,163,145] Studies of COPCs indicate that a host of immuno-inflammatory mediators, both in the bloodstream and in painful peripheral tissues, are altered and play a role in the development and/or maintenance of these conditions in at least a subgroup of patients.[138,25,53,153,24,60,41,152,98] The hypothalamic–pituitary–adrenal (HPA) axis consists of complex interactions among these three endocrine glands that control stress and regulate a wide array of body functions, such as immunity, digestion, emotions, and energy storage. Overall, although study results are inconsistent, HPA axis dysregulation appears to play a role in at least a subset of those with COPCs.[155,26,99,172,133,92,44,120,124,93] This may not be surprising given that baseline and stimulated HPA axis functions are highly dynamic and affected by many factors. One hypothesis is that early dysregulation of the HPA axis results in elevated HPA axis hormone levels, whereas more prolonged dysfunction ultimately leads to blunted cortisol levels because of ineffective HPA axis responsiveness.[80]

Roles of Stress, Behavioral, and Psychological Factors

Adverse childhood experiences, early-life (and/or ongoing) stress, and behavioral and psychological factors are known to play a role in the incidence and maintenance of many chronic illnesses, including type 2 diabetes and heart diseases, as well as some COPCs.[134,20,43,174,66,72,156] Studies demonstrate that the relationship between chronic pain and distress is complex, and that distress can both be an incident factor and a consequence of chronic pain.[129,130] In this latter situation, individuals experience difficulty functioning in their various roles *after* developing COPCs, which can exacerbate symptoms and lead to maladaptive illness behaviors. By using statistical clustering models and other types of research, studies are beginning to identify distinct subgroups of patients with COPCs with similar profiles related to symptom severity, pain/sensory sensitivity, and psychosocial functioning, identifying some groups that appear to be more "resilient" to pain and its biopsychosocial effects, as well as those with more severe symptoms, severe pain, and declined psychosocial functioning.[100,160,56]

TREATMENT OF CHRONIC OVERLAPPING PAIN CONDITIONS

Systematic reviews consistently highlight the poor state of evidence for treatments used to manage each COPC.[7,34,23,48,63,4,21,86,143,36] Recent studies have, however, demonstrated that treatment of one COPC improves that of another.[54,30] As discussed in the previous section, people with multiple pain disorders are thought to have more "centralized pain" (versus PNS-driven pain), and, therefore, it is proposed that those with COPCs will respond more favorably to treatments targeting the CNS, such as tricyclic antidepressants, anticonvulsants, and selective serotonin–norepinephrine

TABLE 8.2 **Mechanistic characterization of chronic pain**

	Peripheral (nociceptive)	Neuropathic	Centralized
Pathogenesis	Primarily due to inflammation or mechanical damage in peripheral tissue	Damage or entrapment of peripheral nerves	Primarily due to abnormal pain processing in the central nervous system although maintenance may require persistent PNS input
Favorable treatment	NSAIDs, opioids, procedures (including surgery)	Pharmacologic therapy targeting peripheral and central nervous systems	Neuroactive compounds affecting the central nervous system (SNRIs, tricyclic antidepressants, anticonvulsants)
Behavioral factors	Minor	N/A	Prominent
Examples	Osteoarthritis, rheumatoid arthritis, cancer pain	Diabetic neuropathy, post-herpetic neuralgia	Chronic overlapping pain conditions

A mechanistic approach to pain requires that clinicians assess whether an individual has nociceptive pain (due to peripheral inflammation or damage), neuropathic pain (due to nerve damage), and/or central pain (due to abnormal sensory processing in the brain and/or spinal cord, i.e., central nervous system), and base treatment on this characterization rather than diagnostic label, for example, headache, fibromyalgia syndrome.

NSAIDs, nonsteroidal anti-inflammatory drugs; SNRIs, selective serotonin–norepinephrine reuptake inhibitors.

reuptake inhibitors (SNRIs), as well as general behavioral approaches found to be helpful in the management of chronic pain, such as cognitive behavioral therapy and pacing (see Table 8.2). No studies, however, have compared the efficacies of certain treatments in those with multiple COPCs versus those with only one COPC. In recent years, the treatment of chronic pain disorders, including COPCs, has shifted to an approach that identifies both pain and non-pain domains that are affected in each person, and then develops a personalized multimodal treatment plan that addresses each. For example, a person with FMS, IBS, and migraine, with a comorbid sleep disorder and cognitive dysfunction, will require and benefit from a different treatment plan than another patient with TMD, vulvodynia, and low back pain with comorbid anxiety disorder, fatigue, and poor physical function.

PUBLICATION TRENDS

Over the past two decades, the number of journal publications specific to the overlap of these conditions has increased 10-fold, from 42 publications in 1995 to 456 in 2015.

TABLE 8.3 **Number of medical journal articles published on various combinations of COPCs between January 2013 and December 2016**

	ENDO	FMS	IBS	IC/PBS	Migraine	cTTH	Vulvodynia	cLBP	TMD
ME/CFS	13	252	107	34	33	4	8	10	23
ENDO		18	27	27	12	1	13	16	4
FMS			136	46	86	11	27	100	71
IBS				59	84	7	23	10	27
IC/PBS					13	2	20	1	10
Migraine						—	3	42	156
cTTH							0	14	54
Vulvodynia								1	10
cLBP									31
TMD									

cLBP, chronic low back pain; COPC, chronic overlapping pain condition; cTTH, chronic tension type headache; ENDO, endometriosis; FMS, fibromyalgia syndrome; IBS, irritable bowel syndrome; IC/PBS, interstitial cystitis/painful bladder syndrome; ME/CFS, myalgic encephalomyelitis/chronic fatigue syndrome; TMD, temporomandibular disorders.

Table 8.3 summarizes the number of journal articles published on various combinations of COPCs over the past 4 years. In this period, 1,291 non-duplicative journal articles were published, most commonly reporting on the relationship between ME/CFS and FMS (128 articles), IBS and FMS (74 articles), migraine and TMD (66 articles), and ME/CFS and IBS (58 articles).

Research Disparities

Tremendous discrepancy exists in the burden of disease and the NIH investment in research for both chronic pain, in general, and COPCs specifically. The 2011 National Academy of Medicine study revealed that 100 million American adults live with chronic pain, at a cost of over $560 billion. In 2015, the NIH invested just $391 million in chronic pain research, an average of $3.91 per affected individual.[112,157] In comparison, heart disease, cancer, and diabetes combined affect the same number of Americans as does chronic pain, yet in 2015, the NIH invested 95% more in research on these three conditions than it did on pain, totaling $7.6 billion or $76 per affected individual.

In 2015 the NIH invested a total of $128 million or $1.18 per affected individual in COPC research.[157] This was slightly increased from a total of $110 million or $1.06 per affected individual in 2014. Individual rates, listed in decreasing order of investment per affected individual, include chronic migraine ($2.86/patient; $20 million total); endometriosis ($1.67/patient; $10 million total); cLBP ($1.50/patient; $30 million total); CFS ($1.50/patient; $6 million total); FMS ($1.33/patient; $8 million total); IC ($1.25/patient; $10 million); IBS ($0.55/patient; $24 million total); vulvodynia ($0.50/patient; $3 million total); TMDs ($0.46/patient; $16 million); and chronic tension-type headache ($0.14/patient; $1 million total).

Promising National Studies

Although the NIH investment for individual COPCs, as described earlier, is meager and stagnant, the agency has invested a considerable amount in just a few well-designed, innovative, prospective, multisite studies investigating the overlap of these disorders. Conducting basic, translational, and clinical research for COPCs in this manner is a more holistic, cost-effective, and patient-centric approach and is beginning to parse out both commonalities and uniqueness among COPC subgroups. These studies, which are in various stages of development, execution, and publication, have been the frontrunners in multidisciplinary, phenotype-based research and are described in the following sections.

Multidisciplinary Approach to the Study of Chronic Pelvic Pain Research Network

The Multidisciplinary Approach to the Study of Chronic Pelvic Pain (MAPP) Network is an NIH-sponsored multicenter study of urologic chronic pelvic pain syndrome (UCPPS)—a term used to encompass both IC/PBS and chronic prostatitis/chronic pelvic pain syndrome—designed to provide new insights into underlying etiology, natural history, and risk factors for UCPPS. The MAPP Network, initiated in 2008 with a 5-year grant, comprises six Discovery Sites, a Data Coordinating Center, a Tissue and Technology Core, and other units. With the goal of establishing a translational foundation for improved clinical management, the MAPP Network's objective is to advance understanding of disease phenotypes; underlying pathophysiology; treated natural history; and biologic, genetic, and behavioral risk factors for UCPPS. An important aim of this program is to better understand the biologic and behavioral relationships between UCPPS and comorbid non-urologic pain syndromes. Those of primary interest are FMS, IBS, CFS, vulvodynia, and migraine headache. To date, the network has recruited more than 1,000 study participants who have undergone extensive phenotypic characterization through complementary, integrated network protocols. It is important that all clinical data are centrally managed and analyzed by the Data Coordinating Center, allowing integration of multiple scientific domains. A second 5-year funding period began in 2014 for MAPP II. Studies broadly focus on predictors of symptom progression and resolution and on understanding different mechanism-based phenotypic subgroups that respond differently to treatment. To date, MAPP has published more than 30 manuscripts describing the project and its methodology, as well as symptoms, patient subsets, biomarkers, and structural/functional neuroimaging results.[111,85] Additional information, including a list of MAPP publications, can be found at www.mappnetwork.org.

Orofacial Pain: Prospective Evaluation and Risk Assessment (OPPERA) Study

In 2006, the NIH funded a first-of-its-kind comprehensive program project at the University of North Carolina Center for Neurosensory Disorders—a multidisciplinary research team of accomplished pain clinicians and researchers, psychophysiologists, molecular and cellular geneticists, biostatisticians, and epidemiologists. The Orofacial Pain, Prospective Evaluation, and Risk Assessment (OPPERA) study—a 7-year, four site, cross-disciplinary, prospective investigation of TMDs—sought to identify putative physiologic and psychological risk factors, clinical characteristics, and related genetic mechanisms that influence the development of chronic orofacial pain associated with TMD. Additionally, it aimed to characterize the biological pathways through which genetic variations causally influence TMD risk. Investigators enrolled and monitored 2,700 men and women aged 18 to 44 years, 260 of whom developed TMD in the 3-year follow-up period.[146]

Moreover, the findings will be of direct benefit for clinicians and for their patients, elucidating mechanisms underlying chronic and idiopathic pain in people with TMD.[146] Additional information on the OPPERA studies can be found at www.nidcr.nih.gov/Research/ResearchResults/InterviewsOHR/TIS012006.htm and http://projectreporter.nih.gov/project_info_description.cfm?aid=8525386&icde=19436520&ddparam=&ddvalue=&ddsub=&cr=1&csb=default&cs=ASC.

Complex Persistent Pain Conditions: Unique and Shared Pathway of Vulnerability

This NIH program project, funded in 2011 by the NIH, expands upon OPPERA I and II to specifically study four prevalent pain conditions that frequently co-occur with TMD: vulvodynia, IBS, episodic migraine, and FMS. Fundamental to the aims and goals of this study are that the etiology of these COPCs is multifactorial and their clinical manifestations are diverse. Furthermore, a unifying hypothesis integrating this study is that multiple genetic factors, when coupled with environmental exposures (e.g., injury, infections, physical and psychological stress), increase the susceptibility to COPCs by enhancing pain sensitivity and/or increasing psychological distress. This project seeks to identify risk factors, clusters, and associated genetic polymorphisms that influence pain amplification and psychological distress in study participants who have established COPCs. Additionally, investigators aim to characterize the biological pathways through which these genetic variations causally influence COPCs. Their analyses will characterize clusters of patients within each condition that varies significantly according to disease manifestation and non-pain domains (e.g., fatigue, sleep). It is important that the team expects some clusters of patients to be more alike across COPCs than within any single COPC diagnosis. Additional information can be found at http://projectreporter.nih.gov/project_info_description.cfm?aid=8457063&icde=19436520.

Pain and Interoception Imaging Network Repository

The Pain and Interoception Imaging Network (PAIN) Repository seeks to improve the understanding of the brain's role in chronic pain states. In 2013, the NIH provided a grant to the UCLA Center for Neurobiology of Stress to pioneer the development of this first large repository of well-characterized multimodal brain images from patients with various pain disorders, including those with COPCs. Currently, imaging data from those with FMS, chronic migraine headache, IBS, vulvodynia, and cLBP are included. Fifteen sites in North America and Europe are participating in this groundbreaking project, which aims to collect and store standardized brain images of 1,000 well-characterized patients, including standardized clinical, behavioral, and genetic metadata. Additional information can be found at https://www.painrepository.org/repositories.

Future Direction

Rigorous COPCs studies, such as those described earlier, are advancing a comprehensive scientific approach to the epidemiology, pathophysiology, and treatment of COPCs, yielding valuable information that can be translated into improved care and quality of life for COPC patients. As high-quality science in this field advances, additional pain and non-pain comorbidities will no doubt be identified. A coordinated basic, translational, and clinical research effort that addresses the complexity and interplay of all pain and non-pain comorbidities is needed. Furthermore, collaborative initiatives—throughout the clinical research and development process—that include academia, industry, government agencies, service and reimbursement sectors, clinical care, nonprofits, and philanthropy are required to translate scientific discoveries into meaningful clinical changes for the affected. Taking into account the valuable information that COPC research has yielded to date, Table 8.4 summarizes the much-needed paradigm shift that has begun to take place across these sectors.

TABLE 8.4 **Paradigm shift needed to improve health and quality of life in COPC patients**

	Past concept	Future direction
Scientific understanding	Each condition is distinct with its own disease mechanisms at the painful body site.	Altered neural, immune, and endocrine mechanisms are common across disorders.
Diagnosis	Individual disorders with separate diagnostic labels that can coexist.	One universal disorder with multiple presentations (e.g., subgroups/ phenotypes)
Medical management	All pain is due to peripheral damage or inflammation in specific body areas and will respond to treatments used for acute pain (e.g., interventions, surgery, opioids).	Some pain conditions are ultimately due to dysregulation of the neural, immune, and endocrine systems, and will not respond favorably to treatments for acute pain, which may worsen pain or cause harm
	Medical care is fragmented by disparate specialists, typically determined by physical location of pain (e.g., rheumatology for fibromyalgia syndrome, urology for interstitial cystitis).	Patient-centered medical home with team-based interdisciplinary approach to treatment
	Palliative treatment that only abates symptoms to various degrees	Selection of treatment regimen is guided by individual's pathophysiology/underlying mechanisms of disease (e.g., personalized medicine)
	Treatment is based on trial and error and draws upon findings from better researched disorders.	Treatment is based on scientific evidence, showing proven efficacy in specific mechanism-based subtypes.
	Treatment of most painful symptom or body part	Recognition that multiple domains of health and quality of life are affected, and that integrated care is guided by the development of an individualized treatment plan of all affected domains and contributing factors (e.g., sleep, mood, pain interference)
	Fee-for-service model often does not benefit patients and can contribute to worsening the patient's health.	Quality- and performance-based reimbursement focused on effectiveness and quality of care received
Research efforts	Disorders are researched separately by diagnostic label or body site, with similar lines of study duplicated across conditions (e.g., brain imaging, genetics, sensory testing).	Disorders are researched collectively to assess common underlying mechanisms, as well as unique features of each condition in different patient subgroups/ phenotypes.

(*Continued*)

TABLE 8.4 **Paradigm shift needed to improve health and quality of life in COPC patients (*Continued*)**

	Past concept	Future direction
Translation of evidence	Evidence not widely disseminated or translated into improved clinical tools or medical care	Heavy focus on translation of scientific findings into improved tools and clinical care
Systemic federal research agency issues	Federal research agencies remain structured such that conditions are researched in isolation or silo, and efforts to approve therapies are fragmented and not to the patient's benefit.	Patient-centered research focus, where federal research agencies work collaboratively to address patient needs and cross-agency mission, with the goal of translating scientific discoveries into therapeutic solutions

COPC, chronic overlapping pain condition.

REFERENCES

1. Aaron LA, Arguelles LM, Ashton S, et al. Health and functional status of twins with chronic regional and widespread pain. *J Rheumatol*. 2002;**29**(11):2426–2434.
2. Aaron LA, Herrell R, Ashton S, et al. Comorbid clinical conditions in chronic fatigue: a co-twin control study. *J Gen Intern Med*. 2001;**16**(1):24–31.
3. Adeyemo MA, Spiegel BM, Chang L. Meta-analysis: do irritable bowel syndrome symptoms vary between men and women? *Aliment Pharmacol Ther*. 2010;**32**(6):738–755.
4. AHRQ. Evidence Report. Treatment for fibromyalgia in adult subgroups. 2015. https://effective healthcare.ahrq.gov/topics/fibromyalgia/research. Accessed August 31, 2017.
5. Allen-Brady K, Norton PA, Cannon-Albright L. Risk of associated conditions in relatives of subjects with interstitial cystitis. *Female Pelvic Med Reconstr Surg*. 2015;**21**(2):93–98.
6. Andresen V, Bach DR, Poellinger A, et al. Brain activation responses to subliminal or supraliminal rectal stimuli and to auditory stimuli in irritable bowel syndrome. *Neurogastroenterol Motil*. 2005;**17**(6):827–837.
7. Andrews JC. Vulvodynia interventions—systematic review and evidence grading. *Obstet Gynecol Surv*. 2011;**66**(5):299–315.
8. Apkarian AV, Sosa Y, Sonty S, et al. Chronic back pain is associated with decreased prefrontal and thalamic gray matter density. *J Neurosci*. 2004;**24**(46):10410–10415.
9. Arnold LD, Bachmann GA, Rosen R, Kelly S, Rhoads GG. Vulvodynia: characteristics and associations with comorbidities and quality of life. *Obstet Gynecol*. 2006;**107**(3):617–624.
10. Arnold LM, Fan J, Russell IJ, et al. The fibromyalgia family study: a genome-wide linkage scan study. *Arthritis Rheum*. 2013;**65**(4):1122–1128.
11. Arnold LM, Hudson JI, Hess EV, et al. Family study of fibromyalgia. *Arthritis Rheum*. 2004;**50**(3): 944–952.
12. Bair E, Gaynor S, Slade GD, et al. Identification of clusters of individuals relevant to temporomandibular disorders and other chronic pain conditions: the OPPERA study. *Pain*. 2016;**157**(6):1266–1278.
13. Bair E, Ohrbach R, Fillingim RB, et al. Multivariable modeling of phenotypic risk factors for first-onset TMD: the OPPERA prospective cohort study. *J Pain*. 2013;**14**(12 suppl):T102–T115.
14. Bair E, Simmons E, Hartung J, Desia K, Maixner W, Zolnoun D. Natural history of comorbid orofacial pain among women with vestibulodynia. *Clin J Pain*. 2015;**31**(1):73–78.

15. Bendtsen L, Jensen R, Olesen J. Decreased pain detection and tolerance thresholds in chronic tension-type headache. *Arch Neurol.* 1996;**53**(4):373–376.
16. Birder LA, Wolf-Johnston AS, Chib MK, Buffington CA, Roppolo JR, Hanna-Mitchell AT. Beyond neurons: involvement of urothelial and glial cells in bladder function. *Neurourol Urodyn.* 2010;**29**(1):88–96.
17. Biurrun Manresa JA, Neziri AY, Curatolo M, Arendt-Nielsen L, Andersen OK. Reflex receptive fields are enlarged in patients with musculoskeletal low back and neck pain. *Pain.* 2013;**154**(8):1318–1324.
18. Boneva RS, Lin JM, Unger ER. Early menopause and other gynecologic risk indicators for chronic fatigue syndrome in women. *Menopause.* 2015;**22**(8):826–834.
19. Brooks JC, Tracey I. The insula: a multidimensional integration site for pain. *Pain.* 2007;**128**(1–2):1–2.
20. Brown DW, Anda RF, Felitti VJ, et al. Adverse childhood experiences are associated with the risk of lung cancer: a prospective cohort study. *BMC Public Health.* 2010;**10**:20.
21. Brown J, Farguhar C. Endometriosis: an overview of Cochrane Reviews. *Cochrane Database Syst Rev.* 2014;3:CD009590.
22. Cathcart S, Winefield AH, Lushington K, Rolan P. Noxious inhibition of temporal summation is impaired in chronic tension-type headache. *Headache.* 2010;**50**(3):403–412.
23. Chambers D, Bagnall AM, Hempel S, Forbes C. Interventions for the treatment, management and rehabilitation of patients with chronic fatigue syndrome/myalgic encephalomyelitis: an updated systematic review. *J R Soc Med.* 2006;**99**(10):506–520.
24. Chang H, Israel H. Analysis of inflammatory mediators in temporomandibular joint synovial fluid lavage samples of symptomatic patients and asymptomatic controls. *J Oral Maxillofac Surg.* 2005;**63**(6):761–765.
25. Chang L, Adeyemo M, Karagiannides I, et al. Serum and colonic mucosal immune markers in irritable bowel syndrome. *Am J Gastroenterol.* 2012;**107**(2):262–272.
26. Chang L, Sundaresh S, Elliott J, et al. Dysregulation of the hypothalamic-pituitary-adrenal (HPA) axis in irritable bowel syndrome. *Neurogastroenterol Motil.* 2009;**21**(2):149–159.
27. Cioffi I, Perrotta S, Ammendola L, et al. Social impairment of individuals suffering from different types of chronic orofacial pain. *Prog Orthod.* 2014;**15**(1):27.
28. Colaco M, Koslov DS, Keys T, et al. Correlation of gene expression with bladder capacity in interstitial cystitis/bladder pain syndrome. *J Urol.* 2014;**192**(4):1123–1129.
29. Cook DB, O'Connor PJ, Lange G, Steffener J. Functional neuroimaging correlates of mental fatigue induced by cognition among chronic fatigue syndrome patients and controls. *Neuroimage.* 2007;**36**(1):108–122.
30. Costantini R, Affaitati G, Wesselmann U, Czakanski P, Giamberardino MA. Visceral pain as a triggering factor for fibromyalgia symptoms in comorbid patients. *Pain.* 2017;158(10):1925–1937.
31. Craft RM. Modulation of pain by estrogens. *Pain.* 2007;**132(suppl 1)**:S3–12.
32. Creed FH, Tomenson B, Chew-Graham C, et al. Multiple somatic symptoms predict impaired health status in functional somatic syndromes. *Int J Behav Med.* 2013;**20**(2):194–205.
33. de Siqueira SR, Teixeira MJ, de Siqueira JT. Orofacial pain and sensory characteristics of chronic patients compared with controls. *Oral Surg Oral Med Oral Pathol Oral Radiol.* 2013;**115**(6):e37–e45.
34. de Souza RF, Lovato da Silva CH, Nasser M, Fedorowicz Z, Al-Muharraqi MA. Interventions for the management of temporomandibular joint osteoarthritis. *Cochrane Database Syst Rev.* 2012;(4):CD007261.
35. Del Valle-Pinero AY, Sherwin LB, Anderson EM, Caudle RM, Henderson WA. Altered vasoactive intestinal peptides expression in irritable bowel syndrome patients and rats with trinitrobenzene sulfonic acid-induced colitis. *World J Gastroenterol.* 2015;**21**(1):155–163.
36. Deyo RA, Dworkin SF, Amtmann D, et al. Report of the NIH Task Force on research standards for chronic low back pain. *J Pain.* 2014;15(6):569–585.
37. Diatchenko L, Fillingim RB, Smith SB, Maixner W. The phenotypic and genetic signatures of common musculoskeletal pain conditions. *Nat Rev Rheumatol.* 2013;**9**(6):340–350.

38. Diatchenko L, Nackley AG, Slade GD, Fillingim RB, Maixner W. Idiopathic pain disorders—pathways of vulnerability. *Pain*. 2006;**123**(3):226–230.
39. Diatchenko L, Nackley AG, Tchivileva IE, Shabalina SA, Maixner W. Genetic architecture of human pain perception. *Trends Genet*. 2007;**23**(12):605–613.
40. Docampo E, Escaramís G, Gratacòs M, et al. Genome-wide analysis of single nucleotide polymorphisms and copy number variants in fibromyalgia suggest a role for the central nervous system. *Pain*. 2014;**155**(6):1102–1109.
41. Domingues RB, Duarte H, Rocha NP, Teixeira AL. Increased serum levels of interleukin-8 in patients with tension-type headache. *Cephalalgia*. 2015;**35**(9):801–806.
42. Donaldson RL, Meana M. Early dyspareunia experience in young women: confusion, consequences, and help-seeking barriers. *J Sex Med*. 2011;**8**(3):814–823.
43. Dong M, Giles WH, Felitti VJ, et al. Insights into causal pathways for ischemic heart disease: adverse childhood experiences study. *Circulation*. 2004;**110**(13):1761–1766.
44. Ehrström S, Kornfeld D, Rylander E, Bohm-Starke N. Chronic stress in women with localised provoked vulvodynia. *J Psychosom Obstet Gynaecol*. 2009;**30**(1):73–79.
45. Faresjö Å, Grodzinsky E, Hallert C, Timpka T. Patients with irritable bowel syndrome are more burdened by co-morbidity and worry about serious diseases than healthy controls—eight years follow-up of IBS patients in primary care. *BMC Public Health*. 2013;**13**:832.
46. Fernández-de-las-Peñas C, Peñacoba-Puente C, Cigarán-Méndez M Díaz-Rodríguez L, Rubio-Ruiz B, Arroyo-Morales M. Has catechol-O-methyltransferase genotype (Val158Met) an influence on endocrine, sympathetic nervous and humoral immune systems in women with fibromyalgia syndrome? *Clin J Pain*. 2014;**30**(3):199–204.
47. Fillingim RB, King CD, Ribeiro-Dasilva MC, Rahim-Williams B, Riley JL III. Sex, gender, and pain: a review of recent clinical and experimental findings. *J Pain*. 2009;**10**(5):447–485.
48. Ford AC, Talley NJ. Irritable bowel syndrome. *BMJ*. 2012;**345**:e5836.
49. Fourquet J, Sinaii N, Stratton P, et al. Characteristics of women with endometriosis from the USA and Puerto Rico. *J Endometr Pelvic Pain Disord*. 2015;**7**(4):129–135.
50. Fuoco MB, Irvine-Bird K, Curtis Nickel J. Multiple sensitivity phenotype in interstitial cystitis/bladder pain syndrome. *Can Urol Assoc J*. 2014;**8**(11–12):E758–E761.
51. Gass JJ, Glaros AG. Autonomic dysregulation in headache patients. *Appl Psychophysiol Biofeedback*. 2013;**38**(4):257–263.
52. Geisser ME, Strader Donnell C, Petzke F, Gracely RH, Clauw DJ, Williams DA. Comorbid somatic symptoms and functional status in patients with fibromyalgia and chronic fatigue syndrome: sensory amplification as a common mechanism. *Psychosomatics*. 2008;**49**(3):235–242.
53. Gerber S, Bongiovanni AM, Ledger WJ, Witkin SS. Defective regulation of the proinflammatory immune response in women with vulvar vestibulitis syndrome. *Am J Obstet Gynecol*. 2002; **186**(4):696–700.
54. Giamberardino MA, Affaitati G, Martelletti P, et al. Impact of migraine on fibromyalgia symptoms. *J Headache Pain*. 2015;**17**:28.
55. Giesecke J, Reed BD, Haefner HK, Giesecke T, Clauw DJ, Gracely RH. Quantitative sensory testing in vulvodynia patients and increased peripheral pressure pain sensitivity. *Obstet Gynecol*. 2004; **104**(1):126–133.
56. Giesecke T, Williams DA, Harris RE, et al. Subgrouping of fibromyalgia patients on the basis of pressure-pain thresholds and psychological factors. *Arthritis Rheum*. 2003;**48**(10):2916–2922.
57. Gockel M, Lindholm H, Niemistö L, Hurri H. Perceived disability but not pain is connected with autonomic nervous function among patients with chronic low back pain. *J Rehabil Med*. 2008;**40**(5):355–358.
58. Greenspan JD, Slade GD, Bair E, et al. Pain sensitivity and autonomic factors associated with development of TMD: the OPPERA prospective cohort study. *J Pain*. 2013;**14**(12 suppl):T63–74.e1.
59. Greenspan JD, Slade GD, Bair E, et al. Pain sensitivity risk factors for chronic TMD: descriptive data and empirically identified domains from the OPPERA case control study. *J Pain*. 2011;**12**(11 suppl):T61–T74.

60. Güzel I, Tasdemir N, Celik Y. Evaluation of serum transforming growth factor ß1 and C-reactive protein levels in migraine patients. *Neurol Neurochir Pol.* 2013;**47**(4):357–362.
61. Hampson JP, Reed BD, Clauw DJ, et al. Augmented central pain processing in vulvodynia. *J Pain.* 2013;**14**(6):579–589.
62. Hanevik K, Wensaas KA, Rortveit G, Eide GE, Mørch K, Langeland N. Irritable bowel syndrome and chronic fatigue 6 years after Giardia infection: a controlled prospective cohort study. *Clin Infect Dis.* 2014;**59**(10):1394–1400.
63. Hanno PM, Burks DA, Clemens JQ, et al.; Interstitial Cystitis Guidelines Panel of the American Urological Association Education and Research, Inc. AUA guideline for the diagnosis and treatment of interstitial cystitis/bladder pain syndrome. *J Urol.* 2011;**185**(6):2162–2170.
64. Harris RE, Napadow V, Huggins JP, et al. Pregabalin rectifies aberrant brain chemistry, connectivity, and functional response in chronic pain patients. *Anesthesiology.* 2013;**119**(6):1453–1464.
65. Hassan S, Muere A, Einstein G. Ovarian hormones and chronic pain: a comprehensive review. *Pain.* 2014;**155**(12):2448–2460.
66. Häuser W, Kosseva M, Üceyler N, Klose P, Sommer C. Emotional, physical, and sexual abuse in fibromyalgia syndrome: a systematic review with meta-analysis. *Arthritis Care Res.* 2011;**63**(6):808–820.
67. Heddini U, Bohm-Starke N, Grönbladh A, Nyberg F, Nilsson KW, Johannesson U. Serotonin receptor gene (5HT-2A) polymorphism is associated with provoked vestibulodynia and comorbid symptoms of pain. *J Sex Med.* 2014;**11**(12):3064–3071.
68. Ichesco E, Quintero A, Clauw DJ, et al. Altered functional connectivity between the insula and the cingulate cortex in patients with temporomandibular disorder: a pilot study. *Headache.* 2012;**52**(3):441–454.
69. Ilgen MA, Kleinberg F, Ignacio RV, et al. Noncancer pain conditions and risk of suicide. *JAMA Psychiatry.* 2013;**70**(7):692–697.
70. Jensen KB, Srinivasan P, Spaeth R, et al. Overlapping structural and functional brain changes in patients with long-term exposure to fibromyalgia pain. *Arthritis Rheum.* 2013;**65**(12):3293–3303.
71. Johannesson U, de Boussard CN, Brodda Jansen G, Bohm-Starke N. Evidence of diffuse noxious inhibitory controls (DNIC) elicited by cold noxious stimulation in patients with provoked vestibulodynia. *Pain.* 2007;**130**(1–2):31–39.
72. Juang KD, Yang CY. Psychiatric comorbidity of chronic daily headache: focus on traumatic experiences in childhood, post-traumatic stress disorder and suicidality. *Curr Pain Headache Rep.* 2014;**18**(4):405.
73. Junqueira DR, Ferreira ML, Refshauge K, et al. Heritability and lifestyle factors in chronic low back pain: results of the Australian twin low back pain study (The AUTBACK study). *Eur J Pain.* 2014;**18**(10):1410–1418.
74. Kairys AE, Schmidt-Wilcke T, Puiu T, et al. Increased brain gray matter in the primary somatosensory cortex is associated with increased pain and mood disturbance in patients with interstitial cystitis/painful bladder syndrome. *J Urol.* 2015;**193**(1):131–137.
75. Karabulut GS, Beser OF, Erginöz E, Kutlu T, Cokugras FÇ, Erkan T. The incidence of irritable bowel syndrome in children using the Rome III criteria and the effect of trimebutine treatment. *J Neurogastroenterol Motil.* 2013;**19**(1):90–93.
76. Kato K, Sullivan PF, Evengård B, Pedersen NL. A population-based twin study of functional somatic syndromes. *Psychol Med.* 2009;**39**(3):497–505.
77. Kilpatrick LA, Kutch JJ, Tillisch K, et al. Alterations in resting state oscillations and connectivity in sensory and motor networks in women with interstitial cystitis/painful bladder syndrome. *J Urol.* 2014;**192**(3):947–955.
78. Kim J, Loggia ML, Cahalan CM, et al. The somatosensory link: S1 functional connectivity is altered by sustained pain and associated with clinical/autonomic dysfunction in fibromyalgia. Arthritis Rheumatol. 2015;**67**(5):1395–1405.
79. Kim J, Loggia ML, Cahalan CM, et al. The somatosensory link in fibromyalgia: functional connectivity of the primary somatosensory cortex is altered by sustained pain and is associated with clinical/autonomic dysfunction. *Arthritis Rheumatol.* 2015;**67**(5):1395–1405.

80. Kim SE, Chang L. Overlap between functional GI disorders and other functional syndromes: what are the underlying mechanisms? *Neurogastroenterol Motil.* 2012;**24**(10):895–913.
81. King CD, Wong F, Currie T, Mauderli AP, Fillingim RB, Riley JL III. Deficiency in endogenous modulation of prolonged heat pain in patients with irritable bowel syndrome and temporomandibular disorder. *Pain.* 2009;**143**(3):172–178.
82. Klumpp DJ, Rudick CN. Summation model of pelvic pain in interstitial cystitis. *Nat Clin Pract Urol.* 2008;**5**(9):494–500.
83. Kobayashi H, Higashiura Y, Shigetomi H, Kajihara H. Pathogenesis of endometriosis: the role of initial infection and subsequent sterile inflammation (review). *Mol Med Rep.* 2014;**9**(1):9–15.
84. Kosek E, Hansson P. Modulatory influence on somatosensory perception from vibration and heterotopic noxious conditioning stimulation (HNCS) in fibromyalgia patients and healthy subjects. *Pain.* 1997;**70**(1):41–51.
85. Kriefer JN, Stephens AJ, Landis JR, et al. Relationship between chronic nonurological associated somatic syndromes and symptom severity in urological chronic pelvic pain syndromes: baseline evaluation of the MAPP study. *J Urol.* 2015;**193**(4):1254–1262.
86. Krishnan A, Silver N. Headache (chronic tension-type). *BMJ Clin Evid.* 2009;**2009**:1205. https://www.ncbi.nlm.nih.gov/pmc/articles/PMC2907789/. Accessed August 31, 2017.
87. Labus JS, Gupta A, Coveleskie K, et al. Sex differences in emotion-related cognitive processes in irritable bowel syndrome and healthy control subjects. *Pain.* 2013;**154**(10):2088–2099.
88. Lackner JM, Ma CX, Keefer L, et al. Type, rather than number, of mental and physical comorbidities increases the severity of symptoms in patients with irritable bowel syndrome. *Clin Gastroenterol Hepatol.* 2013;**11**(9):1147–1157.
89. Lai HH, Gardner V, Ness TJ, Gereau RW IV. Segmental hyperalgesia to mechanical stimulus in interstitial cystitis/bladder pain syndrome: evidence of central sensitization. *J Urol.* 2014;**191**(5):1294–1299.
90. Lai HH, Jemielita T, Sutcliffe S, et al.; MAPP Research Network. Characterization of whole body pain in urological chronic pelvic pain syndrome at baseline: a MAPP Research Network Study. *J Urol.* 2017;**198**(3):622–631.
91. Lai HH, North CS, Andriole GL, et al. Urological symptoms in a subset of patients with urological chronic pelvic pain syndrome and a polysymptomatic, polysyndromic pattern of presentation. *J Urol.* 2014;**191**(6):1802–1807.
92. Lambert CA, Sanders A, Wilder RS, et al. Chronic HPA axis response to stress in temporomandibular disorder. *J Dent Hyg.* 2014;**88(suppl 1)**:5–12.
93. Leistad RB, Stovner LJ, White LR, Nilsen KB, Westgaard RH, Sand T. Noradrenaline and cortisol changes in response to low-grade cognitive stress differ in migraine and tension-type headache. *J Headache Pain.* 2007;**8**(3):157–166.
94. Letzen JE, Craggs JG, Perlstein WM, Price DD, Robinson ME. Functional connectivity of the default mode network and its association with pain networks in irritable bowel patients assessed via lidocaine treatment. *J Pain.* 2013;**14**(10):1077–1087.
95. Light AR, Bateman L, Jo D, et al. Gene expression alterations at baseline and following moderate exercise in patients with chronic fatigue syndrome and fibromyalgia syndrome. *J Intern Med.* 2012;**271**(1):64–81.
96. Light KC, White AT, Tadler S, Iacob E, Light AR. Genetics and gene expression involving stress and distress pathways in fibromyalgia with and without comorbid chronic fatigue syndrome. *Pain Res Treat.* 2012;**2012**:427869.
97. Lin CS. Brain signature of chronic orofacial pain: a systematic review and meta-analysis on neuroimaging research of trigeminal neuropathic pain and temporomandibular joint disorders. *PLoS ONE.* 2014;**9**(4):e94300.
98. Luchting B, Rachinger-Adam B, Zeitler J, et al. Disrupted TH17/Treg balance in patients with chronic low back pain. *PLoS ONE.* 2014;**9**(8):e104883.

99. Lutgendorf SK, Kreder KJ, Rothrock NE, et al. Diurnal cortisol variations and symptoms in patients with interstitial cystitis. *J Urol*. 2002;**167**(3):1338–1343.
100. Maixner W. *Orofacial Pain: Prospective Evaluation and Risk Assessment (OPPERA)*. Paper presented at: 202nd Meeting of the National Advisory Dental and Craniofacial Research Council, National Institutes of Health; 2013; Bethesda, MD. www.irss.unc.edu/content/pdf/OPPERA_NIDCR_Council.pdf. Accessed August 31, 2017.
101. Malkin I, Williams FM, LaChance G, Spector T, MacGregor AJ, Livshits G. Low back and common widespread pain share common genetic determinants. *Ann Hum Genet*. 2014;**78**(5):357–366.
102. Mao C, Wei L, Zhang Q, Liao X, Yang X, Zhang M. Differences in brain structure in patients with distinct sites of chronic pain: A voxel-based morphometric analysis. *Neural Regen Res*. 2013;**8**(32):2981–2990.
103. Markkula R, Järvinen P, Leino-Arjas P, Koskenvuo M, Kalso E, Kaprio J. Clustering of symptoms associated with fibromyalgia in a Finnish twin cohort. *Eur J Pain*. 2009;**13**(7):744–750.
104. Martin VT. Ovarian hormones and pain response: a review of clinical and basic science studies. *Gend Med*. 2009;**6(suppl 2)**:168–192.
105. Martínez-Martínez LA, Mora T, Vargas A, Fuentes-Iniestra M, Martínez-Lavín M. Sympathetic nervous system dysfunction in fibromyalgia, chronic fatigue syndrome, irritable bowel syndrome, and interstitial cystitis: a review of case-control studies. *J Clin Rheumatol*. 2014;**20**(3):146–150.
106. McInnis OA, Matheson K, Anisman H. Living with the unexplained: coping, distress, and depression among women with chronic fatigue syndrome and/or fibromyalgia compared to an autoimmune disorder. *Anxiety Stress Coping*. 2014;**27**(6):601–618.
107. Molana A, Mehrpour M, Vousooghi N, Hajighasem MR, Joghataei MT. Effect of NOS3 gene polymorphism on response to tricyclic antidepressants in migraine attacks. *Iran J Neurol*. 2014;**13**(3):154–159.
108. Moshiree B, Price DD, Robinson ME, Gaible R, Verne GN. Thermal and visceral hypersensitivity in irritable bowel syndrome patients with and without fibromyalgia. *Clin J Pain*. 2007;**23**(4):323–330.
109. Nahman-Averbuch H, Granovsky Y, Coghill RC, Yarnitsky D, Sprecher E, Weissman-Fogel I. Waning of "conditioned pain modulation": a novel expression of subtle pronociception in migraine. *Headache*. 2013;**53**(7):1104–1115.
110. Nakamura Y, Nojiri K, Yoshihara H, et al. Significant differences of brain blood flow in patients with chronic low back pain and acute low back pain detected by brain SPECT. *J Orthop Sci*. 2014;**19**(3): 384–389.
111. Naliboff BD, Stephens AJ, Lai HH, et al.; MAPP Research Network. Clinical and psychosocial predictors of urological chronic pelvic pain symptom change in 1 year: a prospective study from the MAPP Research Network. *J Urol*. 2017;**198**(4):848–857.
112. National Academy of Medicine Report from the Committee on Advancing Pain Research, Care, and Education. *Relieving Pain in America, A Blueprint for Transforming Prevention, Care, Education and Research*. Washington, DC: The National Academies Press; 2011.
113. National Institutes of Health. A workshop on chronic overlapping pain conditions. 2012. http://wayback.archive-it.org/1170/20161005013556/https://www.ninds.nih.gov/news_and_events/events/meeting-summary-chronic-pain.htm. Accessed August 31, 2017.
114. Ness TJ, Lloyd LK, Fillingim RB. An endogenous pain control system is altered in subjects with interstitial cystitis. *J Urol*. 2014;**191**(2):364–370.
115. Nguyen RH, Ecklund AM, Maclehose RF, Veasley C, Harlow BL. Co-morbid pain conditions and feelings of invalidation and isolation among women with vulvodynia. *Psychol Health Med*. 2012;**17**(5):589–598.
116. Nielsen CS, Knudsen GP, Steingrímsdóttir ÓA. Twin studies of pain. *Clin Genet*. 2012;**82**(4):331–340.
117. Nielsen CS, Knudsen GP, Steingrímsdóttir ÓA. Twin studies of pain. *Clin Genet*. 2012;**82**(4):331–340.
118. Nunes FR, Ferreira JM, Bahamondes L. Prevalence of fibromyalgia and quality of life in women with and without endometriosis. *Gynecol Endocrinol*. 2014;**30**(4):307–310.
119. Persico AM, Verdecchia M, Pinzone V, Guidetti V. Migraine genetics: current findings and future lines of research. *Neurogenetics*. 2015;**16**(2):77–95.

120. Petrelluzzi KF, Garcia MC, Petta CA, Grassi-Kassisse DM, Spadari-Bratfisch RC. Salivary cortisol concentrations, stress and quality of life in women with endometriosis and chronic pelvic pain. *Stress.* 2008;**11**(5):390–397.
121. Pielsticker A, Haag G, Zaudig M, Lautenbacher S. Impairment of pain inhibition in chronic tension-type headache. *Pain.* 2005;**118**(1–2):215–223.
122. Plesh O, Noonan C, Buchwald DS, Goldberg J, Afari N. Temporomandibular disorder-type pain and migraine headache in women: a preliminary twin study. *J Orofac Pain.* 2012;**26**(2):91–98.
123. Ploner M, Lee MC, Wiech K, Bingel U, Tracey I. Prestimulus functional connectivity determines pain perception in humans. *Proc Natl Acad Sci USA.* 2010;**107**(1):355–360.
124. Powell DJ, Liossi C, Moss-Morris R, Schlotz W. Unstimulated cortisol secretory activity in everyday life and its relationship with fatigue and chronic fatigue syndrome: a systematic review and subset meta-analysis. *Psychoneuroendocrinology.* 2013;**38**(11):2405–2422.
125. Price DD, Craggs JG, Zhou Q, Verne GN, Perlstein WM, Robinson ME. Widespread hyperalgesia in irritable bowel syndrome is dynamically maintained by tonic visceral impulse input and placebo/nocebo factors: evidence from human psychophysics, animal models, and neuroimaging. *Neuroimage.* 2009;**47**(3):995–1001.
126. Price DD, Staud R, Robinson ME, Mauderli AP, Cannon R, Vierck CJ. Enhanced temporal summation of second pain and its central modulation in fibromyalgia patients. *Pain.* 2002;**99**(1–2):49–59.
127. Puri BK, Jakeman PM, Agour M, et al. Regional grey and white matter volumetric changes in myalgic encephalomyelitis (chronic fatigue syndrome): a voxel-based morphometry 3 T MRI study. *Br J Radiol.* 2012;**85**(1015):e270–e273.
128. Rahmioglu N, Nyholt DR, Morris AP, Missmer SA, Montgomery GW, Zondervan KT. Genetic variants underlying risk of endometriosis: insights from meta-analysis of eight genome-wide association and replication datasets. *Hum Reprod Update.* 2014;**20**(5):702–716.
129. Raphael KG, Chandler HK, Ciccone DS. Is childhood abuse a risk factor for chronic pain in adulthood? *Curr Pain Headache Rep.* 2004;**8**(2):99–110.
130. Raphael KG, Widom CS. Post-traumatic stress disorder moderates the relation between documented childhood victimization and pain 30 years later. *Pain.* 2011;**152**(1):163–169.
131. Reeder JE, Byler TK, Foster DC, et al. Polymorphism in the SCN9A voltage-gated sodium channel gene associated with interstitial cystitis/bladder pain syndrome. *Urology.* 2013;**81**(1):210.e1–210.e4.
132. Ren K, Dubner R. Interactions between the immune and nervous systems in pain. *Nat Med.* 2010;**16**(11):1267–1276.
133. Riva R, Mork PJ, Westgaard RH, Rø M, Lundberg U. Fibromyalgia syndrome is associated with hypocortisolism. *Int J Behav Med.* 2010;**17**(3):223–233.
134. Roberts AL, Agnew-Blais JC, Spiegelman D, et al. Posttraumatic stress disorder and incidence of type 2 diabetes mellitus in a sample of women: a 22-year longitudinal study. *JAMA Psychiatry.* 2015;**72**(3):203–210.
135. Rocca MA, Ceccarelli A, Falini A, et al. Brain gray matter changes in migraine patients with T2-visible lesions: a 3-T MRI study. *Stroke.* 2006;**37**(7):1765–1770.
136. Ropponen A, Svedberg P, Kalso E, Koskenvuo M, Silventoinen K, Kaprio J. A prospective twin cohort study of disability pensions due to musculoskeletal diagnoses in relation to stability and change in pain. *Pain.* 2013;**154**(10):1966–1972.
137. Sales Pinto LM, de Carvalho JJ, Cunha CO, Dos Santos Silva R, Fiamengui-Filho JF, Rodrigues Conti PC. Influence of myofascial pain on the pressure pain threshold of masticatory muscles in women with migraine. *Clin J Pain.* 2013;**29**(4):362–365.
138. Schrepf A, O'Donnell M, Luo Y, Bradley CS, Kreder K, Lutgendorf S; Multidisciplinary Approach to the Study of Chronic Pelvic Pain (MAPP) Research Network. Inflammation and inflammatory control in interstitial cystitis/bladder pain syndrome: associations with painful symptoms. *Pain.* 2014;**155**(9):1755–1761.
139. Schwedt TJ, Chiang CC, Chong CD, Dodick DW. Functional MRI of migraine. *Lancet Neurol.* 2015;**14**(1):81–91.

140. Schwedt TJ, Schlaggar BL, Mar S, et al. Atypical resting-state functional connectivity of affective pain regions in chronic migraine. *Headache*. 2013;**53**(5):737–751.
141. Schweinhardt P, Kuchinad A, Pukall CF, Bushnell MC. Increased gray matter density in young women with chronic vulvar pain. *Pain*. 2008;**140**(3):411–419.
142. Seminowicz DA, Shpaner M, Keaser ML, et al. Cognitive-behavioral therapy increases prefrontal cortex gray matter in patients with chronic pain. *J Pain*. 2013;**14**(12):1573–1584.
143. Shamliyan TA, Kane RL, Taylor FR. *Migraine in Adults: Preventive Pharmacologic Treatments* [Internet]. Rockville, MD: Agency for Healthcare Research and Quality (US); 2013. Report No.: 13-EHC068-EF. AHRQ Comparative Effectiveness Reviews.
144. Sinaii N, Cleary SD, Ballweg ML, Nieman LK, Stratton P. High rates of autoimmune and endocrine disorders, fibromyalgia, chronic fatigue syndrome and atopic diseases among women with endometriosis: a survey analysis. *Hum Reprod*. 2002;**17**(10):2715–2724.
145. Skaper SD, Facci L, Giusti P. Mast cells, glia and neuroinflammation: partners in crime? *Immunology*. 2014;**141**(3):314–327.
146. Slade GD, Ohrbach R, Greenspan JD, et al. Painful temporomandibular disorder: decade of discovery from OPPERA Studies. *J Dent Res*. 2016;**95**(10):1084–1092.
147. Smith SB, Reenilä I, Männistö PT, et al. Epistasis between polymorphisms in COMT, ESR1, and GCH1 influences COMT enzyme activity and pain. *Pain*. 2014;**155**(11):2390–2399.
148. Smorgick N, Marsh CA, As-Sanie S, Smith YR, Quint EH. Prevalence of pain syndromes, mood conditions, and asthma in adolescents and young women with endometriosis. *J Pediatr Adolesc Gynecol*. 2013;**26**(3):171–175.
149. Smorgick N, Marsh CA, As-Sanie S, Smith YR, Quint EH. Prevalence of pain syndromes, mood conditions, and asthma in adolescents and young women with endometriosis. *J Pediatr Adolesc Gynecol*. 2013;**26**(3):171–175.
150. Snekkevik H, Eriksen HR, Tangen T, Chalder T, Reme SE. Fatigue and depression in sick-listed chronic low back pain patients. *Pain Med*. 2014;**15**(7):1163–1170.
151. Staud R, Nagel S, Robinson ME, Price DD. Enhanced central pain processing of fibromyalgia patients is maintained by muscle afferent input: a randomized, double-blind, placebo-controlled study. *Pain*. 2009;**145**(1–2):96–104.
152. Stringer EA, Baker KS, Carroll IR, et al. Daily cytokine fluctuations, driven by leptin, are associated with fatigue severity in chronic fatigue syndrome: evidence of inflammatory pathology. *J Transl Med*. 2013;**11**:93.
153. Sturgill J, McGee E, Menzies V. Unique cytokine signature in the plasma of patients with fibromyalgia. *J Immunol Res*. 2014;**2014**:938576.
154. Suskind AM, Berry SH, Suttorp MJ, et al. Health-related quality of life in patients with interstitial cystitis/bladder pain syndrome and frequently associated comorbidities. *Qual Life Res*. 2013;**22**(7): 1537–1541.
155. Tak LM, Cleare AJ, Ormel J, et al. Meta-analysis and meta-regression of hypothalamic-pituitary-adrenal axis activity in functional somatic disorders. *Biol Psychol*. 2011;**87**(2):183–194.
156. Tietjen GE, Peterlin BL. Childhood abuse and migraine: epidemiology, sex differences, and potential mechanisms. *Headache*. 2011;**51**(6):869–879.
157. Totals derived from NIH Research Portfolio Online Reporting Tools (RePORT) Research, Condition, and Disease Categorization (RCDC) & NIH Project RePORTER. 180Washington, DC: National Institutes of Health; 2017. https://report.nih.gov/categorical_spending.aspxand https://projectreporter.nih.gov/. August 2, 2017.
158. Traub RJ, Cao DY, Karpowicz J, et al. A clinically relevant animal model of temporomandibular disorder and irritable bowel syndrome comorbidity. *J Pain*. 2014;**15**(9):956–966.
159. Tunitsky E, Barber MD, Jeppson PC, Nutter B, Jelovsek JE, Ridgeway B. Bladder pain syndrome/interstitial cystitis in twin sisters. *J Urol*. 2012;**187**(1):148–152.
160. Turk DC, Okifuji A, Sinclair JD, Starz TW. Pain, disability, and physical functioning in subgroups of patients with fibromyalgia. *J Rheumatol*. 1996;**23**(7):1255–1262.

161. van Tilburg MA, Zaki EA, Venkatesan T, Boles RG. Irritable bowel syndrome may be associated with maternal inheritance and mitochondrial DNA control region sequence variants. *Dig Dis Sci.* 2014;**59**(7):1392–1397.
162. Vehof J, Zavos HM, Lachance G, Hammond CJ, Williams FM. Shared genetic factors underlie chronic pain syndromes. *Pain.* 2014;**155**(8):1562–1568.
163. Verma V, Sheikh Z, Ahmed AS. Nociception and role of immune system in pain. *Acta Neurol Belg.* 2015;**115**(3):213–220.
164. Visscher CM, Lobbezoo F. TMD pain is partly heritable. A systematic review of family studies and genetic association studies. *J Oral Rehabil.* 2015;**42**(5):386–399.
165. Wang J, Huang Q, Li N, Tan G, Chen L, Zhou J. Triggers of migraine and tension-type headache in China: a clinic-based survey. *Eur J Neurol.* 2013;**20**(4):689–696.
166. Wang P, Du H, Chen N, et al. Regional homogeneity abnormalities in patients with tension-type headache: a resting-state fMRI study. *Neurosci Bull.* 2014;**30**(6):949–955.
167. Warren JW, Clauw DJ, Wesselmann U, Howard FM, Gallicchio L, Morozov V. Functional somatic syndromes as risk factors for hysterectomy in early bladder pain syndrome/interstitial cystitis. *J Psychosom Res.* 2014;**77**(5):363–367.
168. Warren JW, Langenberg P, Clauw DJ. The number of existing functional somatic syndromes (FSSs) is an important risk factor for new, different FSSs. *J Psychosom Res.* 2013;**74**(1):12–17.
169. Warren JW, Morozov V, Howard FM, et al. Before the onset of interstitial cystitis/bladder pain syndrome, the presence of multiple non-bladder syndromes is strongly associated with a history of multiple surgeries. *J Psychosom Res.* 2014;**76**(1):75–79.
170. Weiner DK, Sakamoto S, Perera S, Breuer P. Chronic low back pain in older adults: prevalence, reliability, and validity of physical examination findings. *J Am Geriatr Soc.* 2006;**54**(1):11–20.
171. Weissman-Fogel I, Sprecher E, Granovsky Y, Yarnitsky D. Repeated noxious stimulation of the skin enhances cutaneous pain perception of migraine patients in-between attacks: clinical evidence for continuous sub-threshold increase in membrane excitability of central trigeminovascular neurons. *Pain.* 2003;**104**(3):693–700.
172. Wingenfeld K, Heim C, Schmidt I, Wagner D, Meinlschmidt G, Hellhammer DH. HPA axis reactivity and lymphocyte glucocorticoid sensitivity in fibromyalgia syndrome and chronic pelvic pain. *Psychosom Med.* 2008;**70**(1):65–72.
173. Witkin SS, Gerber S, Ledger WJ. Differential characterization of women with vulvar vestibulitis syndrome. *Am J Obstet Gynecol.* 2002;**187**(3):589–594.
174. Xu X, Bao H, Strait K, et al. Sex differences in perceived stress and early recovery in young and middle-aged patients with acute myocardial infarction. *Circulation.* 2015;**131**(7):614–623.
175. Yang W, Chu B, Yang J, Yu Y, Wu J, Yu S. Elevated audiovisual temporal interaction in patients with migraine without aura. *J Headache Pain.* 2014;**15**:44.
176. Yim YR, Lee KE, Park DJ, et al. Identifying fibromyalgia subgroups using cluster analysis: relationships with clinical variables. *Eur J Pain.* 2017;**21**(2):374–384.
177. Yoon MS, Manack A, Schramm S, et al. Chronic migraine and chronic tension-type headache are associated with concomitant low back pain: results of the German Headache Consortium study. *Pain.* 2013;**154**(3):484–492.
178. Young EE, Lariviere WR, Belfer I. Genetic basis of pain variability: recent advances. *J Med Genet.* 2012;**49**(1):1–9.
179. Younger JW, Shen YF, Goddard G, Mackey SC. Chronic myofascial temporomandibular pain is associated with neural abnormalities in the trigeminal and limbic systems. *Pain.* 2010;**149**(2):222–228.
180. Yu R, Gollub RL, Spaeth R, Napadow V, Wasan A, Kong J. Disrupted functional connectivity of the periaqueductal gray in chronic low back pain. *Neuroimage Clin.* 2014;**6**:100–108.
181. Yunus MB. The prevalence of fibromyalgia in other chronic pain conditions. *Pain Res Treat.* 2012; **2012**:584573.

182. Yunus MB. The prevalence of fibromyalgia in other chronic pain conditions. *Pain Res Treat*. 2012; **2012**:584573.
183. Zhou Q, Imbe H, Dubner R, Ren K. Persistent Fos protein expression after orofacial deep or cutaneous tissue inflammation in rats: implications for persistent orofacial pain. *J Comp Neurol*. 1999; **412**(2):276–291.
184. Zhou Q, Price DD, Callam CS, Woodruff MA, Verne GN. Effects of the N-methyl-D-aspartate receptor on temporal summation of second pain (wind-up) in irritable bowel syndrome. *J Pain*. 2011;**12**(2):297–303.

CHAPTER 9

Mental Disorders

Winfried Häuser

Summary Points

- Mental disorders (anxiety disorders, depressive disorders, and posttraumatic stress disorder [PTSD]) are frequently associated with fibromyalgia syndrome (FMS).
- The association of FMS and these mental disorders can be explained by symptom overlap and shared biologic (e.g., genes) and psychological (e.g., childhood adversities) mechanisms.
- Mental disorders have a negative impact on the clinical outcome of FMS patients.
- Every FMS patient should be screened for mental disorder.
- Severe mental disorder requires the collaboration with a mental health care specialist.

The main symptom of FMS is chronic widespread pain (CWP). The American College of Rheumatology (ACR) 1990 classification criteria also included a demonstration of tenderness.[35] Recently, revised diagnostic criteria have delegated the sign of tenderness to a list of symptoms that include fatigue, lack of refreshing sleep, cognitive impairments, abdominal discomfort, headache, and depression.[32,33] Therefore, some authors argue that depression and anxiety are such an essential part of the clinical phenomenon of FMS that they cannot be meaningfully separated.[30] The author takes the position that there is a substantial overlap of FMS and mental disorders. However, they should be separated for theoretical and clinical reasons. FMS should not be equated with a mental disorder.

FIBROMYALGIA SYNDROME AND DEPRESSION

The incidence of depressive disorders in FMS ranges from 20% to 70% and the lifetime prevalence between 62% and 86%.[1] The incidence and prevalence rates are higher if self-reports and questionnaires than structured interviews are used and in tertiary than primary care settings, respectively.[6]

The overlap of FMS and depressive disorders can be explained as follows:

- Both disorders have common symptoms such as fatigue and sleep problems. A part of the cognitive complaints of FMS patients can be attributed to depression.[7]
- Both disorders share common predisposing, precipitating, and perpetuating factors.[8] 5-HT2A receptor 102T/C polymorphism confers susceptibility to FMS[19] and depression.[16] Childhood adversities such as emotional, physical, and sexual abuse increase vulnerability to FMS and depression.[22] Psychosocial stress (traumatic and major life events, chronic daily hassles) has been described as precipitating factors in depression and FMS.[8] Once triggered, both depression and FMS involve several similar physiologic mechanisms that likely perpetuate these disorders. Alterations of the hypothalamic–pituitary–adrenal function, altered serotoninergic and noradrenergic function, and altered function of systems that involve substance P, neurosteroids, and cytokines.[8]

These are the reasons to separate FMS from depression:

- Not every patient with FMS is depressed and not every patient with depression reports (widespread) pain. In the National Health Interview Survey, 62.7% of persons meeting FMS criteria self-reported a diagnosis of depression.[31] Widespread pain is not a diagnostic feature of depressive disorder and some patients with depressive disorder do not report any pain at all.[14]
- There is a bidirectional temporal association between depression and FMS. An analysis of the Taiwan National Health Insurance Research Database with 25,969 patients with FMS and without any psychiatric disorder and 17,142 patients with depression and without FMS between 2000 and 2008 and separately compared with age- and sex-matched control groups showed that the patients with FMS were associated with an increased risk (hazard ratio [HR] 7.5, 95% confidence interval [CI] 6.8 to 8.2) of subsequent depression and that those with depression were associated with an increased risk (HR 6.3, 95% CI 5.7 to 7.0) of subsequent FMS.[2]
- Depressive symptoms are not related to pain sensitivity or cerebral processing of pain in FMS.[15]
- Classic analgesic studies of amitriptyline suggest that the pain-relieving mechanism is independent of the antidepressant effects. Pain relief is accomplished at a much smaller dose (25 mg) than those used for depression (100 to 150 mg), and analgesic effects are observed after 1 week of treatment while antidepressant effects were usually observed after 2 to 4 weeks of treatment.[8] A recent secondary analysis of four clinical trials of duloxetine in FMS explored treatment effects in patients who were comorbid with major depression. This analysis demonstrated the relative independence of major depression and FMS in that the baseline level of 1 did not affect the treatment efficacy of the other. A path analysis also found predominant direct effects of treatment on mood and pain. These results suggest that the effects of the duloxetine on pain and major depression were mediated by independent mechanisms. However,

the path analyses also showed indirect effects in which improved mood resulted in improved pain and improved pain resulted in improved mood.[23]

FIBROMYALGIA SYNDROME AND ANXIETY DISORDERS

The frequency of the anxiety disorder ranged from 13% to 64% in studies.[6] In the National Health Interview Survey, 65% of persons meeting FMS criteria self-reported being "often anxious."[31] The reasons for overlap are probably the same as with FMS and depression. Muscle pain, difficulty concentrating, and sleep disturbances are symptoms of FMS and generalized anxiety disorder. Childhood adversities are predisposing factors of FMS[12] and anxiety disorder.[31]

FIBROMYALGIA SYNDROME AND POSTTRAUMATIC STRESS DISORDER

The prevalence of PTSD in FMS patients reported by different studies ranged from 8% to 57%.[9] The prevalence rates were higher in case of a questionnaire-based diagnosis and lower in case of clinical interview–based diagnosis of PTSD.

The overlap of FMS and PTSD can be explained as follows:

- Overlap of FMS and PTSD symptoms: Two symptoms of the D-criterion of PTSD, namely sleeping and concentration problems are main symptoms of FMS. The PTSD rate in the German multicentre study sample decreased from 45% to 39% after removing the sleeping and concentration problems and one additional depression item (loss of interest) from the algorithm of the PTSD.[11]
- Catastrophizing: Catastrophizing is defined as a set of cognitive and emotional processes leading to a tendency to misinterpret and exaggerate situations that may be threatening.[5] Pain-related catastrophizing is broadly conceived as a set of exaggerated and negative cognitive and emotional schema brought to bear during actual or anticipated painful stimulation.[25] Catastrophizing encompasses not only pain, but also major life events in FMS patients.[11] FMS patients tend to experience chronic stress (e.g., working place conflicts) and major life events (e.g., loss of job) to be traumatic and report PTSD symptoms such as nightmares and hyperarousal related to these events that do not meet the criteria of a trauma from a clinician's point of view.[9] These data support the view that PTSD represents a marker of stress vulnerability rather than a particular set of biologic reactions caused by exposure to a trauma.[27]
- Common antecedent traumatic events: In the German multicentre study, 70.3% of patients reported at least one traumatic event. In 66% of these patients, traumatic life events preceded the onset of CWP. In 30% of these patients, traumatic life events and PTSD symptoms followed the onset of CWP. In 4% of these patients, traumatic

life events, PTSD symptoms, and CWP occurred in the same year.[11] These data further support the hypothesis, that traumatic experiences and PTSD increase the risk of developing FMS,[27] as most FMS patients with PTSD reported that CWP developed after both the traumatic event and the onset of PTSD symptoms. PTSD also moderated the relationship between childhood victimization and pain 30 years later in a prospective follow-up of a cohort study of individuals with court-documented early childhood abuse/neglect.[26] PTSD, but not major depressive disorder, mediated the relationship between rape and FMS in a community-based US sample.[3] It appears likely that the particulars of major life events alone do not increase the risk of FMS, but rather that the event is experienced to be traumatic.

Reasons for separating FMS and PTSD:

- There are FMS patients without any traumatic experience.[11]
- PTSD is both a potential risk factor for developing FMS and vice versa.[27] The relationship between CWP and PTSD is bidirectional. Pain can serve as a provocative traumatic stimulus for the development of PTSD, and the hyperarousal, stress intolerance, and selective attention typical of PTSD may exacerbate or perpetuate pain.[11]
- Tranquilizers are not effective to reduce pain and fatigue in FMS.[28]

FIBROMYALGIA SYNDROME AND SUICIDALITY

Suicidal ideation in FMS patients is frequent and closely related to comorbid depression, anxiety, and to a higher impact of the disease in daily life.[29] Treatment with antiepileptic drugs might increase the risk of suicidality.[24] Two large retrospective cohort studies conducted in the United States[34] and Denmark[4] demonstrated an increased risk of suicide in FMS patients compared to the general population.

CONSEQUENCES FOR CLINICAL CARE

Systematic reviews demonstrated that depressive disorder and PTSD have a negative impact on the clinical outcome of FMS. FMS patients with these comorbid mental disorder report more somatic and psychological symptoms and more disability. They respond worse to multidisciplinary treatment compared to FMS patients without depression[18] and apply more frequently for disability pension than FMS patients without these disorders.[11] Because of the importance of mental health problems in FMS, some authors have recently suggested to define an FMS subgroup with significant mental health problems.[13]

The German guideline recommends that every FMS patient should be screened for psychological distress,[17] for example, using the questions of the Patient Health Questionnaire 4.[20] In case of a positive screening, a detailed examination by a mental health care specialists is recommended. The German guideline[17] and the updated

European League Against Rheumatism (EULAR)[21] recommendations for the management of FMS recommend co-therapy of mental health care specialists including psychopharmacologic treatment in case of severe anxiety and/or depressive disorders.

Current cognitive behavioral therapies approaches including acceptance-based therapies focus on pain-related thoughts, emotions, and behaviors. The augmentation of these pain-centered approaches by psychotherapeutic treatments tailored to comorbid mental disorders is a major task for research.[10] Potential targets for tailored psychological treatments are as follows:

Interpersonal therapy or cognitive behavioral therapies for major depression

Cognitive behavioral therapies (e.g., prolonged exposure and cognitive processing therapy), Eye Movement Desensitization and Reprocessing (EMDR), or narrative therapy for PTSD

Emotional awareness and expression therapy (EAET) or psychodynamic therapy for unresolved emotional conflicts

REFERENCES

1. Alciati A, Sgiarovello P, Atzeni F, et al. Psychiatric problems in fibromyalgia: clinical and neurobiological links between mood disorders and fibromyalgia. *Reumatismo*. 2012;**64**(4):268–274.
2. Chang MH, Hsu JW, Huang KL, et al. Bidirectional association between depression and fibromyalgia syndrome: a nationwide longitudinal study. *J Pain*. 2015;**16**(9):895–902.
3. Ciccone DS, Elliott DK, Chandler HK, et al. Sexual and physical abuse in women with fibromyalgia syndrome: a test of the trauma hypothesis. *Clin J Pain*. 2005;**21**(5):378–386.
4. Dreyer L, Kendall S, Danneskiold-Samsøe B, et al. Mortality in a cohort of Danish patients with fibromyalgia: increased frequency of suicide. *Arthritis Rheum*. 2010;**62**(10):3101–3108.
5. Edwards RR, Bingham CO 3rd, Bathon J, et al. Catastrophizing and pain in arthritis, fibromyalgia, and other rheumatic diseases. *Arthritis Rheum*. 2006;**55**(2):325–332.
6. Fietta P, Fietta P, Manganelli P. 6.Fibromyalgia and psychiatric disorders. *Acta Biomed*. 2007;**78**(2):88–95.
7. Gelonch O, Garolera M, Valls J, Rosselló L, Pifarré J. Cognitive complaints in women with fibromyalgia: are they due to depression or to objective cognitive dysfunction? *J Clin Exp Neuropsychol*. 2017;**39**:1–13.
8. Gracely RH, Ceko M, Bushnell MC. Fibromyalgia and depression. *Pain Res Treat*. 2012;**2012**:486590.
9. Häuser W, Ablin J, Walitt B. PTSD and fibromyalgia syndrome: focus on prevalence, mechanisms, and impact. In: Martin CR, Preedy VR, Patel VB, eds. Comprehensive Guide to Post-Traumatic Stress Disorder. Zürich, Switzerland: Springer International Publishing; 2016:563–577.
10. Häuser W, Bernardy K. Psychotherapeutic procedures for fibromyalgia syndrome. *Z Rheumatol*. 2015;**74**(7):584–590.
11. Häuser W, Galek A, Erbslöh-Möller B, et al. Posttraumatic stress disorder in fibromyalgia syndrome: prevalence, temporal relationship between posttraumatic stress and fibromyalgia symptoms, and impact on clinical outcome. *Pain*. 2013;**154**(8):1216–1223.
12. Häuser W, Kosseva M, Üceyler N, et al. Emotional, physical, and sexual abuse in fibromyalgia syndrome: a systematic review with meta-analysis. *Arthritis Care Res*. 2011;**63**(6):808–820.
13. Häuser W, Perrot S, Fitzcharles MA, Clauw D. Unravelling fibromyalgia—steps towards individualized management. *J Pain*. 2018;**19**(2):125–134.
14. Häuser W, Schild S, Kosseva M, et al. Validation of the German version of the Regional Pain Scale for the diagnosis of fibromyalgia syndrome. *Schmerz*. 2010;**24**(3):226–235.

15. Jensen KB, Petzke F, Carville S, et al. Anxiety and depressive symptoms in fibromyalgia are related to poor perception of health but not to pain sensitivity or cerebral processing of pain. *Arthritis Rheum.* 2010;**62**(11):3488–3495.
16. Khait VD, Huang YY, Zalsman G, et al. Association of serotonin 5-HT2A receptor binding and the T102C polymorphism in depressed and healthy Caucasian subjects. *Neuropsychopharmacology.* 2005;**30**(1):166–172.
17. Köllner V, Bernardy K, Greiner W, et al. Psychotherapy and psychological procedures for fibromyalgia syndrome: Updated guidelines 2017 and overview of systematic review articles. *Schmerz.* 2017;**31**(3):266–273.
18. Lange M, Petermann F. Influence of depression on fibromyalgia: a systematic review. *Schmerz.* 2010;**24**(4):326–333.
19. Lee YH, Choi SJ, Ji JD, et al. Candidate gene studies of fibromyalgia: a systematic review and meta-analysis. *Rheumatol Int.* 2012;**32**(2):417–426.
20. Löwe B, Wahl I, Rose M, et al. A 4-item measure of depression and anxiety: validation and standardization of the Patient Health Questionnaire-4 (PHQ-4) in the general population. *J Affect Disord.* 2010;**122**(1–2):86–95.
21. Macfarlane GJ, Kronisch C, Dean LE, et al. EULAR revised recommendations for the management of fibromyalgia. *Ann Rheum Dis.* 2017;**76**(2):318–328.
22. Marackova M, Prasko J, Matousek S, et al. The impact of childhood adversities on anxiety and depressive disorders in adulthood. *Neuro Endocrinol Lett.* 2016;**37**(7):478–484.
23. Marangell LB, Clauw DJ, Choy E, et al. Comparative pain and mood effects in patients with comorbid fibromyalgia and major depressive disorder: secondary analyses of four pooled randomized controlled trials of duloxetine. *Pain.* 2011;**152**(1):31–37.
24. Pereira A, Gitlin MJ, Gross RA, et al. Suicidality associated with antiepileptic drugs: implications for the treatment of neuropathic pain and fibromyalgia. *Pain.* 2013;**154**(3):345–349.
25. Quartana PJ, Campbell CM, Edwards RR. Pain catastrophizing: a critical review. *Expert Rev Neurother.* 2009;**9**(5):745–758.
26. Raphael KG, Janal MN, Nayak S, et al. Psychiatric comorbidities in a community sample of women with fibromyalgia. *Pain.* 2006;**124**(1–2):117–125.
27. Raphael KG, Janal MN, Nayak S. Comorbidity of fibromyalgia and posttraumatic stress disorder symptoms in a community sample of women. *Pain Med.* 2004;**5**(1):33–41.
28. Sommer C, Alten R, Bär KJ, et al. Drug therapy of fibromyalgia syndrome: Updated guidelines 2017 and overview of systematic review articles. *Schmerz.* 2017;**31**(3):274–284.
29. Triñanes Y, González-Villar A, Gómez-Perretta C, et al. Suicidality in chronic pain: predictors of suicidal ideation in fibromyalgia. *Pain Pract.* 2015;**15**(4):323–332.
30. Walitt B, Ceko M, Khatiwada M, et al. Characterizing "fibrofog": subjective appraisal, objective performance, and task-related brain activity during a working memory task. *Neuroimage Clin.* 2016;**11**:173–180.
31. Walitt B, Nahin RL, Katz RS, et al. The Prevalence and Characteristics of Fibromyalgia in the 2012 National Health Interview Survey. *PLoS ONE.* 2015;**10**(9):e0138024.
32. Wolfe F, Clauw DJ, Fitzcharles MA, et al. The American College of Rheumatology preliminary diagnostic criteria for fibromyalgia and measurement of symptom severity. *Arthritis Care Res.* 2010;**62**(5):600–610.
33. Wolfe F, Clauw DJ, Fitzcharles MA, et al. Fibromyalgia criteria and severity scales for clinical and epidemiological studies: a modification of the ACR Preliminary Diagnostic Criteria for Fibromyalgia. *J Rheumatol.* 2011;**38**(6):1113–1122.
34. Wolfe F, Hassett AL, Walitt B, et al. Mortality in fibromyalgia: a study of 8,186 patients over thirty-five years. *Arthritis Care Res.* 2011;**63**(1):94–101.
35. Wolfe F, Smythe HA, Yunus MB, et al. The American College of Rheumatology 1990 Criteria for the Classification of Fibromyalgia. Report of the Multicenter Criteria Committee. *Arthritis Rheum.* 1990;**33**(2):160–172.

CHAPTER 10

Functional Impairment

Winfried Häuser

Summary Points

- On an average, physical fitness, cognitive function, sexual function, and workability of patients with fibromyalgia syndrome (FMS) are lower than that of healthy controls.
- Patients with FMS differ in their degree of functional impairment.
- Functional impairment is associated with somatic and psychological symptom burden.
- "Fibro fog" might be perhaps better defined as a distressing intrusiveness of subjective cognitive symptoms rather than a clinically relevant cognitive deficit.

FIBROMYALGIA SYNDROME PATIENTS DIFFER IN THE AMOUNT OF PHYSICAL IMPAIRMENT

FMS is diagnosed by a report of chronic widespread pain and of impairment by, unrefreshed sleep, physical and mental fatigue, and by additional somatic and psychological symptoms.[20,21] These diagnostic criteria define FMS as a syndrome that is associated with functional impairment that is variable and diminished health-related quality of life (HRQOL).[7]

FMS can be conceptualized as the end of a continuum of biopsychosocial symptom burden (distress).[8] However, persons meeting FMS criteria can differ in the degree of somatic and psychological symptom severity and in the extent of impairment of daily functioning. Mild, moderate, and severe forms of FMS with variable functional impairment may be defined according to values obtained for generic instruments such as the Patient Health Questionnaire 15 (PHQ 15)[9] and disease-specific instruments such as the Fibromyalgia Impact Questionnaire (FIQ).[16] Nearly, all patients in clinical studies meet the criteria for moderate or severe forms of FMS. In contrast, mild forms of FMS are more commonly reported in population-based studies.[9] The heterogeneity of FMS with regard to symptom burden and functional impairment can also be demonstrated by cluster analysis. Yim et al.[24] identified four groups of FMS patients: Group 1 was characterized by high pain, severe physical and mental impairment, and low social support. Group 2 had moderate pain and physical impairment, mild mental impairment, and moderate social support. Group 3 had moderate pain, low physical and moderate mental impairment, and low social support. Group 4 had low pain, nearly normal physical and mental function, and high social support.

When reading the following sections that report average data for mostly heterogeneous cohort samples, the reader should keep in mind the aforementioned variability in degree of severity of FMS as well as the subgroupings of FMS patients.

Physical Impairment

It is likely that the relationship between reduced physical activity/fitness and FMS is bidirectional. Low physical activity combined with obesity predicted FMS development in one longitudinal study.[12] Physical fitness (aerobic capacity, muscle strength) is reduced in FMS patients when compared to healthy controls. Both subjective and objective physical function are reduced in FMS, with a greater perception of impaired subjective function. An explanation for this discordance may be catastrophizing cognitions.[5] In addition, reduced physical fitness is associated with anxiety.[4]

Ability to Work

FMS can be associated with the inability to engage in gainful employment. Major differences exist among studies in reported disability, decreased muscle strength, and endurance, all factors that influence work capacity. However, 34% to 77% of women with FMS work.[10] A systematic review found that symptom severity influenced workability of persons with FMS. Physically demanding jobs and work tasks were especially troublesome and were reported to constitute higher risks of work disability. Working people with FMS at risk of work overload may initiate adjustment strategies such as a career change, working part time, and developing personal skills were necessary for managing work. The support of management and colleagues enabled people with FMS to manage the risk of overload at work.[13]

Cognitive Impairment

Perceived cognitive dysfunction ("fibrofog") is now recognized as a diagnostic feature of FMS.[20,21] The most common complaints include the ability to focus, concentrate, remember, use language, multitask, and organize information. Some of these cognitive functions are summarized in the construct of an executive function, an overarching term used to describe the outcome of goal-directed, coordinated activation of multiple cognitive processes that allow a person to respond to a nonroutine situation in an effective, adaptable manner.[2] Dyscognition contributes significantly to both functional and work disability in FMS.[18]

It is disappointing to note that the entire body of science on dyscognition in FMS comprises only about 20 publications comparing cognitive testing in small populations of FMS patients to controls.[2,1] The quality of the methodology of most studies is low for numerous reasons including poorly described methods of recruitment, lack of a priori calculation of sample size that would allow for adequate power, and lack of report of reliability and validity of the test(s) used. In summary, objective differences of small effect sizes have been demonstrated in performance on some neuropsychological tests of attention, executive function, and memory. However, these findings often required experimental provocation (i.e., distraction, stress) to demonstrate effects that are frequently not identified with standard cognitive tests.[2,18] Another important consideration is that moderators of executive function, such as medication and depression, were seldom controlled for in studies of executive function performance.[2] A recent study demonstrated that depression scores, everyday physical functioning, and working memory performance were most strongly associated with subjective cognitive complaints.[6] It is notable that these cognitive deficits may not be overtly obvious to medical observation, certainly far less than those seen in pathologically defined neuropsychiatric dementias such as Alzheimer's disease. Objective differences noted on cognitive testing also correlate poorly with self-perception of cognitive deficits.[18,17] The cognitive impairment of FMS patients ("fibro fog") might therefore be better defined by a concept of distressing intrusiveness of subjective cognitive symptoms rather than by a clinically relevant cognitive deficit.[18]

Sexual Dysfunction

A Spanish study found that the frequency of sexual dysfunction was significantly higher in patients with FMS than in controls for both females (86.9% vs. 23.6%) and males (76.5% vs. 6.7%).[15] A systematic review identified decreased sexual desire and arousal, decreased experience of orgasm, and in some studies an increase in genital pain in female FMS patients. The psychological aspects, together with the stress related to the constant presence of chronic widespread pain, fatigue, and sleep disturbances, are regarded as major factors that adversely affect the sexuality of the patient with FMS. Moreover, the drugs that are most commonly used for the treatment of symptoms of FMS may adversely affect sexuality and sexual function in many patients.[3]

Health-Related Quality of Life

HRQOL burden for FMS is generally poorer when compared with findings in many other diseases. Tools to measure HRQOL include the quality-adjusted life year (QALY) and the EuroQol (EQ-5D) scores. Both instruments score perfect health as 1 and death as 0, which enables comparison across diseases. In FMS, QALY scores have been estimated to be 0.56[11] and EQ-5D scores range between 0.44 and 0.61.[14,22] These scores tend to be lower (more compromising of HRQOL) than the scores generally seen with other rheumatic, somatic, and psychological disorders, such as inflammatory arthritis (0.66), lower back pain (0.63 to 0.79), gout (0.77), osteoarthritis (0.70), irritable bowel syndrome (0.66), migraine (0.81), menopause (0.73), depression (0.73), and neurotic disorders (0.74).[3,22] The reduction of HRQOL in FMS approaches scores seen in blindness or low vision (0.69) and renal failure (0.65).[23]

The HRQOL burden of FMS can also be considered from a population viewpoint. This has been measured using HRQOL instruments that are normalized to the population, particularly the Short Form-36 Health Survey (SF-36). The SF-36 scores the HRQOL of the population mean as 50, with increments of 10 corresponding to a standard deviation from the population mean. SF-36 scores for the physical component in patients with FMS range between 1.5 and 2 SDs below the population mean (the bottom 5% to 10%), whereas scores for the mental component are generally 1 SD lower (the bottom 33%). FMS patients report feeling considerably worse than a large majority of the general population.[7]

This poorer HRQOL for FMS patients is stable over time. Prospective population studies of FMS patients have reported this stability of HRQOL levels over time, as well as levels far below population norms, regardless of therapy.[19,23] However, this stability is based on average scores, with the knowledge that FMS symptoms can be expected to fluctuate. Meaningful improvements in symptoms, typically defined as ≥25% to 30% improvement in symptom measurements (such as the Visual Analogue Scale for pain or the FIQ) have been shown to occur in 25% of people with FMS. Conversely, symptom severity worsened in 36% of individuals with FMS in the same prospective study.[19]

REFERENCES

1. Ambrose KR, Gracely RH, Glass JM. Fibromyalgia dyscognition: concepts and issues. *Reumatismo.* 2012;**64**:206–215.
2. Berryman C, Stanton TR, Bowering KJ, Tabor A, McFarlane A, Moseley GL. Do people with chronic pain have impaired executive function? A meta-analytical review. *Clin Psychol Rev*. 2014;**34**:563–579.
3. Brazier J, Roberts J, Tsuchiya A, Busschbach J. A comparison of the EQ-5D and SF-6D across seven patient groups. *Health Econ*. 2004;**13**:873–884.
4. Córdoba-Torrecilla S, Aparicio VA, Soriano-Maldonado A, et al. Physical fitness is associated with anxiety levels in women with fibromyalgia: the al-Ándalus project. *Qual Life Res*. 2016;**25**:1053–1058.
5. Estévez-López F, Álvarez-Gallardo IC, Segura-Jiménez V, et al. The discordance between subjectively and objectively measured physical function in women with fibromyalgia: association with catastrophizing and self-efficacy cognitions. The al-Ándalus project. *Disabil Rehabil*. 2018;**40**:329–337.
6. Gelonch O, Garolera M, Valls J, Rosselló L, Pifarré J. Cognitive complaints in women with fibromyalgia: are they due to depression or to objective cognitive dysfunction? *J Clin Exp Neuropsychol*. 2017;**39**:1013–1025.
7. Häuser W, Ablin J, Fitzcharles MA, et al. Fibromyalgia. *Nat Rev Dis Primers*. 2015;**1**:15022.
8. Häuser W, Schmutzer G, Brähler E, Glaesmer H. A cluster within the continuum of biopsychosocial distress can be labeled "fibromyalgia syndrome"0020014;evidence from a representative German population survey. *J Rheumatol*. 2009;**36**:2806–2812.

9. Häuser W, Schmutzer G, Brähler E, Wolfe F. Patient Health Questionnaire 15 as a generic measure of severity in fibromyalgia syndrome: surveys with patients of three different settings. *J Psychosom Res.* 2014;**76**:307–311.
10. Henriksson CM, Liedberg GM, Gerdle B. Women with fibromyalgia: work and rehabilitation. *Disabil Rehabil.* 2005;**27**:685–694.
11. Moore RA, Straube S, Paine J, Phillips CJ, Derry S, McQuay HJ. Fibromyalgia: moderate and substantial pain intensity reduction predicts improvement in other outcomes and substantial quality of life gain. *Pain.* 2010;**149**:360–364.
12. Mork PJ, Vasseljen O, Nilsen TI. Association between physical exercise, body mass index, and risk of fibromyalgia: longitudinal data from the Norwegian Nord-Trøndelag Health Study. *Arthritis Care Res.* 2010;**62**:611–617.
13. Palstam A, Mannerkorpi K. Work ability in fibromyalgia: an update in the 21st century. *Curr Rheumatol Rev.* 2017;**13**:180–187.
14. Perrot S, Schaefer C, Knight T, Hufstader M, Chandran AB, Zlateva G. Societal and individual burden of illness among fibromyalgia patients in France: association between disease severity and OMERACT core domains. *BMC Musculoskelet Disord.* 2012;**13**:22.
15. Rico-Villademoros F, Calandre EP, Rodríguez-López CM, et al. Sexual functioning in women and men with fibromyalgia. *J Sex Med.* 2012;**9**:542–549.
16. Schaefer C, Chandran A, Hufstader M, et al. The comparative burden of mild, moderate and severe fibromyalgia: results from a cross-sectional survey in the United States. *Health Qual Life Outcomes.* 2011;**9**:71.
17. Tesio V, Torta DM, Colonna F. Are fibromyalgia patients cognitively impaired? Objective and subjective neuropsychological evidence. *Arthritis Care Res.* 2015;**67**:143–150.
18. Walitt B, Čeko M, Khatiwada M, et al. Characterizing “fibrofog”: subjective appraisal, objective performance, and task-related brain activity during a working memory task. *Neuroimage Clin.* 2016;**11**:173–180.
19. Walitt B, Fitzcharles MA, Hassett AL, Katz RS, Häuser W, Wolfe F. The longitudinal outcome of fibromyalgia: a study of 1555 patients. *J Rheumatol.* 2011;**38**:2238–2246.
20. Wolfe F, Clauw DJ, Fitzcharles MA, et al. The American College of Rheumatology preliminary diagnostic criteria for fibromyalgia and measurement of symptom severity. *Arthritis Care Res.* 2010;**62**:600–610.
21. Wolfe F, Clauw DJ, Fitzcharles MA, et al. Fibromyalgia criteria and severity scales for clinical and epidemiological studies: a modification of the ACR preliminary diagnostic criteria for fibromyalgia. *J Rheumatol.* 2011;**38**:1113–1122.
22. Wolfe F, Michaud K, Li T, Katz RS. EQ-5D and SF-36 quality of life measures in systemic lupus erythematosus: comparisons with rheumatoid arthritis, noninflammatory rheumatic disorders, and fibromyalgia. *J Rheumatol.* 2010;**37**:296–304.
23. Wolfe F, Walitt BT, Katz RS, Lee YC, Michaud KD, Häuser W. Longitudinal patterns of analgesic and central acting drug use and associated effectiveness in fibromyalgia. *Eur J Pain.* 2013;**17**:581–586.
24. Yim YR, Lee KE, Park DJ, et al. Identifying fibromyalgia subgroups using cluster analysis: relationships with clinical variables. *Eur J Pain.* 2017;**21**:374–384.

SECTION 3

Epidemiology and Social Impact

CHAPTER 11

Epidemiology

Winfried Häuser

Summary Points

- The population prevalence of fibromyalgia syndrome (FMS) established by FMS criteria is approximately 2%.
- The administrative prevalence (people diagnosed with FMS by chart records or billing codes of health insurance companies) in the general population is lower (0.3% to 1%).
- FMS prevalence increases with age.
- FMS is more frequently diagnosed in women in clinical settings with a gender ratio of 8 to 10:1.
- FMS is likely underdiagnosed in men in clinical settings.

FMS is a common disorder, which occurs in all populations worldwide. Three recent systematic reviews summarized the results of studies reporting on the prevalence of FMS.

In the first review of 26 studies worldwide, although not identifying the dates and the databases searched, Queiroz reported a global prevalence of FMS as 2.7%. FMS was more prevalent in women, in patients older than 50 years, in subjects with low education level, with low socioeconomic status, living in rural areas, and possibly in obese women[11,3] (see Table 11.1).

Marques et al.[8] conducted a bibliographic survey from 2005 to 2014 in MEDLINE and Web of Science. FMS prevalence in the general population ranged between 0.2% and 6.6%, in women between 2.4% and 6.8%, in urban areas between 0.7% and 11.4%, in rural areas between 0.1% and 5.2%, and in special populations between 0.6% and 15%.

Heidari et al. searched PubMed, Web of Sciences, Ovid, Ebsco, Scopus, and Cochrane library databanks and Google scholar up to December 2016. They identified 81 studies addressing prevalence of FMS among 3,609,810 subjects from both the general population and specific groups. The overall prevalence (95% confidence intervals) of FMS in the general population was 1.8% (1.6, 1.9), in women 4.0% (2.8, 5.2), in men 0.01% (−0.04, 0.06), in patients referred to rheumatology and internal medicine

TABLE 11.1 **Prevalence of fibromyalgia syndrome in the general population**

Country	Case definition	*n*	Age (years)	Overall prevalence (%)	Female prevalence (%)	Male prevalence (%)
Tunisia	LFESSQ	1,000	≥15	9.3	NR	NR
Brazil	COPCORD	3,038	≥16	2.5	3.9	0.1
Canada	1990 ACR	3,395	≥16	3.3	4.9	1.6
Canada	Self-reported	1,31,535	≥12	1.1	1.8	0.3
United States	1990 ACR	3,006	≥18	2.2	3.4	0.5
United States	Research	3,410	≥21	6.4	7.7	4.9
Bangladesh	COCPCORD	5,211	≥15	3.6	6.2	0.9
China	1990 ACR	1,467	NR	0.8	NR	NR
Israel	LFESSQ + 1990 ACR	1,019	≥18	2.0	2.8	1.1
Japan	Research	20,407	≥20	2.1	NR	NR
Malaysia	COCPCORD	2,594	≥15	0.9	1.5	0.2
Pakistan	COCPCORD	1,997	≥15	2.1	NR	NR
Thailand	2010 ACR	1,000	NR	0.6	NR	NR
Turkey	1990 ACR	600	NR	8.8	12.5	5.1
Denmark	1990 ACR	1,219	≥18	0.7	NR	NR
France	LFESSQ + 1990 ACR	1,014	≥15	1.4	2.0	0.7
France	LFESSQ + 1990 ACR	3,081	≥18	1.6	NR	NR
Finland	Yunus	7,217	≥30	0.8	1.0	0.5

Germany	LFESSQ + 1990 ACR	1,002	≥15	3.2	3.9	2.5
Germany	Research	2,445	≥14	2.1	2.4	1.8
Greece	1990 ACR	8,740	≥19	0.4	NR	NR
Italy	1990 ACR	2,155	≥18	2.2	NR	NR
Italy	LFESSQ + 1990 ACR	1,002	≥15	3.7	5.5	1.6
Portugal	LFESSQ + 1990 ACR	500	≥15	3.6	5.2	1.8
Scotland	1990 ACR	1,604	≥18	1.7	Women/men 13.7	
	2010 ACR			1.2	Women/men 4.8	
	Research			5.4	Women/men 2.3	
Spain	LFESSQ + 1990 ACR	1,001	≥15	2.3	3.3	1.3
Spain	1990 ACR	2,192	≥20	2.4	4.2	0.2
Sweden	1990 ACR	2,425	≥20	1.3	2.4	0.0

ACR, American College of Rheumatology; COPCORD, Community Oriented Program for the Control of Rheumatic Diseases; LFESSQ, London Fibromyalgia Screening Questionnaire; NR, not reported.

Research criteria: Modified ACR 2010 diagnostic criteria. The table was modified from Refs. 1 and 3.

From Queiroz LP. Worldwide epidemiology of fibromyalgia. *Curr Pain Headache Rep*. 2013;17(8):356; Häuser W, Ablin J, Fitzcharles MA, et al. Fibromyalgia. *Nat Rev Dis Primers*. 2015;1:15022.

clinics 15.2% (13.6, 16.9), in patients with irritable bowel syndrome (IBS) 12.9% (12.7, 13.1), in hemodialysis patients 6.3% (4.6, 7.9), and those with type 2 diabetes 14.8% (11.1, 18.4).[6]

Identification of the true incidence of FMS is problematic. A study examined a US-based large insurance claims database for "new" FMS cases and found that the age-adjusted (to the US population) rate for "new" FMS was 6.88 cases per 1,000 person-years for men and 11.28 cases per 1,000 person-years for women.[13] The incidence of new physician-diagnosed FMS, based on self-reports of mainly female Finnish hospital employees, was 1% within 1 year.[7]

The prevalence of people diagnosed with FMS ("administrative prevalence") is probably lower than the 2% to 4% prevalence rates reported in epidemiologic population studies. In a Japanese study, only 2.5% of the individuals meeting the 2011 criteria[15] reported to be diagnosed with FMS.[10] A US study found an age-adjusted and sex-adjusted prevalence of people diagnosed with FMS documented by clinical records to be 1.1% and of potential FMS, diagnosed by the modified 2010 American College of Rheumatology (ACR) diagnostic criteria,[15] to be 6.4%.[12] The 1-year prevalence of people with FMS defined by at least one billing case with the code for FMS of a German health insurance company with 7 million insured individuals was 0.3%.[9]

When the 1990 ACR classification criteria[16] are used for clinical surveys, women are more frequently diagnosed with the disorder. Using these criteria, the female-to-men ratio has ranged from 8:1 to 30:1 in patients studied in clinical institutions and surveys.[1,2,4] However, when criteria for FMS that do not use tender point examination are applied, the sex ratio can be close to equal. The sex ratio has ranged from 4:1 to 1:1 in studies that were conducted in the general population using the 2011 FMS criteria.[15,10,12,14] Most probably, FMS is underdiagnosed in men in clinical studies when the ACR 1990 classification criteria with tender point examination[16] are applied.[5] In addition, FMS is regarded as a "female disease" and therefore it is likely a neglected diagnostic consideration in the evaluation of men with chronic widespread pain.[5]

REFERENCES

1. Bennett RM, Jones J, Turk DC, Russell IJ, Matallana L. An internet survey of 2,596 people with fibromyalgia. *BMC Musculoskelet Disord.* 2007;**8**:27.
2. Galek A, Erbslöh-Möller B, Köllner V, et al. Mental disorders in patients with fibromyalgia syndrome: screening in centres of different medical specialties. *Schmerz.* 2013;**27**(3):296–304.
3. Häuser W, Ablin J, Fitzcharles MA, et al. Fibromyalgia. *Nat Rev Dis Primers.* 2015;**1**:15022.
4. Häuser W, Jung E, Erbslöh-Möller B, et al. The German fibromyalgia consumer reports—a cross-sectional survey. *BMC Musculoskelet Disord.* 2012;**13**:74.
5. Häuser W, Kühn-Becker H, von Wilmoswky H, Settan M, Brähler E, Petzke F. Demographic and clinical features of patients with fibromyalgia syndrome of different settings: a gender comparison. *Gend Med.* 2011;**8**(2):116–125.
6. Heidari F, Afshari M, Moosazadeh M. Prevalence of fibromyalgia in general population and patients, a systematic review and meta-analysis. *Rheumatol Int.* 2017;**37**(9):1527–1539.

7. Kivimäki M, Leino-Arjas P, Virtanen M, et al. Work stress and incidence of newly diagnosed fibromyalgia: prospective cohort study. *J Psychosom Res.* 2004;**57**(5):417–422.
8. Marques AP, Santo AS, Berssaneti AA, et al. Prevalence of fibromyalgia: literature review update. *Rev Bras Rheumatol.* 2017;**57**(4):356–363.
9. Marschall U, Arnold B, Häuser W. Treatment and healthcare costs of fibromyalgia syndrome in Germany: analysis of the data of the Barmer health insurance (BEK) from 2008–2009. *Schmerz.* 2011;**25**:402–404, 406–410.
10. Nakamura I, Nishioka K, Usui C, et al. An epidemiologic internet survey of fibromyalgia and chronic pain in Japan. *Arthritis Care Res.* 2014;**66**(7):1093–1101.
11. Queiroz LP. Worldwide epidemiology of fibromyalgia. *Curr Pain Headache Rep.* 2013;**17**(8):356.
12. Vincent A, Lahr BD, Wolfe F, et al. Prevalence of fibromyalgia: a population-based study in Olmsted County, Minnesota, utilizing the Rochester Epidemiology Project. *Arthritis Care Res.* 2013;**65**(5):786–792.
13. Weir PT, Harlan GA, Nkoy FL, et al. The incidence of fibromyalgia and its associated comorbidities: a population-based retrospective cohort study based on International Classification of Diseases, 9th Revision codes. *J Clin Rheumatol.* 2006;**12**(3):124–128.
14. Wolfe F, Brähler E, Hinz A, Häuser W. Fibromyalgia prevalence, somatic symptom reporting, and the dimensionality of polysymptomatic distress: results from a survey of the general population. *Arthritis Care Res.* 2013;**65**(5):777–785.
15. Wolfe F, Clauw DJ, Fitzcharles MA, et al. Fibromyalgia criteria and severity scales for clinical and epidemiological studies: a modification of the ACR Preliminary Diagnostic Criteria for Fibromyalgia. *J Rheumatol.* 2011;**38**(6):1113–1122.
16. Wolfe F, Smythe HA, Yunus MB, et al. The American College of Rheumatology 1990 Criteria for the Classification of Fibromyalgia. Report of the Multicenter Criteria Committee. *Arthritis Rheum.* 1990;**33**(2):160–172.

CHAPTER 12

Social and Economic Impact

Winfried Häuser

Summary Points

- A significant economic burden on society and on individuals is associated with fibromyalgia syndrome (FMS).
- There are substantial differences in direct health care costs among patients.
- The economic burden of illness is associated with the severity of FMS.
- Probably, health costs of FMS patients do not differ from those of osteoarthritis patients.

The economic burden associated with FMS can be divided into direct and indirect costs. Direct costs include the money spent (by individuals and health insurance companies) for the treatment of FMS and associated comorbidities such as sleep disturbances and mental disorders. Indirect costs involve losses in productivity, reduced work hours, absenteeism, disability, unemployment, early retirement, informal care, and other out-of-pocket costs. Due to the differences between national health care systems, direct comparisons between countries should be regarded with caution.

DIRECT HEALTH COSTS

Adjusted annual direct costs per subject for FMS were significantly higher in the United States ($7,087) than in France ($481) or Germany ($2,417).[11] Another study reported that in France direct annual costs were €910 and in Germany €1,765.[21] In a Japanese study, direct costs of FMS were nearly six times as high (¥1,941,118 [ca. $19,410] vs. ¥335,140 [ca. $3,351) as of matched controls.[13] A Canadian study found annual average direct health costs of $3,804. The purchase of prescribed medications led to the highest costs (mean: $329, SD: $321), followed by consultations to health care professionals other than physicians (mean: $129, SD: $222) and physicians consultations (mean: $98, SD: $116). Results further showed a high economic burden for patients themselves, aside from costs covered by public or private insurers.[12] The standard deviations reported by the Canadian study highlight that there are substantial differences of direct health care costs of patients. In a German study, the annual direct health costs were 3,602 € (SD 6,097 €; minimum 229 €, maximum 32.738 €).[16] In a US study with FMS patients recruited from primary care physicians, direct health costs increased with FMS severity measured by the Fibromyalgia Impact Questionnaire: Mean 3-month total direct costs (including payer costs for health resource use and out-of-pocket costs for medical and nonmedical services) were $1,213, $1,415, and $2,329 for subjects with mild, moderate, and severe FMS, respectively.[3] However, health costs associated with FMS might not differ from other noninflammatory rheumatic diseases. In a US study, total health benefit costs for FMS were $8,452 versus $11,253 for osteoarthritis and $4,013 for no FMS.[10]

INDIRECT COSTS

FMS patients report that limited physical capacity and an increased need of rest made it difficult to manage the physical, psychosocial, and organizational work demands.[14] Lack of adjustment of the work tasks and work environment[17] as well as workplace bullying can enhance the decision of FMS patients to apply for early disability retirement. FMS and disability adjudication are a medicolegal challenge and a controversial issue.[6,8] In a study involving patients at six rheumatology centers in the United States, 26.5% were receiving disability payments.[22] Twenty-six percent of the French and 28% of the German patients recruited from physician offices reported early retirement or unemployment due to FMS.[21] In a Scottish tertiary care center, 46.8% of patients with FMS reported that they had lost their job because of this condition, compared with 14.1% of those without FMS.[1] In a Canadian community study, 26% of FMS cases were receiving some form of disability payment.[20] In a Spanish study, 23% of FMS patients recruited Primary Health Care Centers had some degree of permanent work disability pension.[5] In a Finnish prospective twin study, cumulative incidence of early disability retirement at 14-year follow-up was 9.5% among individuals with no or few symptoms at baseline, and 26% in individuals with FMS-like symptoms at baseline. The individuals with FMS-like symptoms at baseline had a 43% (95% CI 17% to 75%) increased overall mortality risk, which was fully accounted for by adjustment of lifestyle factors, mainly smoking.[15] A Canadian study with patients of a tertiary health care center observed associations of disability compensation with subjective reports of symptom severity, increased use of medications, and previous employment in more physically demanding jobs.[7]

Adjusted mean annual indirect costs per subject for FMS were lower in the United States ($6,431) than in France ($8,718) or Germany ($10,001) in one study.[11] In France, indirect costs were €6,990 and €5,491 in Germany.[21] In a study with a representative Japanese population sample, indirect costs of individuals with FMS were more than twice as high (¥2,826,395 [ca. $ 28,264) vs. ¥1,201,547 [ca. $ 12,015) as of matched controls.[13]

THE IMPACT OF DIAGNOSIS OF FIBROMYALGIA SYNDROME ON HEALTH COSTS

Most patients report "a long journey" to FMS diagnosis including ineffective diagnostic and therapeutic procedures.[4] Preliminary evidence suggests that health costs do not substantially increase or decrease after the diagnosis of FMS.[9,19,18,2] If early diagnosis of FMS combined with appropriate patient education on self-management and appropriate drug use helps to reduce health costs, it needs to be tested.

REFERENCES

1. Al-Allaf AW. Work disability and health system utilization in patients with fibromyalgia syndrome. *J Clin Rheumatol.* 2007;**13**(4):199–201.
2. Berger A, Sadosky A, Dukes EM, Edelsberg J, Zlateva G, Oster G. Patterns of healthcare utilization and cost in patients with newly diagnosed fibromyalgia. *Am J Manag Care.* 2010;**16**(5 Suppl):S126–S137.
3. Chandran A, Schaefer C, Ryan K, Baik R, McNett M, Zlateva G. The comparative economic burden of mild, moderate, and severe fibromyalgia: results from a retrospective chart review and cross-sectional survey of working-age U.S. adults. *J Manag Care Pharm.* 2012;**18**(6):415–426.
4. Choy E, Perrot S, Leon T, et al. A patient survey of the impact of fibromyalgia and the journey to diagnosis. *BMC Health Serv Res.* 2010;**10**:102.
5. Collado A, Gomez E, Coscolla R, et al. Work, family and social environment in patients with Fibromyalgia in Spain: an epidemiological study: EPIFFAC study. *BMC Health Serv Res.* 2014;**14**:513.
6. Fitzcharles MA, Ste-Marie PA, Mailis A, Shir Y. Adjudication of fibromyalgia syndrome: challenges in the medicolegal arena. *Pain Res Manag.* 2014;**19**(6):287–292.
7. Fitzcharles MA, Ste-Marie PA, Rampakakis E, Sampalis JS, Shir Y. Disability in fibromyalgia associates with symptom severity and occupation characteristics. *J Rheumatol.* 2016;**43**(5):931–936.
8. Harth M, Nielson WR. Fibromyalgia and disability adjudication: no simple solutions to a complex problem. *Pain Res Manag.* 2014;**19**(6):293–299.
9. Hughes G, Martinez C, Myon E, Taïeb C, Wessely S. The impact of a diagnosis of fibromyalgia on health care resource use by primary care patients in the UK: an observational study based on clinical practice. *Arthritis Rheum.* 2006;**54**(1):177–183.
10. Kleinman N, Harnett J, Melkonian A, Lynch W, Kaplan-Machlis B, Silverman SL. Burden of fibromyalgia and comparisons with osteoarthritis in the workforce. *J Occup Environ Med.* 2009;**51**(12):1384–1393.
11. Knight T, Schaefer C, Chandran A, Zlateva G, Winkelmann A, Perrot S. Health-resource use and costs associated with fibromyalgia in France, Germany, and the United States. *Clinicoecon Outcomes Res.* 2013;**5**:171–180.
12. Lacasse A, Bourgault P, Choinière M. Fibromyalgia-related costs and loss of productivity: a substantial societal burden. *BMC Musculoskelet Disord.* 2016;**17**:168.
13. Lee LK, Ebata N, Hlavacek P, DiBonaventura M, Cappelleri JC, Sadosky A. Humanistic and economic burden of fibromyalgia in Japan. *J Pain Res.* 2016;**9**:967–978.
14. Mannerkorpi K, Gard G. Hinders for continued work among persons with fibromyalgia. *BMC Musculoskelet Disord.* 2012;**13**:96.
15. Markkula R, Kalso E, Huunan-Seppälä A, et al. The burden of symptoms predicts early retirement: a twin cohort study on fibromyalgia-associated symptoms. *Eur J Pain.* 2011;**15**(7):741–747.
16. Marschall U, Arnold B, Häuser W. Treatment and healthcare costs of fibromyalgia syndrome in Germany: analysis of the data of the Barmer health insurance (BEK) from 2008-2009. *Schmerz.* 2011;**25**:402–404, 406–410.

17. Palstam A, Mannerkorpi K. Work ability in fibromyalgia: an update in the 21st century. *Curr Rheumatol Rev.* 2017;**13**(3):180–187.
18. Sanchez RJ, Uribe C, Li H, et al. Longitudinal evaluation of health care utilization and costs during the first three years after a new diagnosis of fibromyalgia. *Curr Med Res Opin.* 2011;**27**(3):663–671.
19. White KP, Nielson WR, Harth M, Ostbye T, Speechley M. Does the label "fibromyalgia" alter health status, function, and health service utilization? A prospective, within-group comparison in a community cohort of adults with chronic widespread pain. *Arthritis Rheum.* 2002;**47**(3):260–265.
20. White KP, Speechley M, Harth M, Ostbye T. Comparing self-reported function and work disability in 100 community cases of fibromyalgia syndrome versus controls in London, Ontario: the London Fibromyalgia Epidemiology Study. *Arthritis Rheum.* 1999;**42**(1):76–83.
21. Winkelmann A, Perrot S, Schaefer C, et al. Impact of fibromyalgia severity on health economic costs: results from a European cross-sectional study. *Appl Health Econ Health Policy.* 2011;**9**(2):125–136.
22. Wolfe F, Anderson J, Harkness D, et al. Work and disability status of persons with fibromyalgia. *J Rheumatol.* 1997;**24**(6):1171–1178.

CHAPTER 13

A Patient's Perspective

Kathy Longley

Summary Points

- Fibromyalgia syndrome (FMS) affects every aspect of day-to-day life.
- Education of medical professionals, politicians, and social security workers is of utmost importance.
- Symptoms need to be recognized more readily so that a prompt diagnosis can be made.
- Access to treatment and the range of treatment on offer needs to be improved.
- Physical therapy needs to be approached with gentleness and encouragement.
- Patient support groups are important as they can offer friendship and support from those who truly understand and provide information about FMS.

IMPACT ON QUALITY OF LIFE

Day-to-Day Life

FMS has an impact on every area of life. The constant aching in the muscles, which feels like you have a flu or have been run over by a bus the day before, together with the ceaseless bone-weary fatigue can make each day a struggle. Everyday activities require more time and effort, from dragging yourself out of bed in the morning and having a shower to trying to summon the energy to do household chores or decide what to cook for dinner. Mobility can be seriously affected and the level of pain can ebb and flow from day-to-day meaning that you never quite know what state you will be in and therefore what you will be able to do, making planning activities quite a challenge. We often feel guilty at having to cancel preplanned events and get frustrated when we cannot look after ourselves and those we love.

Our brains do not seem to function properly anymore, with missing words and thoughts, which were very clear one moment, disappearing into the ether while we stand there blank-faced wondering what we were saying. It can feel like living in a fog, where what we want to express is always just out of reach. Then there is the sensitivity to noise, smell, temperature, and light, which can make social activities a bit of an ordeal. Noise at the cinema or theater can be overwhelming, and the cold can keep you inside, avoiding other people's houses or cafes/restaurants that are not heated to the necessary level for comfort. All this can cause isolation and the associated feelings of loneliness and depression.

One strange aspect of FMS is the way we almost always look well. This can be an advantage or disadvantage depending on the situation. It can be an advantage at a social event when you do not want to talk about your symptoms, but simply enjoy the evening without people asking you lots of questions about your health. But of course, it can also be a disadvantage when you need people to understand how you are feeling, and how this affects you. Symptoms can often be dismissed or not noticed by those around you as you look at blooming health. People assume you have now recovered as you look fine, and struggle to get to grips with the chronic nature of FMS. This can be extremely frustrating because there is always the need to explain what you feel you can and cannot do and why you are still feeling so exhausted all the time.

Relationships

Living with someone with FMS is also not an easy task, and pressures show in family relationships. A partner can either feel that he or she has been put upon to do many of the household chores and childcare, which were previously shared, or feel helpless to know what to do to make the situation better. The person with FMS can become withdrawn or very emotional as they struggle to come to terms with their situation and communication can break down leading to possible resentment or feelings of helplessness on both sides. Therapies such as cognitive behavioral therapy can prove helpful in learning to deal with all these emotions and how to communicate your feelings with other members of the family. Feelings of helplessness and guilt can be overwhelming, and it is like going through the process of grief. FMS does not go away and patients and their families need help to adapt and move forward.

The pain and fatigue of FMS can also interfere in a couple's sexual relationship. Fatigue can zap all motivation, making sex the last thing on your mind; and then the pain can make you recoil at your partner's touch. Muscle pain can also result in painful intercourse, making sex even less attractive. These problems need to be taken seriously and openly discussed so that solutions can be found to enable a couple to remain intimate in their relationship. On a general level, couples need to be encouraged to communicate honestly with each other; to perhaps find a time in the week to schedule a sexual encounter so that the person with FMS can save up their energy and take painkillers in advance; or to start with a warm bath, to help reduce pain and spark intimacy. However, if intercourse is very painful, then medical solutions need to be found, such as for women the regular use of dilators to help keep the vaginal muscles stretched or application of lidocaine gel in the vagina before intercourse.

Case Study

When Carol was first diagnosed, the impact on her and her family was huge, but taking part in the UK Expert Patient Programme helped her and her family to move forward.

I was fearful for my family and had all these things going round in my head like: Will my husband leave me? I am no good anymore, I'm useless. They were terrible feelings, almost like grief. My husband became really quiet and I don't think he really knew how to deal with me. There were days when he could see I wasn't feeling well but simply didn't know what to say or what to do, and that is where the frustration and anger came in. He went off and did his own thing, almost burying himself in his own life as a way of dealing with the situation, but unfortunately, it made me feel as though I was being left to deal with everything on my own, which made me feel lonely and frightened. I became angry and bitter, and very jealous of other people as I kept thinking they can do that and I can't.

The course enabled me to change the way I see things so that I was able to look at things more positively and as a couple, we were able to talk problems throughmore constructively. I was able to say things in different ways so that my husband could actually understand what help I needed. Before I simply wouldn't ask for help, but the course gave me the courage to turn around and simply say, look I can't do this will you help me. I feel I have my life back and I'm very grateful. If I have a bad day I always try to think that tomorrow will be better.

Work

The pain and fatigue can also have a serious impact on work. The energy required to do a full-time job is simply no longer there, and sitting at a desk or being on your feet all day can make the pain overwhelming. This can feel particularly scary, as many people's identity is in their work and having to scale back or even giving up can have a major psychological impact. Receiving encouragement and guidance on how jobs can be adapted can make all the difference. Some people have no choice but to continue working as they have a family to support, whereas others love their work and want to find a way to keep on working within the restrictions of the pain and fatigue. Understanding that help is out there, that work situations can be adapted or that there are other options that can make a considerable difference, and help patients cope with the stresses of fear of losing their job and financial insecurity or the guilt of not being able to perform as they used to in their work.

Case Study

Jenny found that moving from employment to self-employment allowed her more control to manage her symptoms during the working day.

I found the symptoms of fibromyalgia limited the number of hours I could work and the type of work I could do. It was a struggle to find a job that suited me, as I needed something I could physically do that was flexible enough to give me the time I needed to rest and manage my pain. Self-employment gave me that flexibility to organise my own time so that I could rest in the morning and work in the afternoon, or the reverse, depending on how I felt. Also, it meant I could work from home and not have to travel, which in itself uses up lots of energy. I also learnt about technology that could help me in my work and decided to use voice dictation software, which removed the pain caused by the repetitive activity of typing, and meant I could work for longer hours.

Difficulties Obtaining a Diagnosis

Obtaining a diagnosis is very important, and can lead to a huge sense of relief after years of struggling with unexplained pain and fatigue. Patient groups from around Europe have reported that the length of time it takes to get a diagnosis has improved over the past 10 years, but education within the medical profession is still urgently needed, as situations where patients' symptoms are ignored or encounters where doctors say that FMS does not exist still occur today. It can still take years to obtain a diagnosis, with patients being passed from doctor to doctor without any resolution and symptoms being dismissed when tests come back negative. This can lead to frustration and anger and a complete lack of faith in the medical profession, therefore this needs to be addressed.

A diagnosis is usually made by a general practitioner, a rheumatology consultant, a neurologist, or pain clinic, although some patients are still referred to a psychiatrist as the primary referral due to a lack of knowledge in the field of general medicine. When a patient is finally diagnosed, it is important to give them as much information as possible so that they can begin to understand what is going on in their bodies and to appreciate that FMS is a syndrome and has many associated symptoms in addition to pain and fatigue. Understanding that irritable bowel syndrome, irritable bladder, and numbness and tingling, for example, are all associated with FMS can reduce anxiety and prevent further medical investigations.

A lack of diagnosis and education among medical professionals can also make it very difficult for patients to access help through social services and welfare agencies.

Some doctors who work as assessors in the welfare system still do not recognize FMS as a disability, leading to patients being rejected for social services help and financial benefits. Education of the medical profession is still seen as a major priority from the patient's point of view.

Treatment Aspects

Access to treatment can vary depending on where you live. In many European countries, it is generally straightforward to access pharmacologic medication, such as antidepressants, anticonvulsants, muscle relaxants, and some pain medications, because doctors are now more willing to prescribe them and they are covered by general health insurance; but access to physical therapy and pain clinics is much harder to gain. FMS is best treated using a multidisciplinary approach, but waiting lists for pain clinics can be up to a year, and even then they are not always suitable for people with FMS or are not covered by health insurance. In Serbia, for example, health insurance only covers medication, whereas other treatments need to be paid for; and in Sweden, there are only a few pain clinics with specialist knowledge about FMS, and this is the same in the United Kingdom.

Increasing access to physiotherapy and pain clinics with specialist knowledge of FMS would allow patients to become better educated about FMS and how to manage it. Many patients do not want to take lots of long-term medication due to the side effects and often minimal efficacy. They want to play an active role in their own treatment and need the medical profession to listen to them and to work with them to achieve the best possible outcome. Learning to pace through the day, how to gradually build up an exercise program, and how to reduce stress caused by constant pain and fatigue can make a massive difference to patient quality-of-life. These management programs work best when they are individualized, as different patients can respond differently to therapies and they need to work out what works best for them.

Although patients are obviously keen to be treated, receiving treatment, especially physical therapy, can be frightening. The thought of exercising when you are so tired and in lots of pain can just feel insurmountable, and medical professionals need to be aware of this and work gently with patients to encourage them to build up an exercise routine gradually over time. Exercising can feel like walking a tightrope: If you do not do enough you feel stiff and sore, but if you do too much your body can react resulting in a flare-up of pain throughout your whole body or intense myofascial pain in one area. Flare-ups as a result of exercise occur as a patient works with their physical therapist to work out a suitable exercise program, and patients need to understand that their pain levels probably increase at first, and need encouragement and reassurance to keep going. Exercise boundaries need to be pushed, but this must be done gently to minimize flares and discouragement. Finding a form of exercise that the patient enjoys, and actually wants to do, can be half the battle.

This lack of access to treatment can lead patients to spend a lot of money on other alternative, holistic therapies in their search for relief from pain and improvement in their quality-of-life. Some of these therapies can be beneficial, although there is often limited evidence to support their use, but sometimes patients can fall prey to unscrupulous therapists with very little knowledge about what they are treating, and can cause more harm than good.

Mobility aids can be severely frowned on by the medical profession when it comes to managing FMS, but some patients gain real benefit from using these aids to allow them to pace themselves through their day. For example, using a wheelchair to go round a shopping mall for a couple of hours allows a patient to save energy for more interesting and beneficial activities like going for a walk outside in the woods or playing with their children in the park. Deciding what to spend your energy on can be challenging when you have many demands on your time and energy, so a mobility aid, whether it is a wheelchair, a walking stick, wrist straps, and so on, can help save energy for more enjoyable activities allowing a patient to do more in a day, feel more in control, and greatly increase their quality-of-life. It is dependence on mobility aids that needs to be avoided, in particular, psychological dependence, but when used correctly, they can be of great benefit.

Case Study

When Rachel was first told that exercise would be an important part of her treatment program she thought her doctor was joking.

I could hardly move without pain, why on earth would I want to invoke even more pain by exercising? The first physiotherapist I encountered met with stonewall resistance and it took a lot of persuasion and quite a few arguments to convince me that my overall health would simply decline if I refused to cooperate. Remoulding my concept of the word exercise proved to be as vital as taking my first tentative step toward my individually tailored regime. When I understood that, at first, walking around the garden several times a day would be classified as a praiseworthy achievement. I began to relax a little and realize that these kinds of goals might just be within my reach. Over time my ability to exercise and the enjoyment I get out of it has gradually increased, although it has not been a simple upward curve. There have been many frustrating steps backward and diversions down blind alleys as I have learned to listen to my body, be more self-aware, and find a programme that works for me. Exercising when you have fibromyalgia is no easy business, but I know from experience that gentle persistence does pay off to give your body more flexibility, strength, and stamina to enable you to achieve your goals in everyday life.

SUPPORT GROUPS

Support groups can be a lifeline for patients. Finally finding someone else who totally understands what you are trying to live with can make such a difference, and as with other illnesses, you learn that you are not alone. They understand without the need for long explanations, and the act of sharing what you are going through can be a release in itself. There is no judgment and no need to justify yourself, people who are just willing to listen and who actually understand. Support groups are also a place where you can access information about FMS, find out what treatments are available in your area, and what other people find helpful in managing their symptoms. Many also offer a social life, organizing fun events and activities such as afternoons out, fundraising events, speakers, coffee mornings, and so on, which can reduce isolation and loneliness, and even lead to lifelong friendships.

Some patients, however, do not want to go to support groups. They do not want to talk about FMS and can feel ashamed of being ill and not being able to do the things they used to do. They do not want help from other patients and prefer to gain information from the Internet themselves and their own doctors. Also, patients who have very supportive family and friends can feel they have no need of additional support. Each patient is different and needs to do what is best for them.

Attending a support group can be difficult for people who live in rural areas. However, many countries have a national association that can offer information in the form of leaflets and booklets to explain about FMS and what help is available. The majority also offer a telephone helpline, which is available for people to phone and talk to another person with FMS, who will listen and share tips and recommendations for self-management if appropriate. Many people just want to be listened to, and this can be a lifeline for people living in remote areas. Some associations, such as in the United Kingdom, also offer a helpline for advice about welfare payments, and can help guide people through the many forms they need to complete or suggest where they can get further impartial advice.

It is important though that medical professionals who diagnose FMS are aware of support groups in their local area and pass on this information to the patients they meet. The opportunity to find support from other people with FMS should always be available, especially as doctors themselves often lack the time to give sufficient information about FMS and help the patient to come to terms with a chronic condition. Medical professionals should also consider offering their support to patient groups, perhaps by offering to give a talk or to be involved in awareness events.

INCLUDING PATIENTS IN RESEARCH DESIGN

Patients feel it is very important to include people who have the condition that is being researched in the design of clinical trials and treatment guidelines right from the offset. Patients who live with FMS day in and day out can offer insights into research that can be overlooked by medical professionals. For example, when deciding which domains to measure in a trial, you need to know which symptoms are most important to the patient you are trying to help. In rheumatoid arthritis research, it was a patient who suggested measuring the domain of fatigue, which was greeted by some surprise by the researchers, but total agreement by all the patients present. This was a symptom that was important to them in their day-to-day lives.

The same is true with treatment guidelines. Patients have a unique perspective to offer as they are the ones who are receiving the treatment. They can offer insights into why some therapies simply do not work in real clinical practice, despite positive clinical trial evidence; explain what side effects people are happy to put up with if it means some release from pain; and what other therapies need to be explored in clinical trials from positive anecdotal evidence. Patients are more than willing to be included and should be regarded as a valuable resource, not just an add-on to gain additional funding.

More information about including patient representatives in scientific research can be found at the European League Against Rheumatism (EULAR) website: http://www.eular.org/pare_patient_research_partners.cfm.

POLITICAL ACTIVITIES

Patient groups work hard to educate both politicians and medical professionals about the impact FMS has on people's lives and on those with whom they live. They want to raise awareness to create a better understanding of FMS within health services and the social security system to improve the services they offer. FMS can still be disregarded by the welfare system and penalized by uneducated welfare assessors, which can lead to financial insecurity, frustration, and anger. Education and awareness are the most important factors to many people with FMS when they are asked what needs to be done in their country.

Some patient groups have an All Party Parliamentary Group to which they can invite politicians and raise specific issues, and these need backing by prominent doctors in the field of FMS. This is where change can happen and patient groups need support in achieving this.

SECTION 4

Diagnosis

CHAPTER 14

Screening Tests and Clinical Diagnosis of Fibromyalgia Syndrome

Serge Perrot

Summary Points

- The American College of Rheumatology (ACR) classification criteria for fibromyalgia syndrome (FMS) are difficult to apply routinely and screening tools for FMS can be useful in daily practice for all physicians.
- Screening tools for FMS, such as Fibromyalgia Rapid Screening Tool (FiRST) and FibroDetect show that FMS can discriminate FMS from other chronic pain conditions, with very high sensitivity and specificity.
- The diagnosis is based on the history of a typical cluster of symptoms (chronic widespread pain [CWP], nonrestorative sleep, physical and/or mental fatigue) that cannot be sufficiently explained by another medical condition.

FMS is a chronic pain syndrome without any diagnostic gold standard, differently characterized according to criteria and authors.[13] In 1990, the ACR classification criteria for FMS[22] integrated spontaneous diffuse pain and pressure-induced pain as the two main criteria. This is close to previous Smythe and Moldofsky[15] criteria that included tender point examination with sleep and fatigue symptoms. Another type of criteria has been developed, including pain and several other symptoms, according to the concept of central sensitization[26,4]: the Yunus criteria[25] but also the ACR 2010,[19] 2011,[20] and 2016[21] ACR criteria include poor sleep, fatigue, and symptoms of other functional disorders such as chronic headache, irritable bowel syndrome, or cystalgia.

All these criteria are difficult to apply in daily practice because they may require either a specific examination of tender points[22,15] that cannot be carried out without some training[6] or because the number of symptoms to assess requires a complex calculation of Symptom Severity Scale.[19,20,21] The FMS symptom/survey questionnaire (FSQ) capturing the ACR 2011 criteria can be completed by the patient within 5 minutes and evaluated by the doctor within 30 seconds.[8] Some authors have suggested to abandon the use of ACR1990 criteria in the clinic.[24] Thus, in clinical practice, especially in primary care practice, criteria are not frequently used and FMS is often diagnosed late, after multiple investigations and consultations. Although rheumatologists, pain specialists, and neurologists play an important role in diagnosing FMS, primary care providers (PCPs) are often the first physicians FMS patients are visiting. This has led to the development of simple and easy-to-fill questionnaires as screening tests for FMS in clinical practice.

THE CORE SET OF FIBROMYALGIA SYNDROME DIAGNOSIS AND ASSESSMENT: OMERACT

A group of clinician/researchers interested in FMS formed a working group in 2003 that proceeded to conduct, through 2008, a series of OMERACT workshops and a module to define a core set of domains for assessment in FMS. It was proposed and ratified at OMERACT 9[9] that the core domains that should be assessed routinely in FMS included pain, tenderness, fatigue, sleep disturbance, patient global response, and multidimensional function. In addition, cognitive dysfunction and depression were considered important, but instruments to appropriately assess these in FMS still required further development and validation for use in FMS.

SCREENING TESTS FOR EPIDEMIOLOGIC STUDIES OF FIBROMYALGIA SYNDROME: THE LONDON FIBROMYALGIA EPIDEMIOLOGY STUDY SCREENING QUESTIONNAIRE

A questionnaire has been specifically developed for epidemiologic studies of FMS: the London Fibromyalgia Epidemiology Study Screening Questionnaire (LFESSQ).[17] This questionnaire includes four pain and two fatigue items. A positive screen was defined in two ways: (a) positive responses to all four items on pain and (b) positive responses to all pain and fatigue items. Studies based on the LFESSQ have been developed in many countries and generated estimates of the prevalence of FMS in the general population as high as 2% in Northern America[16] and in Europe.[2] The FSQ has also been used in epidemiology studies in Japan[10] and Germany.[18]

TESTS FOR RAPID FIBROMYALGIA SYNDROME SCREENING

Multidimensional Health Assessment Questionnaire for Use in Rheumatology Setting

Patients with FMS report high levels of pain and fatigue, and multiple symptoms. These phenomena may be recorded quantitatively on a self-report multidimensional health assessment questionnaire (MDHAQ).[14] Responses to MDHAQ are likely to differ in people with FMS or chronic pain conditions compared with people with an inflammatory rheumatic disease, such as rheumatoid arthritis. Data from the MDHAQ provide clues to the presence of FMS/chronic pain conditions, including patients with inflammatory diseases who also have concomitant FMS/chronic pain conditions.

The Fibromyalgia Syndrome Rapid Screening Tool

This questionnaire was developed for the detection of FMS in patients with diffuse chronic pain (Table. 14.1).[11] The provisional questionnaire was tested in a prospective multicenter study of 162 patients with chronic pain due to FMS (according to 1990 ACR criteria; $n = 92$) compared with a group of patients with chronic diffuse pain due to other rheumatic conditions, including rheumatoid arthritis ($n = 32$), ankylosing spondylitis ($n = 25$), and osteoarthritis ($n = 13$). A cutoff score of 5 (corresponding to the number of positive items) gave the highest rate of correct identification of patients (87.9%), with a sensitivity of 90.5% and a specificity of 85.7%. It has been translated and validated in several languages.[3,27]

The FibroDetect Questionnaire

The FibroDetect questionnaire[1] was developed based on the information provided by literature review, focus groups conducted with clinicians, and face-to-face interviews with FMS patients. A scoring method was created using an iterative process based on statistical and clinical considerations with ACR 1990 FMS$^+$ patients

TABLE 14.1 The Fibromyalgia Rapid Screening Tool (FiRST)[a]

	Yes	No
I have pain all over my body.		
My pain is accompanied by a continuous and very unpleasant general fatigue.		
My pain feels like burns, electric shocks, or cramps.		
My pain is accompanied by other unusual sensations throughout my body, such as pins and needles, tingling, or numbness.		
My pain is accompanied by other health problems such as digestive problems, urinary problems, headaches, or restless legs.		
My pain has a significant impact on my life, particularly on my sleep and my ability to concentrate, making me feel slower generally.		

You have been suffering from joint, muscle, or tendon pain *for the past 3 months at least*. Please answer this questionnaire in order to help your doctor evaluate your pain and symptoms more effectively.

Please fill in this questionnaire by answering either yes or no (only one answer: YES *or* NO) to each of the following statements. Put a cross in the box that corresponds to your answer.

and ACR1990 FMS^- patients (n = 276), and validated with FMS and non-FMS patients (n = 312). Six questions were retained in the final scoring of FibroDetect, with good psychometric qualities. It is available in three languages, but final validation is still needed.

SCREENING TOOLS FOR CONCOMITANT FIBROMYALGIA SYNDROME

Some screening tools have already been used in large epidemiologic studies, to screen for concomitant FMS, especially in rheumatology setting: in rheumatoid arthritis, spondyloarthritis[5] but also systemic sclerosis.[12] In a study of 607 patients with rheumatic diseases (279 rheumatoid arthritis, 271 spondyloarthritis, and 57 connective tissue disease), FiRST questionnaire detected 143 concomitant FMS (24.4%). When assessed against ACR 1990 criteria, FiRST had a sensitivity of 74.5%, a specificity of 80.4%, a positive predictive value of 26.6%, and a negative predictive value (NPV) of 97.1%. When assessed against the rheumatologist's opinion, FiRST had a sensitivity of 75.8%, a specificity of 85.1%, a positive predictive value of 48.3%, and an NPV of 95%.

THE CLINICAL DIAGNOSIS OF FIBROMYALGIA SYNDROME

Screening tools for FMS show that FMS presents with specific clinical characteristics different from those of other painful rheumatologic conditions and that it is possible to discriminate FMS from these chronic pain conditions, with very high sensitivity and specificity, using a questionnaire including only a few items. It is also possible to screen for comorbid or concomitant FMS, not an infrequent condition. These easy-to-use screening tools facilitate the identification of patients with FMS, both in daily clinical practice and in the research setting. These tools can be completed by severity assessment questionnaires like the polysymptomatic distress categories.[23]

By comprehensively assessing the multiple physical and psychological domains and symptoms associated with FMS, the screening tools allow a reduction in the delay before diagnosis and appropriate referral to specialists, ensuring access to the best available care. Skepticism among health professionals regarding the existence of FMS is another factor to be added to the whole FMS detection challenge. One advantage of a standardized detection of FMS as it is proposed by the FibroDetect or FiRST screening tools is to give legitimacy to the patient's feedback, which is essential in this contentious pathologic condition.

Recent evidence- and consensus-based guidelines from Canada, Germany, Israel, and the European League Against Rheumatism aim to support physicians in achieving a comprehensive diagnostic workup of patients with CWP and to assist patients and physicians in shared decision-making on treatment options.[7] Every patient with CWP requires, at the first medical evaluation, a complete history, medical examination, and some laboratory tests (complete blood count, measurement of C-reactive protein, serum calcium, creatine phosphokinase, thyroid-stimulating hormone, and 25-hydroxyvitamin D levels) to screen for metabolic or inflammatory causes of CWP. Any additional laboratory or radiographic testing should depend on red flags suggesting some other medical condition. The diagnosis is based on the history of a typical cluster of symptoms (CWP, nonrestorative sleep, physical and/or mental fatigue) that cannot be sufficiently explained by another medical condition.[7] Optimal management should begin with education of patients regarding the current knowledge of FMS (including written materials).

REFERENCES

1. Baron R, Perrot S, Guillemin I, et al. Improving the primary care physicians' decision making for fibromyalgia in clinical practice: development and validation of the Fibromyalgia Detection (FibroDetect®) screening tool. *Health Qual Life Outcomes.* 2014;**12**:128.
2. Branco JC, Bannwarth B, Failde I, et al. Prevalence of fibromyalgia: a survey in five European countries. *Semin Arthritis Rheum.* 2010;**39**(6):448–453.
3. Collado A, Torres X, Messina OD, et al. The discriminatory ability of the Fibromyalgia Rapid Screening Tool (FiRST): an international study in Spain and four Latin American countries. *Pain Med.* 2016;**17**(5):931–939.
4. Desmeules JA, Cedraschi C, Rapiti E, et al. Neurophysiologic evidence for a central sensitization in patients with fibromyalgia. *Arthritis Rheum.* 2003;**48**(5):1420–1429.
5. Fan A, Tournadre A, Pereira B, et al. Performance of Fibromyalgia Rapid Screening Tool (FiRST) to detect fibromyalgia syndrome in rheumatic diseases. *Rheumatology.* 2016;**55**(10):1746–1750.
6. Harth M, Nielson WR. The fibromyalgia tender points: use them or lose them? A brief review of the controversy. *J Rheumatol.* 2007;**34**(5):914–922.
7. Häuser W, Ablin J, Perrot S, Fitzcharles MA. Management of fibromyalgia: practical guides from recent evidence-based guidelines. *Pol Arch Intern Med.* 2017;**127**(1):47–56.
8. Häuser W, Jung E, Erbslöh-Möller B, et al. Validation of the Fibromyalgia Survey Questionnaire within a cross-sectional survey. *PLoS ONE.* 2012;**7**(5):e37504.
9. Mease P, Arnold LM, Choy EH, et al.; OMERACT Fibromyalgia Working Group. Fibromyalgia syndrome module at OMERACT 9: domain construct. *J Rheumatol.* 2009;**36**(10):2318–2329.
10. Nakamura I, Nishioka K, Usui C, et al. An epidemiologic internet survey of fibromyalgia and chronic pain in Japan. *Arthritis Care Res.* 2014;**66**(7):1093–1101.
11. Perrot S, Bouhassira D, Fermanian J; Cercle d'Etude de la Douleur en Rhumatologie. Development and validation of the Fibromyalgia Rapid Screening Tool (FiRST). *Pain.* 2010;**150**(2):250–256.
12. Perrot S, Peixoto M, Dieudé P, et al. Patient phenotypes in fibromyalgia comorbid with systemic sclerosis or rheumatoid arthritis: influence of diagnostic and screening tests. Screening with the FiRST questionnaire, diagnosis with the ACR 1990 and revised ACR 2010 criteria. *Clin Exp Rheumatol.* 2017;**35**Suppl 105(3):35–42.
13. Perrot S. Fibromyalgia syndrome: a relevant recent construction of an ancient condition? *Curr Opin Support Palliat Care.* 2008;**2**(2):122–127.
14. Pincus T, Hassett AL, Callahan LF. Clues on the MDHAQ to identify patients with fibromyalgia and similar chronic pain conditions. *Rheum Dis Clin North Am.* 2009;**35**(4):865–869, xii.
15. Smythe HA, Moldofsky H. Two contributions to understanding of the "fibrositis" syndrome. *Bull Rheum Dis.* 1977;**28**(1):928–931.

16. White KP, Harth M. Classification, epidemiology, and natural history of fibromyalgia. *Curr Pain Headache Rep*. 2001;**5**(4):320–329.
17. White KP, Speechley M, Harth M, et al. The London Fibromyalgia Epidemiology Study: the prevalence of fibromyalgia syndrome in London, Ontario. *J Rheumatol*. 1999;**26**(7):1570–1576.
18. Wolfe F, Brähler E, Hinz A, et al. Fibromyalgia prevalence, somatic symptom reporting, and the dimensionality of polysymptomatic distress: results from a survey of the general population. *Arthritis Care Res*. 2013;**65**(5):777–785.
19. Wolfe F, Clauw DJ, Fitzcharles MA, et al. The American College of Rheumatology preliminary diagnostic criteria for fibromyalgia and measurement of symptom severity. *Arthritis Care Res*. 2010;**62**(5):600–610.
20. Wolfe F, Clauw DJ, Fitzcharles MA, et al. Fibromyalgia criteria and severity scales for clinical and epidemiological studies: a modification of the ACR Preliminary Diagnostic Criteria for Fibromyalgia. *J Rheumatol*. 2011;**38**(6):1113–1122.
21. Wolfe F, Clauw DJ, Fitzcharles MA, et al. 2016 Revisions to the 2010/2011 fibromyalgia diagnostic criteria. *Semin Arthritis Rheum*. 2016;**46**(3):319–329.
22. Wolfe F, Smythe HA, Yunus MB, et al. The American College of Rheumatology 1990 criteria for the classification of fibromyalgia. Report of the Multicenter Criteria Committee. *Arthritis Rheum*. 1990;**33**(2):160–172.
23. Wolfe F, Walitt BT, Rasker JJ, Katz RS, Häuser W. The use of polysymptomatic distress categories in the evaluation of fibromyalgia (FM) and FM severity. *J Rheumatol*. 2015;**42**(8):1494–1501.
24. Wolfe F. Stop using the American College of Rheumatology criteria in the clinic. *J Rheumatol*. 2003;**30**(8):1671–1672.
25. Yunus MB, Masi AT, Aldag JC. Preliminary criteria for primary fibromyalgia syndrome (PFS): multivariate analysis of a consecutive series of PFS, other pain patients, and normal subjects. *Clin Exp Rheumatol*. 1989;**7**(1):63–69.
26. Yunus MB. Fibromyalgia and overlapping disorders: the unifying concept of central sensitivity syndromes. *Semin Arthritis Rheum*. 2007;**36**(6):339–356.
27. Zis P, Brozou V, Stavropoulou E, et al. Validation of the Greek version of the fibromyalgia rapid screening tool. *Pain Pract*. 2017;**17**(7):925–929.

CHAPTER 15

Differential Diagnosis: Diseases Mimicking Fibromyalgia Syndrome

Mary-Ann Fitzcharles

Summary Points

- Although diffuse widespread pain suggests a diagnosis of fibromyalgia syndrome FMS, other conditions may present similarly, requiring that all patients undergo a complete medical history and physical examination.
- The early stages of an inflammatory rheumatic disease may masquerade as FMS prior to the emergence of objective physical or laboratory findings.
- The early stages of various neurologic diseases such as multiple sclerosis (MS), Parkinson's disease (PD), spinal stenosis, and myopathies may present with widespread pain, but astute neurologic evaluation will focus toward a neurologic disease.
- The differential diagnosis should also include various other conditions such as endocrine/metabolic disorders, gastrointestinal diseases, infectious diseases, mental health disorders, and drug-induced pain.

Formulating a differential diagnosis for any health complaint is the hallmark of good clinical practice. Although diagnosis of FMS is the most likely reason for a complaint of chronic widespread pain (CWP), especially in a middle-aged woman, widespread body pain may occur in several clinical settings. First, the patient may truly be presenting with FMS; second, the pain may be a symptom of some other illness; and finally, the patient may previously have suffered from FMS, but may now be presenting with onset of another illness that could erroneously be attributed to FMS.

The first step to establishing any clinical diagnosis is to obtain a comprehensive history. In patients presenting with diffuse body pain, the symptoms commonly associated with FMS should be explored, as well as a full systemic questioning to determine whether there are symptoms present related to any other organ system. The previous medical history, family and psychosocial history, as well as all current medications and substance use are recorded. Thereafter, a physical examination must be done, with particular attention to the musculoskeletal and neurologic examination. Clues gained from the history allow focussing the examination to exclude these other masquerading conditions.

Another scenario that warrants attention is the comorbid association of FMS in the setting of some other disease. It is postulated that the underlying pain condition induces a pain sensitization that persists even when the underlying condition is under control. Diagnostic confusion may result when the pain condition is attributed to the primary illness, rather than recognition of FMS. The comorbid association of FMS has been most commonly recognized in the setting of inflammatory rheumatic diseases, with reports of FMS in 20% to 30% of patients with rheumatoid arthritis (RA), systemic lupus erythematosus, or inflammatory spondyloarthritis (SpA).[28] The importance of recognizing an associated FMS is that the global health status is adversely impacted, treatments may be inappropriately directed to the primary disease rather than to FMS, and health-related quality of life is affected and costs of the underlying disease are increased.[22] Although limited study of increased prevalence of FMS has been reported for some neurologic diseases such as MS, post-polio syndrome, and chronic pain (not specifically FMS) for PD, no study has reported on the impact of pain symptoms on the underlying neurologic disease. Gastrointestinal diseases, especially celiac disease, non-celiac gluten enteropathy, and irritable bowel syndrome have overlap with FMS, and in some instances have been misdiagnosed as FMS, especially in the early stages.

Failure to recognize some illness other than FMS as a cause for body pain will compromise clinical care as these other conditions require a treatment strategy different from that of FMS. Emphasizing the need to always consider a differential diagnosis, all current guidelines for FMS stress the importance of a comprehensive evaluation to identify any clinical features that could point to an alternate diagnosis.[7,1,6,16]

Diagnoses that can be confused with FMS may be broadly grouped into the following categories: rheumatic diseases, neurologic conditions, other medical conditions (endocrinology, gastroenterology, infectious diseases, oncology), mental health disorders, and medication-induced pain conditions.[11] Many of these conditions may in fact strictly fulfill criteria for FMS at the time of presentation, but with time, the underlying illness emerges. This chapter covers the various conditions that can present with generalized pain and cause confusion with FMS and highlight specific features that help to distinguish these conditions from FMS.

RHEUMATIC DISEASES

Inflammatory rheumatic diseases refer to a broad group of diseases that are characterized by systemic features of ill health, often painful and inflamed joints, extra-articular complaints that may involve other organ systems, and with diagnosis supported by abnormality of immunologic parameters as well as various specific investigations such as ultrasound or imaging studies. The common rheumatic conditions are inflammatory polyarthritis of which RA is the most common, but also include other diseases such as psoriatic arthritis (PsA), SpA among others.[19]

Pain is a frequent complaint for almost all rheumatic diseases, but symptoms focused toward the joints rather than diffuse in nature are more common. It can also be anticipated that identifiable physical or laboratory abnormalities develop over time, but a single abnormal laboratory test is generally not sufficient evidence to diagnose an inflammatory rheumatic disease. Although joint swelling is the hallmark of many inflammatory rheumatic diseases, some may have less prominent joint symptoms and rather present with a diffuse pain syndrome, but often with accompanying systemic symptoms or additional clues on the history.

Inflammatory Polyarthritis

Peripheral inflammatory arthritis (IA) is a symptom of various rheumatic conditions including RA, PsA, systemic lupus erythematosus, and others. Recent study has reported that prior to definite changes of joint swelling in RA, a preclinical RA stage can be recognized with symptoms of fatigue, stiffness, and even muscle weakness in addition to pain.[17] The nonspecific presenting symptoms, however, evolve into a definite expression of joint disease over time, but could take several months.

Features that should alert the clinician to an IA include a family member with IA, prolonged morning stiffness, more severe constitutional symptoms such as weight loss, a progressive increase in symptom severity, and pain symptoms focused on the joints. It is also not uncommon for a patient to be able to identify a time of onset of symptoms, within a period of a few weeks or months. As many of these illnesses have involvement of other organ systems, questions focused toward these organ systems should be included. For example, there may be a current or previous skin rash of psoriasis in patient or family to suggest an underlying PsA; questions about sun-sensitive skin rash, Raynaud's phenomenon, hair thinning, or alopecia could direct to a diagnosis of systemic lupus erythematosus; dry mucosal surfaces and salivary gland swelling could suggest Sjogren's syndrome; and prominent bowel symptoms, especially diarrhea could point to an underlying inflammatory bowel disease.

Examination findings that may point toward a diagnosis of IA include tenderness more localized to the joints, especially the joints of hands and feet, skin rashes such as psoriasis, malar rash, livedo reticularis, or vasculitis changes especially at the nail fold regions, adenopathy or salivary gland enlargement for Sjogren's syndrome, or any abnormality on examination of other organ systems. Specific blood testing includes measurement of inflammatory markers such as erythrocyte sedimentation rate (ESR), C-reactive protein (CRP), rheumatoid factor, anti-cyclic citrullinated peptide (anti-CCP) antibodies, and other immunologic parameters such as antinuclear antibody as indicated. When joint swelling is less clinically obvious, ultrasound of joints can show subclinical synovitis and inflammation.

Polymyalgia Rheumatica

In any patient older than 50years presenting with a new onset of body pain, polymyalgia rheumatica (PMR) should always be in the differential diagnosis. PMR is common with an incidence rate of about 50 cases per 100,000 persons aged 50 years and older and is twice as common in women compared to men.[5] Patients may describe a fairly defined time of onset, even going from excellent health to "suddenly becoming very old" over a few weeks. The classical presentation is of shoulder and hip girdle pain, with prominent stiffness, and important night pain and disturbed sleep. There may be associated symptoms of fatigue, weight loss, and poor appetite. The physical examination usually shows symmetrical limitation of range of motion of shoulders, or mild peripheral synovitis. The gait may be slow and patients move slowly and painfully when changing position, that is, standing up or lying down. Blood testing may reveal elevated inflammatory markers, ESR or CRP, although these may be normal in a small proportion of patients. Imaging techniques such as ultrasound examination of the subacromial bursa or the temporal artery or MRI are promising additional studies to demonstrate areas of inflammation. When PMR is suspected, a therapeutic trial of corticosteroids should be given, with expected definitive improvement in symptoms within a few days.

Inflammatory Spondyloarthritis

Ankylosing spondylitis was previously remembered as a disease of men, diagnosed by radiographic findings of sacroiliitis and resulting in a fused or bamboo spine. In the past few years, new classification criteria for SpA have been developed by the Assessment of SpondyloArthritis International Society (ASAS), which allow for diagnosis at a much earlier stage of disease and incorporates peripheral disease parameters such as enthesitis, tenderness at ligamentous insertions into bone at sites such as epicondyles of elbows, iliac crests, and others.[24] SpA is now classified as peripheral and axial disease, with the latter subdivided into non-radiographic axial SpA (nr-axSpa) and radiographic ax-SpA.[24] Allowing for earlier diagnosis of SpA, there are now challenges in differentiating early SpA from FMS.

Inflammatory spinal pain is the hallmark of axial SpA and is defined as spinal pain occurring in a person younger than 45 years, pain in the second half of the night and worse in the early morning, somewhat relieved by exercise, and stiffness in the mornings for longer than an hour. The axial pain of SpA may change location over time giving the impression of a more generalized body pain similar to FMS. For example, pain may move from low back and buttock regions, to cervical, mid-thoracic or anterior chest wall regions. A further challenge to the diagnosis of SpA is that the peripheral forms can be diagnosed when there is predominant enthesitis in some other features such as psoriasis, inflammatory bowel disease, or a family history of SpA. Similar to the variability in axial pain, enthesitis, especially when occurring at multiple sites, can be misinterpreted as diffuse pain. An additional clinical confounder is that SpA patients may experience fatigue, sleep disturbance, and depression, similar to FMS. Further investigation with appropriate imaging, including MRI of the spine and sacroiliac joints, as well as measurement of the human leucocyte antigen-B27 and CRP will serve to support a diagnosis of SpA.

There may be considerable overlap between SpA and FMS. One-third of patients with inflammatory back pain fulfilled criteria for FMS on the basis of tender point examination, demonstrating overlap with enthesopathic sites of tenderness.[21] Alternately, 10% of FMS patients met ASAS criteria for axial SpA, raising the question of either underdiagnosed SpA or SpA with associated FMS.[2]

Noninflammatory Musculoskeletal Conditions

Myofascial pain syndrome (MPS) and hypermobility syndrome (HS) are two conditions that should be considered in the differential diagnosis of CWP. Although MPS is more commonly identified as a regional muscular pain disorder, symptoms may occur at different locations, especially spinal regions, giving the impression of a more generalized pain syndrome. MPS is identified by the latent and active trigger points, which are discrete, focal, hyperirritable areas, usually within a taut band of skeletal muscle or in the muscles fascia. Compared to FMS, the pain in MPS is more pronounced and localized, and especially focused on the neck, shoulder, and low back regions, and associated with "trigger points." The concept of "trigger points," however, remains contentious especially as trigger points are inconsistently assessed and the inter-rater reliability of assessment is of low quality.[20] MPS is common, but similar to FMS is a clinical diagnosis without laboratory or radiographic abnormalities. This overlap has recently been demonstrated by Ge et al. who showed that the tender point sites in FMS patients are actually trigger points and therefore may function as peripheral pain generators.[8]

Joint hyperlaxity is a common variation of normal with various studies reporting prevalence rates between 2% and 50%, and most common in younger females of Asian, Middle Eastern, and African descent.[23] When generalized joint laxity is associated with chronic body pain, as for about 3% of individuals, the term HS is applied. Joint laxity is also a feature of various connective tissue disorders including Marfan's syndrome and Ehlers–Danlos syndrome (EDS), a heritable disorder of connective tissue characterized by skin extensibility and tissue fragility. HS may be diagnosed when generalized joint hypermobility is accompanied by pain in ≥4 joints over a period ≥3 months and in the absence of other conditions that cause chronic pain.[23] There is, however, still debate regarding whether hypermobility and EDS are distinct conditions with frequent misdiagnosis of joint hypermobility as a type of EDS.[3] Similar to FMS, there is an emerging recognition of a high prevalence of psychological distress, psychosocial factors, and psychiatric disorders in persons with benign joint hypermobility and EDS. Therefore, at this time, identification of hypermobility may be a plausible explanation for the pain, but with possible overlap with FMS.

NON-RHEUMATIC MEDICAL CONDITIONS

Endocrine and Metabolic Disorders

Endocrine and metabolic conditions that can mimic FMS include hypothyroidism, hyperparathyroidism, acromegaly, and vitamin D deficiency. All these conditions may present with ill-defined symptoms of body pain and fatigue, but with other clues unique to each condition that can lead to appropriate testing. Patients with hypothyroidism may have a family history of thyroid disease and have weight gain, whereas hyperparathyroidism may be associated with constipation. There is a frequent association of autoimmune thyroid (Hashimoto) disease with and without hypothyroidism and FMS. Excessive growth hormone as a cause of acromegaly, although a rare condition, will be associated with increased size of hands and feet, coarsening of facial features as well as body pain and stiffness. For each of these conditions, specific laboratory testing is available.

Severe vitamin D deficiency is a cause of generalized bone pain due to osteomalacia.[27] Although mostly related to poor sun exposure, vitamin D deficiency may also result from disturbances in phosphate metabolism. Clues to prompt consideration of this diagnosis include muscle weakness recognized as a waddling gait in a person who has had limited sun exposure. This is particularly true for persons wearing clothing that covers most of the body and living in the northern hemisphere.

Gastrointestinal Diseases

Although abdominal pain, bloating, and diarrhea are common symptoms of celiac disease, vague symptoms of ill health, fatigue, and body pain may be misdiagnosed as FMS. A primary diagnosis of FMS was initially given to 9% of celiac patients who responded to an online patient support group survey and 14.9% of celiac patients attending a celiac clinic reported CWP.[30,26] Inflammatory bowel disease, either Crohn's disease or ulcerative colitis, may be associated with SpA, which can mimic FMS. This scenario may occur in the early stage of presentation prior to diagnosis of either the bowel or the spinal disease.

Infectious Diseases

Some infectious disease may have CWP as a component of the symptomatology as for hepatitis C and HIV. Other features of these illnesses with both systemic and organ-specific symptoms prompt further laboratory screening and lead to a definitive diagnosis. Furthermore, a chronic pain syndrome indistinguishable from FMS may follow some viral infections, although a search for a specific infectious etiology is not routinely required. The existence of chronic Lyme disease following infection with Borrelia burgdorferi remains contentious. This poorly defined diagnosis is sometimes given to patients with prolonged, unexplained symptoms, including body pain, but current data do not support the concept that chronic, treatment-refractory infection is responsible for the many subjective symptoms attributed to chronic infection.[14] In a longitudinal study of 100 patients with culture-confirmed Lyme disease, FMS was observed to develop in a single patient, and 19 years after the diagnosis of Lyme disease.[29] Therefore, there is no consistent evidence that Lyme disease specifically is a trigger for FMS. In the setting of fatigue, musculoskeletal pain, and cognitive complaints that persist for 6 months or longer after completion of antibiotic therapy, without persisting infection, the diagnosis of secondary FMS should be considered.

Malignancy

Prior to a diagnosis of a malignancy such as multiple myeloma, metastatic cancer, or leukemia/lymphoma, there may be symptoms of ill health and widespread body pain. Identification of other constitutional symptoms such as fever, weight loss, or night sweats should prompt further investigation.

NEUROLOGIC CONDITIONS

Neurologic Diseases

The early stages of some neurologic conditions may present with CWP that could be confused with FMS. These include MS, PD, and peripheral neuropathies (PNPs). Clues to a diagnosis of MS include a fluctuating course and paroxysmal symptoms, gait difficulties, visual disturbances, prominent sensory symptoms, and bowel or bladder dysfunction. PD in the early stages, prior to the more prominent symptoms of tremor and rigidity, may present with diffuse pain in up to two-thirds of patients, with moderate severity pain associated with sleep disturbance, depressed mood, and compromised activities of daily living. The stiffness that can occur in the early stages of PD may be interpreted as pain and could have features of a diffuse pain syndrome.[25] Neuropathy is usually recognized as the causing pain in the distal extremities, but small fiber neuropathy has many overlapping features with FMS, raising the question of whether these are two distinct conditions, or whether the neuropathy may be an underlying pathogenic mechanism for some persons with FMS.[4]

Spinal Stenosis and Myelopathy

A diagnosis of spinal stenosis is clinically suspected when a patient presents with symptoms of claudication, but has patent peripheral blood vessels. Some older patients can have difficulty describing the fluctuating pain of spinal stenosis, especially when there is involvement of the cervical region causing a more widespread character to the pain.[18] Spinal stenosis may occur in the setting of degenerative disc disease, facet joint osteoarthritis as well as congenital deformity of the spinal canal. Proliferative bony bridges across at least three vertebral spaces that are seen mostly in the thoracic spine indicate diffuse idiopathic skeletal hyperostosis (DISH), another cause of spinal stenosis. In addition, the enthesopathy associated with DISH may also be a cause of CWP. Imaging studies such as MRI or CT identify spinal canal stenosis. As imaging studies generally correlate poorly with clinical symptoms, the clinical context requires careful evaluation.

Myopathies and Myositis

CWP associated with muscle weakness should suggest the diagnosis of a myopathy, which may be classified as congenital, metabolic, drug-induced, and inflammatory. In the setting of myopathy, muscle weakness is the most prominent symptom, with patients complaining of functional difficulties such as difficulty climbing stairs, or standing from a seated position, even with normal muscle power on physical examination. Features to be explored on history include a family history of muscle disease, symptoms aggravated by exercise or carbohydrate intake, or associated symptoms suggesting a connective tissue disease such as skin rash in a heliotrope pattern on the face, "mechanics hands," Raynaud's phenomenon, skin tightening, or respiratory symptoms. Myositis as a paraneoplastic phenomenon must be remembered, especially for those with dermatomyositis.

Various inherited myopathies may present with muscle pain and mimic FMS. Increased muscle pain following exercise should suggest an inherited myopathy such as McArdle disease, or muscle complaints with only mild elevation of creatine kinase (CK) suggest late-onset Pompe disease.[10,15] In the setting of proximal weakness of the legs, myotonia, and modest elevation of CK, myotonic dystrophy type 2 (DM2) is a diagnostic consideration.[9] Although muscle fasciculations may occur in FMS, their presence should suggest a diagnosis of neuromyotonia.

MENTAL DISORDERS

Because chronic pain and mental health disorders occur commonly in the general population, it is reasonable to expect overlap of these conditions. Moreover, there is increasing evidence for shared neurobiologic mechanisms operative within these disorders leading to a hypothesis of a bidirectional relationship. Pain is indeed accepted as one of the diagnostic criteria of generalized anxiety disorder and somatoform pain disorder. This bidirectional relationship is further supported by increased prevalence rates of mental health disorders across all chronic pain conditions. Major depressive disorder occurs in up to 61%, generalized anxiety disorder in 1% to 10%, and substance abuse disorder in up to 25% of patients with chronic pain.[13] Alternately, prevalence of mental health disorders such as anxiety, depression, and posttraumatic stress disorder is as high as 80% for patients with FMS. Therefore, in assessing a patient with a chronic pain complaint, attention should be given to examine for an underlying mental health disorder that is presenting with a somatic symptom.

MEDICATION-INDUCED PAIN CONDITIONS

Medications that can be associated with body pain include statins, opioids, some chemotherapeutic agents, aromatase inhibitors, and bisphosphonates. Myalgia usually occurs early in treatment with statins in 2% to 10% of patients, and may be sufficiently severe-to-warrant treatment discontinuation with resolution within 2 months. Opioids, often used to treat pain, may induce a hyperalgesic state that can present with diffuse pain.[12] Opioid-induced pain may be burning in nature and can occur even with low-dose opioid treatment. Particular consideration of opioid-induced hyperalgesia should be given to FMS patients receiving opioids as a factor in perpetuation of FMS symptoms. Chemotherapy-induced neuropathy, although mostly recognized as neuropathic symptoms in a glove and stocking distribution, can be a cause of a more generalized pain syndrome. Anecdotally, it has also been observed that some patients with a previous background of low-grade FMS may develop a more severe exacerbation of diffuse pain with neuropathic qualities following chemotherapy. Other medications that can cause body pain include the aromatase inhibitors in up to 50% of women treated for breast cancer, bisphosphonates, and proton pump inhibitors.

CONCLUSION

Physicians must always consider a differential diagnosis in the assessment of a patient presenting with CWP. Clues to the cause of a diffuse pain syndrome may be gleaned from a comprehensive medical and psychosocial history and a full clinical examination. FMS still remains the most common reason for a complaint of CWP, but failure to recognize some other cause will compromise patient care. With laboratory and various technical diagnostics mostly of lesser importance than a sound clinical evaluation, the assessment of CWP exemplifies the essence of practicing the "art of medicine." Therefore, diagnosis of FMS is reliant on a history of a typical cluster of symptoms, a physical examination without findings indicating some other disease and normal basic laboratory testing without need for specialist referral. Various conditions that may mimic FMS have been described, with highlighting of features that can help to differentiate them from FMS. By categorizing these conditions as systemic inflammatory rheumatic diseases, noninflammatory musculoskeletal conditions, non-rheumatic medical conditions, neurologic disorders, mental health disorders, and medication-related pain conditions, health care professionals should be more alert to other diagnostic possibilities in the setting of CWP.

REFERENCES

1. Ablin JN, Amital H, Ehrenfeld M, et al. Guidelines for the diagnosis and treatment of the fibromyalgia syndrome. *Harefuah.* 2013;**152**(12):742–747, 751, 750.
2. Ablin JN, Eshed I, Berman M, et al. Prevalence of axial spondyloarthropathy among patients suffering from fibromyalgia: an MRI study with application of the ASAS classification criteria. *Arthritis Care Res.* 2016;**69**(5):724–729.
3. Beighton P, De Paepe A, Steinmann B, Tsipouras P, Wenstrup RJ. Ehlers-Danlos syndromes: revised nosology, Villefranche, 1997. Ehlers-Danlos National Foundation (USA) and Ehlers-Danlos Support Group (UK). *Am J Med Genet.* 1998;**77**(1):31–37.
4. Caro XJ, Winter EF. The role and importance of small fiber neuropathy in fibromyalgia pain. *Curr Pain Headache Rep.* 2015;**19**(12):55.
5. Dasgupta B, Cimmino MA, Maradit-Kremers H, et al. 2012 Provisional classification criteria for polymyalgia rheumatica: a European League Against Rheumatism/American College of Rheumatology collaborative initiative. *Ann Rheum Dis.* 2012;**71**(4):484–492.
6. Eich W, Häuser W, Arnold B, et al.; Arbeitsgemeinschaft der Wissenschaftlichen Medizinischen Fachgesellschaften. Fibromyalgia syndrome. Definition, classification, clinical diagnosis and prognosis. *Schmerz.* 2012;**26**(3):247–258.
7. Fitzcharles MA, Ste-Marie PA, Goldenberg DL, et al. Canadian Pain Society and Canadian Rheumatology Association recommendations for rational care of persons with fibromyalgia: a summary report. *J Rheumatol.* 2013;**40**(8):1388–1393.
8. Ge HY, Wang Y, Danneskiold-Samsøe B, Graven-Nielsen T, Arendt-Nielsen L. The predetermined sites of examination for tender points in fibromyalgia syndrome are frequently associated with myofascial trigger points. *J Pain.* 2010;**11**(7):644–651.
9. George A, Schneider-Gold C, Reiners K, Sommer C. Musculoskeletal pain as the most prominent feature in myotonic dystrophy type 2. *Schmerz.* 2006;**20**(5):388, 390–384, 396.
10. Gesquière-Dando A, Attarian S, Maues De Paula A, Pouget J, Salort-Campana E. Fibromyalgia-like symptoms associated with irritable bowel syndrome: a challenging diagnosis of late-onset Pompe disease. *Muscle Nerve.* 2015;**52**(2):300–304.
11. Goldenberg DL. Diagnosis and differential diagnosis of fibromyalgia. *Am J Med.* 2009;**122**(12 Suppl):S14–S21.
12. Hayhurst CJ, Durieux ME. Differential opioid tolerance and opioid-induced hyperalgesia: a clinical reality. *Anesthesiology.* 2016;**124**(2):483–488.
13. Hooten WM. Chronic pain and mental health disorders: shared neural mechanisms, epidemiology, and treatment. *Mayo Clin Proc.* 2016;**91**(7):955–970.
14. Lantos PM. Chronic Lyme disease. *Infect Dis Clin North Am.* 2015;**29**(2):325–340.
15. Lucia A, Nogales-Gadea G, Pérez M, Martín MA, Andreu AL, Arenas J. McArdle disease: what do neurologists need to know? *Nat Clin Pract Neurol.* 2008;**4**(10):568–577.
16. Macfarlane GJ, Kronisch C, Dean LE, et al. EULAR revised recommendations for the management of fibromyalgia. *Ann Rheum Dis.* 2017;**76**(2):318–328.
17. Mankia K, Emery P. Preclinical rheumatoid arthritis: progress toward prevention. *Arthritis Rheumatol.* 2016;**68**(4):779–788.
18. Melancia JL, Francisco AF, Antunes JL. Spinal stenosis. *Handb Clin Neurol.* 2014;**119**:541–549.
19. Perrot S, Dieudé P, Pérocheau D, Allanore Y. Comparison of pain, pain burden, coping strategies, and attitudes between patients with systemic sclerosis and patients with rheumatoid arthritis: a cross-sectional study. *Pain Med.* 2013;**14**(11):1776–1785.
20. Quintner JL, Bove GM, Cohen ML. A critical evaluation of the trigger point phenomenon. *Rheumatology.* 2015;**54**(3):392–399.

21. Roussou E, Ciurtin C. Clinical overlap between fibromyalgia tender points and enthesitis sites in patients with spondyloarthritis who present with inflammatory back pain. *Clin Exp Rheumatol.* 2012;**30**(6 Suppl 74):24–30.
22. Sarzi-Puttini P, Atzeni F, Clauw DJ, Perrot S. The impact of pain on systemic rheumatic diseases. *Best Pract Res Clin Rheumatol.* 2015;**29**(1):1–5.
23. Scheper MC, de Vries JE, Verbunt J, Engelbert RH. Chronic pain in hypermobility syndrome and Ehlers-Danlos syndrome (hypermobility type): it is a challenge. *J Pain Res.* 2015;**8**:591–601.
24. Sepriano A, Landewé R, van der Heijde D, et al.; ASAS. Predictive validity of the ASAS classification criteria for axial and peripheral spondyloarthritis after follow-up in the ASAS cohort: a final analysis. *Ann Rheum Dis.* 2016;**75**(6):1034–1042.
25. Toda K, Harada T. Prevalence, classification, and etiology of pain in Parkinson's disease: association between Parkinson's disease and fibromyalgia or chronic widespread pain. *Tohoku J Exp Med.* 2010;**222**(1):1–5.
26. Tovoli F, Giampaolo L, Caio G, et al. Fibromyalgia and coeliac disease: a media hype or an emerging clinical problem? *Clin Exp Rheumatol.* 2013;**31**(6 Suppl 79):S50–S52.
27. Wintermeyer E, Ihle C, Ehnert S, et al. Crucial role of vitamin D in the musculoskeletal system. *Nutrients.* 2016;**8**(6):pii: E319.
28. Wolfe F, Clauw DJ, Fitzcharles MA, et al. Fibromyalgia criteria and severity scales for clinical and epidemiological studies: a modification of the ACR Preliminary Diagnostic Criteria for Fibromyalgia. *J Rheumatol.* 2011;**38**(6):1113–1122.
29. Wormser GP, Weitzner E, McKenna D, et al. Long-term assessment of fibromyalgia in patients with culture-confirmed Lyme disease. *Arthritis Rheumatol.* 2014;**67**(3):837–839. doi:10.1002/art.38972.
30. Zipser RD, Patel S, Yahya KZ, Baisch DW, Monarch E. Presentations of adult celiac disease in a nationwide patient support group. *Dig Dis Sci.* 2003;**48**(4):761–764.

SECTION 5

Pathophysiologic Concepts

CHAPTER 16

Genetics

Jacob N. Ablin

Summary Points

- Fibromyalgia syndrome (FMS) is a complex disorder with a strong familial aggregation, implicating an underlying genetic predisposition.
- Candidate gene studies, though laborious to perform, have identified several genetic markers associated with FMS.
- Genetic markers associated with the sympathetic nervous system as well as with additional pain-related neurotransmitters are appealing candidates.
- More recent techniques such as genome-wide association studies (GWAS) have extended our understanding of FMS genetics.
- Epigenetic modifications, such as microRNA signature, offer a novel way to study FMS and to link between the syndrome and the triggers that have long been implicated.

Even though the concept of FMS continues to evolve, the genetics of FMS in particular and chronic pain in general continue to pose a challenge to both geneticists and clinicians. Although the strong familial association of FMS has long been recognized[2] and ascribed to a genetic underpinning, the growing complexity of both chronic pain in general and the broadening scope of genetic technology has made it imperative to incorporate genetic data into a wider matrix of information, rather than restricting the focus to markers associated with a diagnosis of FMS per se. An intriguing point of reference in this aspect can be gained from scrutinizing the Research Domain Criteria (RDoC) of the National Institute of Mental Health (NIMH)[18]—an ambitious project attempting to piece together data from fields such as genetics, networks, hormones, as well as social factors—into the understanding of complex disorders involving the central nervous system (CNS), such as psychiatric disorders. A similar approach may become eventually conceivable regarding the understanding of complex chronic pain conditions such as FMS. It is noteworthy that in the process of this evolution, just as the *Diagnostic and Statistical Manual of Mental Disorders* (*DSM*) definitions may be replaced or updated based on emerging RDoC findings, the very concept of FMS may change and evolve into more precise as well as individualized definitions of chronic pain, which might dramatically change the way we address these patients. Moreover, progress in the field of pharmacogenetics may further enhance our ability to offer personalized treatment more effectively to patients currently diagnosed with FMS and treated on a largely empirical basis. For the time being, it remains our obligation to make the most of the clinical as well as genetic evidence available, and to treat patients with a clinical diagnosis of FMS as best we can, taking into consideration what genetics has to offer. In the current section, we have attempted to provide a current appraisal of where the genetics of FMS stands today.

FAMILIAL AGGREGATION IN FIBROMYALGIA SYNDROME

Familial aggregation of FMS and chronic pain has long been recognized on the basis of clinical observations among both siblings and parents of FMS patients[26] with a significant concordance between mothers and children regarding both the occurrence of FMS and of sleep disorders.[27] Moreover, patients suffering from FMS have been shown to have an increase in rates of additional functional pain syndromes such as irritable bowel syndrome (IBS), temporomandibular joint disorder (TMJD), and so on, among family members.[8]

The most significant family study of FMS has been conducted by Arnold et al.,[3] who studied 533 relatives of 78 FMS probands and 272 relatives of 40 rheumatoid arthritis (RA) probands. A strong familial aggregation of FMS was documented and the odds ratio of FMS in a relative of an FMS proband (compared with that of a relative of an RA proband) was 8.5. A strong aggregation was also observed regarding the quality of tenderness.

Twin studies, a classical tool in investigating genetic traits, have been performed in chronic pain states. Such studies have generally demonstrated a modest genetic influence expressed by a concordance rate of 30% among monozygotic female twins and 16% for dizygotic female twins.[21]

Although the aforementioned studies have convincingly documented a significant familial component in FMS, they obviously do not indicate that FMS is the result of a single genetic trait. As in many other complex disorders that implicate the CNS, it is much more likely to assume that FMS, like chronic pain in general, is a multifactorial and spectrum-like trait. Because we now know that multiple neurotransmitters as well as additional factors are involved in the transmission and processing of pain, it is natural to assume that a large number of genetic traits may likewise be involved in determining the tendency of an individual to ultimately develop FMS. A host of factors that are not intuitively directly related to pain may in fact bear upon this process. Thus, for instance, genetic markers that are related to the autonomic nervous system can also be related to pain processing, but even more tangentially genetic disorder related to hypermobility (e.g., Ehler–Danlos syndromes), which is associated with autonomic dysfunction, can also pose a genetically determined risk of FMS development. Finally, one must keep in mind the fact that FMS is not a congenital disorder but rather develops over years in each affected individual. Some patients deserve a diagnosis of FMS in their teens, while others will not reach this state until well after menopause. Thus, one must assume that the genetic predisposition toward developing FMS is subsequently exposed to and influenced by a host of external triggers to which the individual is exposed throughout his or her life, eventually culminating in the development of FMS.

Understanding the nature of this process, through which a genetically prone individual moves from being asymptomatic to being a fully manifest clinical patient, is a major challenge of modern genetics. Moving from classical genetic research into the fields of epigenetics and gene-expression patterns are fields that are beginning to shed light on these aspects and are discussed subsequently in this chapter.

Candidate Gene Studies

Studying candidate genetic markers for a complex polygenetic trait is often likened to the challenge of finding a needle in a haystack. Although it is tempting to look for polymorphisms in genes, which are related to mediators known to participate in pain processing and modulation, the immense number of possible targets combined with the logistic complexity and cost of conducting such studies has made this metaphor justifiable. Notwithstanding these limitations, the target–gene approach has nonetheless come up in the past with some valuable results that help advance the genetic study of FMS.

Catechol-O-Methyltransferase Gene Polymorphisms and Their Relationship With Fibromyalgia Syndrome

Catechol-*O*-methyltransferase (COMT), an enzyme that plays a major role in the metabolism of catecholamines, has been one of the first targets for genetic analysis in FMS, in view of the presumed role of the autonomic nervous system in the processing of pain. Early studies by Zubieta et al.[31] drew attention to this gene, showing that *COMT* polymorphisms predicted pain thresholds in healthy individuals, as could be demonstrated both through quantitative sensory testing (QST) and functional neuroimaging.

An increased risk of chronic pain has been associated with the Val158Met (rs4680) polymorphism of the *COMT* gene, encoding an enzyme with lower activity.[30] Several additional studies have been conducted relating to *COMT* in chronic pain, including the investigation of haplotypes that modify both expression and activity.[14,13] Tammimäki and Männistö[29] have conducted a systemic review and meta-analysis regarding the role of COMT polymorphisms in chronic pain conditions, including migrainous headache, FMS (or chronic widespread pain [CWP]), and chronic musculoskeletal pain.

Their results indicated that FMS is the only type of chronic pain that could be associated with the *COMT* single-nucleotide polymorphism (SNP) rs4680 (Val158Met), which results in the low-activity variant of *COMT*.[29]

Additional genetic markers linked to the sympathetic nervous system have been studied as target genes for FMS. Thus, Arg16Gly (rs1042713) and Gln27Glu (rs1042714), which are both SNPs within the β2-adrenergic receptor gene (*ADRB2*), have been associated with an increased risk of FMS as well as CWP.[16] Moreover, different haplotypes of the β2 adrenergic receptor, which are associated with either positive or negative imbalance in ADRB2 function, may increase the vulnerability to chronic pain conditions as well as influencing the emotional and hemodynamic response.[12]

Dopamine Receptor–Related Genes

Although the role of the dopaminergic system in FMS and CWP is not sufficiently understood, some research has been performed looking at dopamine-related genetic markers in this condition. Thus, the dopamine D4 receptor exon III repeat polymorphism has been studied and found to be significantly decreased in frequency among FMS patients[10] as well as being associated with a so-called low-novelty-seeking personality trait. As the central role played by the dopaminergic system in stress, reward, and other aspects of neural functional continues to unravel, additional attention is likely to be directed toward dopamine-related genetic markers in the pathogenesis of FMS.

Serotonin-Related Studies

The concept of neurotransmitter dysregulation underlying at least part of the pathogenesis of FMS is a straightforward and appealing one, even if somewhat simplistic. Decreased levels of specific neurotransmitters, such as serotonin (and others), have been documented in the cerebrospinal fluid (CSF) of FMS patients, and medications such as selective serotonin reuptake inhibitors (SSRIs) and serotonin-norepinephrine reuptake inhibitors (SNRIs) are among those most frequently used for the treatment of patients suffering from FMS. Thus, serotonin-related genetic variants were among the first target genes to be scrutinized. The 5-hydroxytryptamine receptor 2A (5HT-2A, encoded by HTR2A) and 5HT transporter (5HTT, or sodium-dependent serotonin transporter, encoded by SLC6A4) are two of these targets. An insertion/deletion polymorphism in the *SLC6A4* gene has been shown to be associated with chronic pain, with the deletion allele ("short allele") shown to increase the risk of FMS. Studying the promoter region of the serotonin transporter gene (*5-HTT*), Offenbaecher et al.[25] demonstrated an increased frequency of the S/S genotype among patients versus controls, a finding which was subsequently confirmed by Cohen et al.[9]

Smith et al.[28] have published the largest candidate–gene study to date, enrolling 496 FMS patients and 348 controls. In this study, genotyping was performed using the Pain Research Panel, a dedicated gene array chip, analyzing >350 genes involved in biologic pathways related to nociception, inflammation, and mood. Significant differences in allele frequencies were observed between cases and controls for three genes: *GABRB3*, *TAAR1*, and *GBP1*. In the second part of this research, a replication study was conducted on an independent cohort of FMS patients and controls, demonstrating an association of FMS with four genes—*TAAR1*, *RGS4*, *CNR1*, and *GRIA4*. One of these genes, the *CNR1*, codes the CB-1 cannabinoid receptor, responsible for the binding of endogenous and exogenous cannabinoids and has previously been associated with the genetics of pain conditions such as migraine.[20] Thus, this large-scale candidate gene approach demonstrates the potential of this methodology to identify relevant associations as well as highlighting that the genetics overlaps between different chronic pain conditions.[22]

Genome-Wide Association Studies on Fibromyalgia Syndrome and Chronic Pain

GWAS have been described as a major breakthrough regarding deciphering the genetic underpinnings of complex human conditions such as chronic pain and pose an intuitively appealing alternative to the Sisyphean effort to study individual genetic markers in the hope of identifying one or more that are significant. This technique has identified hundreds of robustly replicated loci for common traits. GWAS, however, has its limitations and has yet to lead to major clinically significant findings in the context of FMS. Family-based designs appear to be of value in this context and have been utilized by Arnold et al.[1] in order to perform a genome-wide linkage analysis of FMS with 341 microsatellite markers. In this study, Arnold was able to demonstrate evidence of linkage at specific regions within chromosome 17p11.2–q11.2, which coincides with two potential FMS candidate genes—the serotonin transporter gene (*SLC6A4*) and the transient receptor and the vanilloid channel 2 gene (*TRPV2*).

A second large study implemented GWAS methodology as well as evaluation of copy number variations (CNVs) by using genotyping data and array comparative genomic hybridization experiments (aCGH).[15] The researchers selected 313 FMS cases having low comorbidities and 220 controls. No SNP reached GWAS-association threshold; however, while performing a replication analysis, the authors were able to identify an intronic deletion in *NRXN3*, a gene essential for neuronal development, which was associated with female FMS cases. The authors further identified the SNP rs11127292, located in the third intron of *MYT1L*, a gene also involved in neuronal differentiation. The authors thus concluded that both GWAS and aCGH results point to a role for the CNS in FMS genetic susceptibility.

Genome-Wide Expression Profiling

Jones et al.[19] have shifted from the traditional efforts to identify genetic predisposition to FMS toward the approach of looking at gene expression—as a way to both identify an objective biomarker for FMS and exploring the possible roles of specific alterations in gene expression in the pathogenetic process. Using this approach, they analyzed messenger RNA (mRNA) from 70 FMS patients and 70 controls. The results indicated that FMS patients showed differential expression of 421 genes, including genes relevant to pain processing (e.g., glutamine/glutamate) and axonal development. They further demonstrated upregulation of inflammatory pathways and downregulation of pathways related to hypersensitivity and allergy. Finally, this study was able to achieve a diagnostic sensitivity of 95% and a specificity of 96% for the diagnosis of FMS.

MicroRNA Signature

MicroRNAs are short endogenous noncoding RNAs that act as posttranscriptional regulators of gene expression and have been demonstrated to play an important role both in CNS development and in the response to stress.[24] Both circulating and CSF levels of microRNA have been studied in FMS patients in an attempt to identify a specific profile and specific microRNA molecules for those identified, which differed significantly between FMS patients and controls.[5,4] In a recent study published in abstract form, so-called liquid biopsies (i.e., serum and saliva) were used for the determination of a microRNA signature of FMS patients, and six such microRNAs were identified.[17] In view of the emerging recognition of the role of epigenetics in the development of chronic pain,[11,7] microRNAs, which are a key mediator of epigenetics, offer a novel perspective regarding the genetic understanding of FMS and a hope for novel future therapeutic targets. Methylation patterns and differentially methylated sites can be studied in order to identify epigenetic changes occurring during life and have been utilized in FMS, demonstrating some differential patterns of methylation in genes that may be pathogenetically relevant.[23] Notably, progress in epigenetics offers novel insights into the widely recognized link between early childhood adversity and the subsequent development of FMS beyond traditional explanations, such as an effect on the hypothalamic–pituitary–adrenal (HPA) axis. Epigenetic changes such as histone deacetylation or phosphorylation, DNA methylation, and chromatin remodeling lead to stable changes, which can subsequently be transferred across generations but are also potential targets for novel treatments, for example, histone deacetylase inhibitors.[6] Thus, epigenetics may significantly broaden our perspective regarding the interaction between genes and FMS.

CONCLUSION

The genetic study of FMS is an ever-evolving process, which continues to morph and expand because novel techniques and increased efficiency of methods continue to shed light and demystify the underpinnings of this previously elusive condition. The interplay between genetic research and other seemingly unrelated areas, such as functional neuroscience, creates an intriguing matrix of information that eventually may enable a truly holistic understanding of complex CNS-involving conditions such as FMS, and may make it possible to devise much better and more personalized modes of treatment. In addition, the frontiers of epigenetics and neuroplasticity are opening windows toward the prospect of understanding how the CNS of FMS patients may have entered into the zone of centralized pain, often appearing to be related to stress or trauma, and how we might hope to reprogram such changes regardless of the underlying (presumably unchangeable) genetics involved.

REFERENCES

1. Arnold LM, Fan J, Russell IJ, et al. The fibromyalgia family study: a genome-wide linkage scan study. *Arthritis Rheum.* 2013;**65**(4):1122–1128.
2. Arnold LM, Hudson JI, Hess EV, et al. Family study of fibromyalgia. *Arthritis Rheum.* 2004;**50**(3): 944–952.
3. Arnold LM, Hudson JI, Hess EV, et al. Family study of fibromyalgia. *Arthritis Rheum.* 2004;**50**(3): 944–952.
4. Bjersing JL, Bokarewa MI, Mannerkorpi K. Profile of circulating microRNAs in fibromyalgia and their relation to symptom severity: an exploratory study. *Rheumatol Int.* 2015;**35**(4):635–642.
5. Bjersing JL, Lundborg C, Bokarewa MI, Mannerkorpi K. Profile of cerebrospinal microRNAs in fibromyalgia. *PLoS ONE.* 2013;**8**(10):e78762.
6. Burke NN, Finn DP, McGuire BE, Roche M. Psychological stress in early life as a predisposing factor for the development of chronic pain: clinical and preclinical evidence and neurobiological mechanisms. *J Neurosci Res.* 2017;**95**(6):1257–1270.
7. Burri A, Marinova Z, Robinson MD, et al. Are epigenetic factors implicated in chronic widespread pain? *PLoS ONE.* 2016;**11**(11):e0165548.
8. Buskila D, Neumann L, Hazanov I, Carmi R. Familial aggregation in the fibromyalgia syndrome. *Semin Arthritis Rheum.* 1996;**26**(3):605–611.
9. Cohen H, Buskila D, Neumann L, Ebstein RP. Confirmation of an association between fibromyalgia and serotonin transporter promoter region (5- HTTLPR) polymorphism, and relationship to anxiety-related personality traits. *Arthritis Rheum.* 2002;**46**(3):845–847.
10. Dan B, Hagit C, Lily N, Ebstein R. An association between fibromyalgia and the dopamine D4 receptor exon III repeat polymorphism and relationship to novelty seeking personality traits. *Mol. Psychiatry.* 2004;**9**(8):730.
11. Descalzi G, Ikegami D, Ushijima T, Nestler EJ, Zachariou V, Narita M. Epigenetic mechanisms of chronic pain. *Trends Neurosci.* 2015;**38**(4):237–246.
12. Diatchenko L, Anderson AD, Slade GD, et al. Three major haplotypes of the β2 adrenergic receptor define psychological profile, blood pressure, and the risk for development of a common musculoskeletal pain disorder. *Am J Med Genet B Neuropsychiatr.* 2006;**141B**(5):449–462.
13. Diatchenko L, Fillingim RB, Smith SB, Maixner W. The phenotypic and genetic signatures of common musculoskeletal pain conditions. *Nat Rev Rheumatol.* 2013;**9**(6):340–350.
14. Diatchenko L, Slade GD, Nackley AG, et al. Genetic basis for individual variations in pain perception and the development of a chronic pain condition. *Hum Mol Genet.* 2005;**14**(1):135–143.
15. Docampo E, Escaramís G, Gratacòs M, et al. Genome-wide analysis of single nucleotide polymorphisms and copy number variants in fibromyalgia suggest a role for the central nervous system. *Pain.* 2014;**155**(6):1102–1109.

16. Hocking LJ, Smith BH, Jones GT, Reid DM, Strachan DP, Macfarlane GJ. Genetic variation in the beta2-adrenergic receptor but not catecholamine-*O*-methyltransferase predisposes to chronic pain: results from the 1958 British Birth Cohort Study. *Pain.* 2010;**149**(1):143–151.
17. Iannuccelli C, Guzzo M, Baldassarre A, et al. AB0838 A microrna signature in liquid biopsies for the diagnosis of fibromyalgia. *Ann Rheum Dis.* 2016;**75**(suppl 2):1189–1190.
18. Insel TR. The NIMH Research Domain Criteria (RDoC) Project: precision medicine for psychiatry. *Am J Psychiatry.* 2014;**171**(4):395–397.
19. Jones KD, Gelbart T, Whisenant TC, et al. Genome-wide expression profiling in the peripheral blood of patients with fibromyalgia. *Clin Exp Rheumatol.* 2016;**34**(2 suppl 96):S89–S98.
20. Juhasz G, Lazary J, Chase D, et al. Variations in the cannabinoid receptor 1 gene predispose to migraine. *Neurosci Lett.* 2009;**461**(2):116–120.
21. Kato K, Sullivan PF, Evengård B, Pedersen NL. Importance of genetic influences on chronic widespread pain. *Arthritis Rheum.* 2006;**54**(5):1682–1686.
22. Lee YH, Choi SJ, Ji JD, Song GG. Candidate gene studies of fibromyalgia: a systematic review and meta-analysis. *Rheumatol Int.* 2012;**32**(2):417–426.
23. Menzies V, Lyon DE, Archer KJ, et al. Epigenetic alterations and an increased frequency of micronuclei in women with fibromyalgia. *Nurs Res Pract.* 2013;**2013**:795784.
24. Meza-Sosa KF, Valle-García D, Pedraza-Alva G, Pérez-Martínez L. Role of microRNAs in central nervous system development and pathology. *J Neurosci Res.* 2012;**90**(1):1–12.
25. Offenbaecher M, Bondy B, de Jonge S, et al. Possible association of fibromyalgia with a polymorphism in the serotonin transporter gene regulatory region. *Arthritis Rheum.* 1999;**42**(11):2482–2488.
26. Pellegrino MJ, Waylonis GW, Sommer A. Familial occurrence of primary fibromyalgia. *Arch Phys Med Rehabil.* 1989;**70**(1):61–63.
27. Roizenblatt S, Tufik S, Goldenberg J, Pinto LR, Hilario MO, Feldman D. Juvenile fibromyalgia: clinical and polysomnographic aspects. *J Rheumatol.* 1997;**24**(3):579–585.
28. Smith SB, Maixner DW, Fillingim RB, et al. Large candidate gene association study reveals genetic risk factors and therapeutic targets for fibromyalgia. *Arthritis Rheum.* 2012;**64**(2):584–593.
29. Tammimäki A, Männistö PT. Catechol-*O*-methyltransferase gene polymorphism and chronic human pain: a systematic review and meta-analysis. *Pharmacogenet Genomics.* 2012;**22**(9):673–691.
30. Vargas-Alarcón G, Fragoso JM, Cruz-Robles D, et al. Catechol-*O*-methyltransferase gene haplotypes in Mexican and Spanish patients with fibromyalgia. *Arthritis Res Ther.* 2007;**9**(5):R110.
31. Zubieta JK, Heitzeg MM, Smith YR, et al. COMT val158met genotype affects mu-opioid neurotransmitter responses to a pain stressor. *Science.* 2003;**299**(5610):1240–1243.

CHAPTER 17

The Hormonal Perspective

Jacob N. Ablin

Summary Points

- The protean clinical manifestations of fibromyalgia syndrome (FMS) often overlap with those of systemic metabolic–endocrine disorders, which must be considered in the differential diagnosis of FMS.
- The female preponderance of FMS points toward the possible role of sex hormones in pain processing, and multiple studies have analyzed the role of these factors in FMS, although results have not always been consistent.
- The hypothalamic–pituitary–adrenal axis (HPA) axis, which is a major stress-regulating system, is often implicated in FMS and is closely related to the autonomic nervous system.
- The growth hormone (GH)–insulin-like growth factor-1 (IGF-1) axis has been implicated as being deficient in FMS, and treatment with GH replacement appears to be effective at least in a subset of patients.
- Thyroid hormones, endo-cannabinoids, and additional endocrinologic factors have also been studied.
- Neuroendocrine mediators implicated in neuro-inflammation and autoimmunity pose intriguing novel targets for studying the pathogenesis of FMS.

While the pathophysiology of FMS continues to evolve and to add additional aspects and fields of research, it is obvious to all who deal with complex conditions such as FMS that a complex interaction among many different biologic processes is likely to be involved in putting together the puzzle (and indeed puzzling) final phenotype, which we currently describe as FMS. In this chapter, we shall focus on the hormonal aspects of the puzzle—to the extent that they have been partially delineated—and on the intriguing points of connection between the endocrinologic and other fields such as immunology, autoimmunity, genetics, and the autonomic nervous system.

Two aspects of FMS tend to call for immediate attention to the possible role of hormones in its pathogenesis, that is, the strong female preponderance and the relationship with stress, and we shall thus start by addressing these topics.

SEX HORMONES AND FIBROMYALGIA SYNDROME

FMS has been historically considered a condition more prevalent among females than males. In the past, it was estimated that as many as 90% of cases occurred among females, leading to FMS being characterized as a woman's health problem. This conclusion was based to a large degree on the effect of the original, tender point based on the 1990 American College of Rheumatology (ACR) FMS classification criteria, because women are much more likely to satisfy the tender point criteria than men, regardless of symptom severity. Subsequently, it has become apparent that male FMS is by no means rare. Indeed, more recent studies that utilized the up-to-date diagnostic criteria for FMS have actually shown rates of FMS in the general population that were not significantly different between women and men, although women were still much more likely to receive a clinical diagnosis of FMS.[22]

A considerable amount of literature has accumulated regarding the possible role of sex hormones in the processing of chronic pain and the effects of these hormones on central nervous system (CNS) pain processing (see for instance Bartley and Fillingim; for review see Hassan et al.[2]). Sex hormones and their receptors are widely distributed throughout the central and peripheral nervous system and both estrogen and progesterone have been shown to play pro-nociceptive and anti-nociceptive roles in different circumstances,[19] while testosterone usually appears to play an anti-nociceptive role. Moreover, sex hormones have the ability to alter the levels of additional pain-modulating neurotransmitters that are not considered sex hormones, such as substance P, glutamate, and the like, and to increase expression of excitatory synapses in specific CNS areas such as the hippocampus, cerebellum, and cortex.[1] Specifically, extensive research has indicated an interaction between estrogen and γ-amino-butyric acid (GABA), an impotent pain-modulating neurotransmitter, with the synthesis, release, production, as well as the GABA receptor levels all being directly modulated by estrogen levels (see Hassan et al.[9] for a comprehensive review).

In addition to the general role played by sex hormones in FMS and chronic pain, specific attention has been focused on the role of the menstrual cycle and of pregnancy on the clinical manifestations of FMS, issues which are of considerable concern for patients, many of whom are of childbearing age. Several studies have indicated that FMS pain is increased in conditions associated with lower levels of estrogen. Thus, in regularly menstruating patients, more FMS pain was reported in the premenstrual phase compared with the postmenstrual phase, while no change was observed among patients receiving oral contraceptives,[14] and higher levels of pain have been reported among menopausal patients compared with premenopausal ones.[16] Higher pain scores were also reported in the last trimester of pregnancy.

Although FMS has traditionally been singled out among rheumatologists (and often even disputed as to being classified as a rheumatologic entity to begin with), recent research into the mechanisms of chronic pain in general and FMS in particular has started highlighting the role of neuro-immunity in the initiation and propagation of chronic pain. Multiple cells of the innate and adaptive immune system, including microglia, macrophages, astrocytes, as well as $CD4^{+}$Th1 and $CD4^{+}$Th2 cells, take part in the process of neuro-inflammation as a mechanism of chronic pain, thus blurring the historical line between inflammatory and noninflammatory mechanisms of pain. Notably, sex hormones play an important role in the development and function of the immune system, clinically exemplified by the widely disparate frequencies of many autoimmune disorders among males and females. Thus, estrogens can play both pro-inflammatory and anti-inflammatory roles in the functioning of cells such as microglia and astrocytes, and progesterone has also been shown in more limited studies to play diverse roles in this aspect. Finally, testosterone, the male hormone, has also been shown to have both pro- and anti-inflammatory effects on the CNS. Thus, as recently reviewed by Rosen et al.,[17] immune modulation of the CNS by sex hormones is a rapidly evolving field of research, which may eventually explain more of the underlying causes of the sex differences attributed to FMS.

What Is the Role of the Hypothalamic–Pituitary–Adrenal Axis System?

As noted earlier, FMS has often been related to a broad array of stressors, ranging from childhood trauma and adversity all the way through workplace bullying and up to recent exposure to warfare or torture. While there is obviously a tremendous amount of heterogeneity implicit in these associations, taken together, they tend to focus attention on the possibility of the body's stress system, that is, the HPA axis, playing a role in either the etiology and/or the maintenance of the symptoms of FMS. In fact, many studies have attempted to decipher this association, with varying degrees of success. While neuroendocrine perturbations of the HPA axis have been described both for FMS and chronic fatigue syndrome (CFS), conditions that share a considerable amount of clinical overlap, conflicting results have been described.[13] Thus, in humans, cerebrospinal fluid (CSF) levels of corticotropin-releasing factor (CRF) have been shown to correlate with levels of pain, fatigue, and depressive symptoms in FMS patients,[12] but it is not clear whether this represents a cause or an effect of chronic pain. In a meta-analysis performed by Tak et al.,[20] significantly decreased basal cortisol levels could only be found among CFS patients compared with controls, and not among FMS and irritable bowel syndrome (IBS) patients. This meta-analysis however only focused on basal hypocortisolism and did not look at more subtle measures of HPA dysfunction, such as lack of responsiveness to stress, which may be more sensitive attributes of FMS.[23]

In addition, many studies have implicated alterations of the sympathetic nervous system, expressed through parameters such as heart rate variability (HRV) in the pathogenesis,[11] but again a cause-and-effect relationship is difficult to establish. Thus, although some consider FMS to be a largely sympathetically maintained neuropathic pain syndrome, with autonomic dysfunction explaining many of the clinical manifestations besides pain,[10] this concept is not universally accepted.

Growth Hormone as a Target

A number of studies have implicated impairment of the GH axis (i.e., GH insulin-like growth factor-1 [IGF-1]) in the pathogenesis of FMS, an idea that is intuitively appealing in view of the relationship between GH and sleep. Most notably, almost two decades ago, Bennet et al.,[4] in a randomized double-blind placebo-controlled trial, were able to demonstrate a significant improvement in FMS symptoms among female FMS patients with low levels of IGF-1, while a more recent placebo-controlled trial showed that the addition of GH to standard care was effective in reducing FMS symptoms.[6] Moreover, during aerobic exercise, serum IGF-1 levels were shown to be correlated with the CSF levels of substance P, neuropeptide Y (NPY), and pain thresholds, indicating a beneficial role of IGF-1 during exercise in FMS.[5]

Role of Thyroid Hormones in FMS

Thyroid dysfunction, both hypothyroidism and hyperthyroidism, is a metabolic disorder that can manifest in a wide range of clinical symptoms, many of which are relatively nonspecific (e.g., fatigue, dyscognition) and thus are frequently considered within the differential diagnosis of FMS. In addition, a number of studies have attempted to identify specific thyroid disorders among FMS patients in the hope of identifying a treatable disorder. Autoimmune thyroiditis has been found to exist at an increased rate among patients diagnosed as suffering from FMS[3] and was shown to correlate with specific symptom constellations, such as dry eyes, burning, or pain with urination, allodynia, blurred vision, and sore throat. Also, the hypothesis has been raised that FMS might represent a condition of (subclinical) thyroid resistance;[8] because stress is also known to trigger autoimmune thyroid disease, it may partially explain the association with FMS. Further research is warranted in order to identify subtle signs of thyroid dysfunction (e.g., sonographic evidence of pathology) among patients clinically designated as suffering from "primary" FMS, and may identify patients who are candidates for more specific treatment.

An Endocannabinoid Deficiency?

Although not traditionally considered hormones, the endocannabinoid system is increasingly being studied and recognized for its interaction with the endocrine system at diverse sites, from the hypothalamus to the female reproductive tract.[21] The endocannabinoid system is a highly complex system of receptors and endogenous mediators distributed throughout the CNS as well as in peripheral tissues such as joints. This system is increasingly recognized as playing an important role in functions such as pain modulation, appetite, sleep, thermoregulation, stress response, neuroendocrine regulation, and cognitive functions.[15] In view of these accumulating data and in view of anecdotal as well as preliminary data regarding the efficacy of cannabinoids in ameliorating symptoms of FMS,[7] a hypothesis has been proposed regarding the possibility that FMS actually may represent a so-called endocannabinoid deficiency condition.[18] Although this concept is provocative and intriguing, it currently awaits more conclusive evidence in order to be established.

In conclusion, FMS is a highly multivariate disease with a host of symptoms impinging upon various seemingly far-flung aspects of human function, sensation, and behavior. As such, it often clinically overlaps with many aspects of endocrinologic disorders, entities that by nature also have broad and sometimes nonspecific manifestations. Moreover, the clinical association of FMS with stress as well as the female-to-male preponderance emphasize the possibility of endocrine disorders playing a role. While specific classical endocrine disorders, such as thyroid- or GH-related disorders, have all been targets of investigation, more subtle cutting-edge areas such as neuroendocrine biology, inflammation, and autoimmunity, as well as previously under-recognized systems including the endocannabinoid system promise to shed future light on the complex pathogenesis of FMS.

REFERENCES

1. Aloisi AM, Bonifazi M. Sex hormones, central nervous system and pain. *Horm Behav.* 2006;**50**(1):1–7.
2. Bartley EJ, Fillingim RB. Sex differences in pain: a brief review of clinical and experimental findings. *Br J Anaesth.* 2013;**111**(1):52–58.
3. Bazzichi L, Rossi A, Giuliano T, et al. Association between thyroid autoimmunity and fibromyalgic disease severity. *Clin Rheumatol.* 2007;**26**(12):2115–2120.
4. Bennett RM, Clark SC, Walczyk J. A randomized, double-blind, placebo-controlled study of growth hormone in the treatment of fibromyalgia. *Am J Med.* 1998;**104**(3):227–231.
5. Bjersing JL, Dehlin M, Erlandsson M, Bokarewa MI, Mannerkorpi K. Changes in pain and insulin-like growth factor 1 in fibromyalgia during exercise: the involvement of cerebrospinal inflammatory factors and neuropeptides. *Arthritis Res Ther.* 2012;**14**(4):R162.
6. Cuatrecasas G, Alegre C, Fernandez-Solà J, et al. Growth hormone treatment for sustained pain reduction and improvement in quality of life in severe fibromyalgia. *Pain.* 2012;**153**(7):1382–1389.
7. Fiz J, Durán M, Capellà D, Carbonell J, Farré M. Cannabis use in patients with fibromyalgia: effect on symptoms relief and health-related quality of life. *PLoS ONE.* 2011;**6**(4):e18440.
8. Garrison RL, Breeding PC. A metabolic basis for fibromyalgia and its related disorders: the possible role of resistance to thyroid hormone. *Med Hypotheses.* 2003;**61**(2):182–189.
9. Hassan S, Muere A, Einstein G. Ovarian hormones and chronic pain: a comprehensive review. *Pain.* 2014;**155**(12):2448–2460.
10. Martinez-Lavin M. Biology and therapy of fibromyalgia. Stress, the stress response system, and fibromyalgia. *Arthritis Res Ther.* 2007;**9**(4):216.

11. Martínez-Martínez LA, Mora T, Vargas A, Fuentes-Iniestra M, Martínez-Lavín M. Sympathetic nervous system dysfunction in fibromyalgia, chronic fatigue syndrome, irritable bowel syndrome, and interstitial cystitis: a review of case-control studies. *J Clin Rheumatol.* 2014;**20**(3):146–150.
12. McLean SA, Williams DA, Stein PK, et al. Cerebrospinal fluid corticotropin-releasing factor concentration is associated with pain but not fatigue symptoms in patients with fibromyalgia. *Neuropsychopharmacology.* 2006;**31**(12):2776–2782.
13. Neeck G, Crofford LJ. Neuroendocrine perturbations in fibromyalgia and chronic fatigue syndrome. *Rheum Dis Clin North Am.* 2000;**26**(4):989–1002.
14. Ostensen M, Rugelsjøen A, Wigers SH. The effect of reproductive events and alterations of sex hormone levels on the symptoms of fibromyalgia. *Scand J Rheumatol.* 1997;**26**(5):355–360.
15. Pacher P, Bátkai S, Kunos G. The endocannabinoid system as an emerging target of pharmacotherapy. *Pharmacol Rev.* 2006;**58**(3):389–462.
16. Pamuk ON, Cakir N. The variation in chronic widespread pain and other symptoms in fibromyalgia patients. The effects of menses and menopause. *Clin Exp Rheumatol.* 2005;**23**(6):778–782.
17. Rosen S, Ham B, Mogil JS. Sex differences in neuroimmunity and pain. *J Neurosci Res.* 2017;**95**(1–2):500–508.
18. Russo EB. Clinical endocannabinoid deficiency (CECD): can this concept explain therapeutic benefits of cannabis in migraine, fibromyalgia, irritable bowel syndrome and other treatment-resistant conditions? *Neuro Endocrinol Lett.* 2008;**29**(2):192–200.
19. Smith YR, Stohler CS, Nichols TE, Bueller JA, Koeppe RA, Zubieta JK. Pronociceptive and antinociceptive effects of estradiol through endogenous opioid neurotransmission in women. *J Neurosci.* 2006;**26**(21):5777–5785.
20. Tak LM, Cleare AJ, Ormel J, et al. Meta-analysis and meta-regression of hypothalamic-pituitary-adrenal axis activity in functional somatic disorders. *Biol Psychol.* 2011;**87**(2):183–194.
21. Vettor R, Pagotto U, Pagano C, Pasquali R. Here, there and everywhere: the endocannabinoid system. *J Neuroendocrinol.* 2008;**20**(suppl 1):iv–vi.
22. Vincent A, Lahr BD, Wolfe F, et al. Prevalence of fibromyalgia: a population-based study in Olmsted County, Minnesota, utilizing the Rochester Epidemiology Project. *Arthritis Care Res.* 2013;**65**(5):786–792.
23. Wingenfeld K, Heim C, Schmidt I, Wagner D, Meinlschmidt G, Hellhammer DH. HPA axis reactivity and lymphocyte glucocorticoid sensitivity in fibromyalgia syndrome and chronic pelvic pain. *Psychosom Med.* 2008;**70**(1):65–72.

CHAPTER 18

Infections

Jacob N. Ablin

Summary Points

- Various infectious agents have been traditionally linked to the pathogenesis of fibromyalgia syndrome (FMS) or have served as diagnostic confounders.
- Chronic viral infections such as hepatitis C and HIV are among the most established associations.
- Lyme disease has frequently been confused with FMS, but evidence to support a causative link is lacking.
- Antibiotic and antiviral treatment has generally not proven effective for FMS.
- New insights into the role of the gut microbiome and its relationship to the nervous system, including conditions such as FMS, may be elucidated in the future.

Similar to other triggers, which have been phenomenologic or simply temporally linked to FMS, infections have presented from an early stage in the development of the FMS concept as a possible trigger. Almost any clinician dealing with FMS patients should be familiar with the narrative according to which "everything began" right after suffering from an acute febrile illness, or from an ongoing low-grade fever. Specific infectious agents have waxed and waned in popularity as possible causative factors and attracted considerable amounts of public interest and publicity (e.g., Lyme disease). Nonetheless and most importantly, a direct cause and effect between FMS and infection is still largely undocumented, pathogenetic links remain speculative, and most importantly—no antimicrobial treatment has been established as a treatment for FMS. In this chapter, we try to compile existing knowledge regarding the possible links between FMS and infection, and point some attention at the most novel development in this story—the possible role of the gut microbiome.

EPSTEIN–BARR VIRUS AND OTHER MONONUCLEOSIS-LIKE INFECTIONS

The primary symptoms of FMS, muscular pain, and fatigue seem to overlap considerably with those of an extended viral infection and thus it is not surprising that viral agents such as Epstein–Barr virus (EBV) presented as "immediate suspects" in this context.

In one early study, Buchwald et al.[2] described 50 FMS patients displaying symptoms of "chronic Epstein–Barr virus infection," including sore throat, recurrent rash, adenopathy, and recurrent low-grade fever. Notably, all patients related a history of an acute onset characteristic of a viral disease—thus raising the clinical suspicion that FMS was indeed initiated by mononucleosis. Disappointingly, however, antibody titers to EBV were no different among these patients compared to controls. Another study looking for evidence of EBV infection among chronic fatigue syndrome (CFS) patients also failed to document serologic evidence of such infection.[28] On the other hand, Moldofsky,[17] one of the first developers of the FMS concept, reported the effect of acute viral infection on development of sleep disorders considered to be harbingers of FMS, while Glaser et al.[10] reported on the occurrence of stress-related changes in the expression of latent EBV as a possible mechanism for the development of CFS.

In a more recent study, levels of immunoglobulin G (IgG) antibodies against EBV were found to be correlated with pain intensity and associated symptoms in a group of 21 FMS patients while no evidence of IgM antibodies could be found.[21] Thus, taken together the actual evidence linking EBV infection to the development of FMS is rather weak and circumstantial, but as previously noted, clinical experience nonetheless tends to validate the concept that a certain percentage of individuals, exposed to an infectious trigger, will contract ongoing symptoms of pain and fatigue, while most others will not.

HEPATITIS C VIRUS

Hepatitis C virus (HCV) is another viral agent, which has attracted relatively much attention as a possible trigger for the development of FMS. This association was initially demonstrated in a study comparing 90 HCV patients to 128 healthy controls and 32 patients with non-HCV-related cirrhosis.[5] Fourteen HCV patients (16%) met American College of Rheumatology (ACR) FMS criteria as well as one of the cirrhotic patients, compared with none of the controls patients. Higher counts of tender points were also found among HCV patients.

In another study taking a different approach, HCV antibodies were compared between FMS patients and patients suffering from rheumatoid arthritis (RA).[22] HCV antibodies were found in 15.2% of FMS patients compared with 5.3% of RA patients, leading to the conclusion that HCV infection should be screened among patients diagnosed with FMS on a routine basis. FMS has also been included in the spectrum of rheumatologic manifestations of HCV infection, which might lead to an incorrect diagnosis of RA.[14] Thus, HCV workup appears to be called for in the context of various and multiple musculoskeletal symptoms. The association between HCV and FMS has however been disputed by a group from Spain who failed to find an association,[18] while Israeli researchers did find a high prevalence of FMS (16%) among HCV patients.[4] Most recently, Mohammad et al.[16] have reported a surprisingly high prevalence (57%) of FMS among chronic HCV patients; the reasons for this large spectrum of results are unclear and may reflect both geographical/ethnic differences and differences in patient populations and clinical characteristics.

Although the precise mechanisms through which chronic infection such as HCV might lead to hyperalgesia and eventually FMS remains incompletely understood is notable that HCV may act on glial cells as well as influencing various cytokines and cytokine receptors involved in the establishment of chronic pain.[25] As recently reviewed by Yarlott et al., mild cognitive impairment is common among HCV patients, and may be the result of the ability of HCV to cross the blood–brain barrier and causing neuroinflammation. Microglia, astrocytes, and endothelial cells may actually act as minor replication sites for HCV and might mediate some of these effects.[30] On a clinical basis, fatigue is a common and severe symptom of HCV infection and may not be correlated with the degree of viral load.[12] Depression and other psychiatric comorbidities are other well-known and frequent comorbidity of HCV (as well as a side effect of some antiviral medications such as interferon).[11] Last but not the least, inflammatory arthritis is another significant complication of HCV infection, which can lead to widespread pain and fatigue.[9] Thus, multiple pathways may converge in bringing about the link between HCV infection and FMS.

In contrast to the relatively many studies concerning the occurrence of FMS in the context of HCV, little has been reported regarding an association with HBV although one such report has been published.[1]

HIV AND FIBROMYALGIA SYNDROME

The clinical spectrum of HIV infection has evolved dramatically over the decades since its identification, to a large part due to the changes in treatment and survival. Nevertheless, since its initial recognition, HIV has frequently been associated with rheumatologic manifestations and FMS was relatively early on recognized as being part of the spectrum of such expressions. The prevalence of FMS among HIV patients has been estimated variously at rates ranging between 11% and 29%, comprising as much as 41% of musculoskeletal symptoms among these patients.[3,24] Evidently, these numbers stress the importance of recognizing FMS symptoms among HIV patients in order to avoid unnecessary extensive investigations and in order to offer optimal treatment to patients who currently may enjoy a near-normal life expectancy.

Interestingly, high rates of FMS (14% to 17%) continued to be documented among FMS patients even with the introduction of highly active antiretroviral treatment (HAART), associated with a dramatic improvement in prognosis.[15] Moreover, in a recent study, no correlation was found between either CD4 or viral load levels and symptoms of FMS.[8] Similar to the situation with HCV infection, the association between HIV and FMS may be partially mediated by the increased frequency of depression and anxiety among HIV patients.

LYME DISEASE

Lyme disease caused by *Borrelia burgdorferi* has been recognized as a confounder of FMS capable of causing overlapping symptoms such as diffuse pain, discognition, and fatigue. Due to the complex serologic diagnosis of Lyme disease, patients with a clinical presentation compatible with FMS may erroneously be labeled as suffering from chronic Lyme disease, especially in geographic areas where Lyme is endemic (and concerns about the disease are high). This misclassification has often led to patients being repeatedly treated with broad-spectrum antibiotics, in an attempt to eradicate Borreliosis, instead of being treated for FMS. Thus, in a study investigating 100 patients at a Lyme disease clinic, 25 patients were diagnosed with FMS, while only 3 were diagnosed with active Lyme disease and 17 with previous infection.[23] Moreover, in another study, even among patients with supposedly conclusive evidence of Lyme infection, FMS failed to improve in most cases following antibiotic treatment.[6] The relative futility of treating apparent FMS with broad-spectrum antibiotics in the context of suspected "post-Lyme" has been repeatedly demonstrated.

The most convincing evidence for the lack of an etiologic association between Lyme disease and FMS has been reported by Wormser et al.[29] These investigators evaluated 100 patients with a documented history of culture-confirmed Lyme disease and a mean follow-up of 15/4 years, for the occurrence of FMS. Only 1% (i.e., one patient) fulfilled diagnostic criteria for FMS in this cohort, a frequency clearly no higher than that expected in the general population.

Thus, although Lyme disease appears to act as confounder for FMS has frequently been discussed in the literature as a possible trigger, evidence to support such an association is lacking.

OTHER INFECTIONS

Ever-increasing lists of infectious agents have been occasionally and somewhat anecdotally linked to the development or exacerbation of FMS. *Mycoplasma* are agents capable of instigating chronic disease in humans including constitutive symptoms such as fatigue, following a more acute presentation which may include flu-like symptoms, fever, and adenopathy. In one study conducted among patients suffering from either FMS or CFS, PCR was conducted on circulating cells to identify *Mycoplasma pneumonia, Mycoplasma fermentans, Mycoplasma hominis*, and *Mycoplasma penetrans*. In this study, 30.8% of patients showed evidence of double infection and 22% of triple infection, with no control group reported.[19] Another study, however, found no evidence of *Mycoplasma* infection among 34 CFS patients, using *Mycoplasma* species-specific primer pairs for direct amplification of microbes from plasma DNA.[27] Moreover, a well-conducted therapeutic trial, conducted on patients diagnosed with the Gulf war syndrome, a clinical entity with considerable overlap with FMS and CFS failed to demonstrate clinical effectivity of 12 months of antibiotic treatment with doxycycline in patients with detectable blood *Mycoplasma* DNA.[7]

Additional infectious agents such as Parvovirus, Coxsackie, and chlamydia have been occasionally mentioned in the literature as being associated with FMS, but hard evidence is not available.

Building on the hypothesis that latent Herpes virus infection may play a role in the pathogenesis of FMS, presumably being reactivated through stress, Pridgen et al. have recently conducted a double-blind placebo-controlled study testing the efficacy of IMC-1, a combination drug including both a potent antiviral agent (famciclovir) and a cox-2 inhibitor (celecoxib) in the treatment of FMS.[20] In this study conducted on 143 patients, IMC-1 was shown to significantly decrease FMS-related pain and fatigue compared with placebo. Although this result was interpreted by the researchers as indicating the efficacy of antiviral treatment, the possible analgesic contribution of celecoxib is difficult to overlook and no evidence of actual HSV infection was documented. Thus, the actual link between HSV infection and FMS remains speculative.

WHAT ABOUT THE MICROBIOME?

As is evident from the aforementioned discussion, the current links between FMS and specific infection remain somewhat circumstantial and have hitherto not led to major breakthroughs in the treatment of the disorder. Nonetheless, a novel aspect of the relationship between FMS and microbes may be emerging. The gut microbiome is currently receiving huge attention as a possible ecologic system with far-reaching and very incompletely understood influences on many aspects of human biology and pathology. The microbiome is currently being linked to all parts of the nervous system, ranging from the enteric nervous system (ENS) and via the vagus nerve to the central nervous system (CNS) and is being ascribed a role in human behavior and emotion, as well as in pain processing. Irritable bowel syndrome (IBS), a functional disorder with great clinical and epidemiologic overlap with FMS, has recently been postulated to constitute a "microbiome–gut–brain axis disorder"[13] and one provocative case report has even described an FMS patient seemingly cured after self-administered fecal transplantation.[26] Thus, it stands to reason that in the near future, additional and fascinating data become available regarding the role of the gut microbiota in the pathogenesis of FMS and related disorders and the old "FMS-infection" paradigms may receive a substantial face-lift.

REFERENCES

1. Adak B, Tekeoglu I, Ediz L, et al. Fibromyalgia frequency in hepatitis B carriers. *J Clin Rheumatol.* 2005;**11**(3):157–159.
2. Buchwald D, Goldenberg DL, Sullivan JL, et al. The "chronic, active Epstein-Barr virus infection" syndrome and primary fibromyalgia. *Arthritis Rheum.* 1987;**30**(10):1132–1136.
3. Buskila D, Gladman DD, Langevitz P, Urowitz S, Smythe HA. Fibromyalgia in human immunodeficiency virus infection. *J Rheumatol.* 1990;**17**(9):1202–1206.
4. Buskila D, Shnaider A, Neumann L, et al. Musculoskeletal manifestations and autoantibody profile in 90 hepatitis C virus infected Israeli patients. *Semin Arthritis Rheum.* 1998;**28**(2):107–113.
5. Buskila D, Shnaider A, Neumann L, Zilberman D, Hilzenrat N, Sikuler E. Fibromyalgia in hepatitis C virus infection. Another infectious disease relationship. *Arch Intern Med.* 1997;**157**(21):2497–2500.
6. Dinerman H, Steere AC. Lyme disease associated with fibromyalgia. *Ann Intern Med.* 1992; **117**(4):281–285.
7. Donta ST, Engel CC Jr, Collins JF, et al.; VA Cooperative #475 Group. Benefits and harms of doxycycline treatment for Gulf War veterans' illnesses: a randomized, double-blind, placebo-controlled trial. *Ann Intern Med.* 2004;**141**(2):85–94.
8. Dotan I, Riesenberg K, Toledano R, Schlaeffer F, Smolyakov A, Saidel-Odes L. Prevalence and characteristics of fibromyalgia among HIV-positive patients in southern Israel. *Clin Exp Rheumatol.* 2015;34(2 Suppl 96):34–39.
9. Ferucci ED, Choromanski TL, Varney DT, et al. Prevalence and correlates of hepatitis C virus-associated inflammatory arthritis in a population-based cohort. *Semin Arthritis Rheum.* 2017;**47**(3):445–450.
10. Glaser R, Padgett DA, Litsky ML, et al. Stress-associated changes in the steady-state expression of latent Epstein-Barr virus: implications for chronic fatigue syndrome and cancer. *Brain Behav Immun.* 2005;**19**(2):91–103.
11. Häuser W, Holtmann G, Grandt D. Determinants of health-related quality of life in patients with chronic liver diseases. *Clin Gastroenterol Hepatol.* 2004;**2**(2):157–163.
12. Kallman J, O'Neil MM, Larive B, Boparai N, Calabrese L, Younossi ZM. Fatigue and health-related quality of life (HRQL) in chronic hepatitis C virus infection. *Dig Dis Sci.* 2007;**52**(10):2531–2539.
13. Kennedy PJ, Cryan JF, Dinan TG, Clarke G. Irritable bowel syndrome: a microbiome-gut-brain axis disorder? *World J Gastroenterol.* 2014;**20**(39):14105–14125.
14. Lovy MR, Starkebaum G, Uberoi S. Hepatitis C infection presenting with rheumatic manifestations: a mimic of rheumatoid arthritis. *J Rheumatol.* 1997;**23**(6):979–983.
15. Marquez J, Restrepo CS, Candia L, Berman A, Espinoza LR. Human immunodeficiency virus-associated rheumatic disorders in the HAART era. *J Rheumatol.* 2004;**31**(4):741–746.
16. Mohammad A, Carey JJ, Storan E, Scarry M, Coughlan RJ, Lee JM. Prevalence of fibromyalgia among patients with chronic hepatitis C infection: relationship to viral characteristics and quality of life. *J Clin Gastroenterol.* 2012;**46**(5):407–412.
17. Moldofsky H. Nonrestorative sleep and symptoms after a febrile illness in patients with fibrositis and chronic fatigue syndromes. *J Rheumatol Suppl.* 1989;**19**:150–153.
18. Narváez J, Nolla JM, Valverde-García J. Lack of association of fibromyalgia with hepatitis C virus infection. *J Rheumatol.* 2005;**32**(6):1118–1121.
19. Nasralla M, Haier J, Nicolson GL. Multiple mycoplasmal infections detected in blood of patients with chronic fatigue syndrome and/or fibromyalgia syndrome. *Eur J Clin Microbiol Infect Dis.* 1999;**18**(12):859–865.

20. Pridgen WL, Duffy C, Gendreau JF, Gendreau RM. A famciclovir + celecoxib combination treatment is safe and efficacious in the treatment of fibromyalgia. *J Pain Res.* 2017;**10**:451–460.
21. Reshkova V, Kalinova D, Milanov I. Evaluation of antiviral antibodies against Epstein-Barr Virus and neurotransmitters in patients with fibromyalgia. *J Neurol Neurosci.* 2015;**6**(3):1–4.
22. Rivera J, de Diego A, Trinchet M, García Monforte A. Fibromyalgia-associated hepatitis C virus infection. *Br J Rheumatol.* 1997;**36**(9):981–985.
23. Sigal LH. Summary of the first 100 patients seen at a Lyme disease referral center. *Am J Med.* 1990;**88**(6):577–581.
24. Simms RW, Zerbini CA, Ferrante N, Anthony J, Felson DT, Craven DE, Fibromyalgia syndrome in patients infected with human immunodeficiency virus. The Boston City Hospital Clinical AIDS Team. *Am J Med.* 1992;**92**(4):368–374.
25. Thompson ME, Barkhuizen A. Fibromyalgia, hepatitis C infection, and the cytokine connection. *Curr Pain Headache Rep.* 2003;**7**(5):342–347.
26. Thurm T, Ablin J, Buskila D, Maharshak N. Fecal microbiota transplantation for fibromyalgia: a case report and review of the literature. *Open J Gastroenterol.* 2017;**7**(04):131.
27. Vernon SD, Shukla SK, Reeves WC. Absence of Mycoplasma species DNA in chronic fatigue syndrome. *J Med Microbiol.* 2003;**52**(Pt 11):1027–1028.
28. Whelton CL, Salit I, Moldofsky H. Sleep, Epstein-Barr virus infection, musculoskeletal pain, and depressive symptoms in chronic fatigue syndrome. *J Rheumatol.* 1992;**19**(6):939–943.
29. Wormser GP, Weitzner E, McKenna D, Nadelman RB, Scavarda C, Farber S. Brief report: long-term assessment of fibromyalgia in patients with culture-confirmed Lyme disease. *Arthritis Rheum.* 2015;**67**(3):837–839.
30. Yarlott L, Heald E, Forton D. Hepatitis C virus infection, and neurological and psychiatric disorders—a review. *J Adv Res.* 2017;**8**(2):139–148.

CHAPTER 19

Central Nervous System Factors

Daniel J. Clauw

Summary Points

- The cardinal symptoms of fibromyalgia syndrome (FMS) include widespread pain, hyperresponsiveness to other sensory stimuli, as well as fatigue, sleep, memory, and mood disturbances. Some of these symptoms such as widespread pain could theoretically be due to a widespread or systemic effect on nociceptive processing, but the confluence of these symptoms strongly suggests the prominent involvement of the central nervous system (CNS) in FMS.
- Animal models demonstrate that all of the aforementioned symptoms, as well as evidence of central sensitization, can occur following the same types of trauma and adverse life experiences that are known to trigger or exacerbate FMS.
- The neurobiologic correlates of central sensitization including diffuse allodynia/hyperalgesia, hyperresponsiveness to other sensory stimuli, and neural hyperexcitability and hyperresponsiveness are all reproducibly identified in cohorts of individuals with FMS.
- When these CNS changes are targeted with pharmacologic or nonpharmacologic therapies known to be working in the CNS, the subset of individuals who has improvement in the cardinal symptoms of FMS has corresponding improvement in functional, chemical, and structural neuroimaging findings in the CNS. The "CNS theory" of FMS pathogenesis is the only one to have moved from early cross-sectional studies establishing *association* to subsequent longitudinal studies suggesting *causation*.

ANIMAL MODELS OF FIBROMYALGIA SYNDROME

Although few would purport that there is an animal model that mimics all of the key clinical features of FMS, nonetheless animal models can be very helpful in understanding the pathogenesis of this condition. This topic has been covered in depth in a recent review.[19] For example, arguably the biggest controversy in the field of pain is the relative contribution of peripheral versus central factors leading to chronic pain conditions. Some would argue that there must be some type of ongoing peripheral drive or input to cause chronic pain. This is almost certainly not the case. Animals develop the critical features of central sensitization or centralization of pain when exposed to swim stress, neonatal separation from their mothers, and many other non-painful stimuli.[1] All of these animal models can be instructive regarding the pathogenesis of FMS. Features of central sensitization and animal pain behaviors consistent with diffuse pain are also seen when CNS neurotransmitters are purposefully altered in the direction found in FMS. For example, chronic reserpine administration that depletes bioamines lead to features consistent with FMS, as does directly increasing glutamate levels in the insulae. This same model of increasing glutamate in the insulae was recently reverse-translated to show that the findings of FMS as well as "small fiber neuropathy" could be induced simply by increasing CNS insular glutamate, as is known to occur in FMS.[12]

EVIDENCE OF CENTRAL NERVOUS SYSTEM DISTURBANCES IN PAIN AND SENSORY PROCESSING IN FIBROMYALGIA SYNDROME

In humans, the physiologic hallmark of FMS, centralized pain, or central sensitization is augmented central pain processing. This was originally identified in FMS (and still can be clinical) by noting that an individual is diffusely tender to palpation. The scientific terms for this phenomenon are diffuse hyperalgesia (increased pain to normally painful stimuli) and/or allodynia (pain in response to normal nonpainful stimuli). In the absence of an identifiable diffuse "peripheral" inflammatory process involving the body tissues, this strongly suggests that the CNS (i.e., spinal cord and brain) is causing augmented pain processing. In 1990 when the original criteria for FMS were first published, this feature of diffuse tenderness was incorporated into the diagnostic criteria by requiring that an individual had a certain number of tender points (11 or greater) in addition to chronic widespread pain in order to qualify for this diagnosis. Subsequent studies using more sophisticated measures of experimental pain testing showed that individuals with FMS are more tender everywhere in the body, not just in the 18 regions considered to be "tender points."[18] Subsequent experimental pain-testing studies have identified multiple potential mechanisms that may be responsible for pain amplification in FMS, including a decrease in the activity of descending analgesic pathways, and an increase in facilitatory activity.[14]

Many studies have shown that this hyperresponsiveness to pain that is the hallmark of FMS is often or usually accompanied by hypersensitivity to other non-painful sensory stimuli. Gerster and Hadj-Djilani[4] were the first to demonstrate that FMS patients also display a low noxious threshold to auditory tones, and this finding was subsequently replicated by several other groups. However, both these studies used ascending measures of the auditory threshold, so these findings could theoretically be due to expectancy or hypervigilance. A subsequent study by Geisser et al.[3] presented auditory tones in a random and unpredictable manner to mitigate against these effects and showed that the FMS patients were hyperresponsive to auditory tones and that this did not appear to be driven by hypervigilance. This and other studies have also shown that when FMS patients are tested in response to multiple sensory stimuli, there is shared variance in hypersensitivity to these various stimuli, suggesting a common central mechanism. This is one of many findings that strongly suggest that the primary pathology in FMS is central and not peripheral (e.g., small fiber neuropathy), because it is difficult to conceive a peripheral mechanism that would drive these changes. Moreover, the insulae are known to be critical in the processing of all sensory stimuli, and functional, chemical, and structural neuroimaging studies have all suggested that this brain region is playing a key role across FMS and centralized pain states. This region has been noted to play a critical role in sensory integration, with the posterior insula serving a purer sensory role and being a strong indicator of the intensity of pain an individual is experiencing, whereas the anterior insula being associated with the emotional processing of sensations.[20,1]

These initial observations that individuals with FMS were diffusely tender led to subsequent functional, chemical, and structural brain neuroimaging studies that have been among the best "objective" evidence that the pain in FMS and related pain amplification syndrome is "real."[9] These methods such as functional MRI (fMRI) clearly demonstrate that when individuals with FMS are given a mild pressure or heat stimuli that most individuals would feel as "touch" rather than "pain," they experience pain, and similar brain activation patterns in brain areas involved in pain processing.[7]

A more recent advance in the use of fMRI is to look at the extent brain regions are "connected" to each other, that is, simultaneously activated (or deactivated). The advantage of resting state analysis is that it is a window into brain changes associated with chronic, ongoing spontaneous pain. Studies have shown that individuals with FMS have increased connectivity between brain regions involved in increasing pain transmission and neural networks not normally involved in pain such as the default mode network, and the degree of this hyper-connectedness is related to the severity of ongoing pain.[17] A different group has shown that during a painful stimulus, connectivity is decreased between key antinociceptive regions (e.g., the brainstem—the origin of descending analgesic pathways) and a region they had previously identified to be a potential source of dysfunctional pain inhibition in FMS.[13] López-Solà et al.[16] have performed imaging studies confirming quantitative sensory testing (QST) that these individuals are more sensitive to several sensory stimuli other than pain, and that machine learning paradigms can accurately distinguish FMS from non-FMS patients with more than 90% accuracy using these results.

Other imaging techniques have been used to identify the neurotransmitter abnormalities that may be "driving" the pain amplification seen in FMS and other chronic pain disorders. Wood et al.[21] used positron emission tomography (PET) to show that attenuated dopaminergic activity may be playing a role in pain transmission in FMS, and Harris et al.[8] showed evidence of decreased *mu* opioid receptor availability (possibly due to increased release of endogenous *mu* opioids) in FMS. This latter finding as well as previous studies showing increases in endogenous opioids in the cerebrospinal fluid (CSF) of FMS patients has been suggested as evidence of why opioid analgesics appear to not be efficacious in FMS.

Other groups have used proton magnetic resonance spectroscopy (H-MRS) to probe other neurotransmitters. Several groups have shown that there are increases in brain concentrations of the body's major excitatory neurotransmitter, glutamate, in pain-processing regions such as the insula in FMS.[11] This finding has also been noted in the CSF in FMS. Drugs such as pregabalin and gabapentin are likely working in part in FMS by reducing glutamatergic activity. This has been well demonstrated by Harris et al.[10] who showed that individuals with FMS who had the highest pretreatment levels of glutamate in the posterior insula were those most likely to respond to pregabalin. When pregabalin led to improvement in symptoms in these individuals, there was normalization of fMRI and connectivity findings, all suggesting that this neurotransmitter is playing a critical role in the pathogenesis of FMS in some individuals. An even more important finding from this study was the fact that individuals with FMS with normal or low baseline levels of glutamate in their posterior insula did not respond to pregabalin, even though this drug further lowered glutamate levels in these individuals as well. This helps us understand why no single class of CNS analgesic is likely to work in every patient with pain of CNS origin.

Conversely, H-MRS has recently been used to demonstrate low levels of one of the body's major inhibitory neurotransmitters, gamma-aminobutyric acid (γGABA).[2] This likely accounts for the efficacy of drugs such as gamma-hydroxybutyrate in FMS. This finding may also suggest biologic plausibility for the finding that FMS patients who have low alcohol consumption (compared to none or high) have fewer symptoms and better functionality.[15] Functional imaging studies have been instructive regarding how these comorbid mood disorders or cognitions may be influencing pain processing in FMS. fMRI undertaken on 30 FMS patients with variable levels of depression, with additional experimental pain testing investigated how the presence or absence of depression influenced pain report.[5] This study found that the level of depressive symptomatology did not influence the degree of neuronal activation in brain regions responsible for coding for the sensory intensity of pain, the primary and secondary somatosensory cortices. As expected, the depressed individuals did display greater activations in brain regions known to be responsible for the affective or cognitive processing of pain, such as the amygdala and insula. Another study with similar methodology examined how the presence or absence of catastrophizing might influence pain report in FMS.[6] In contrast to the aforementioned results, the presence of catastrophizing was associated with increased neuronal activations in the sensory coding regions. These studies thus provide empirical evidence for the value of treatments such as cognitive behavioral therapy. This is especially the case if individuals exhibit cognitions such as catastrophizing which, independent of other factors, may be capable of increasing pain intensity.

CONCLUSION

There is overwhelming evidence that the CNS is involved in the pathogenesis of FMS. Many if not most of the symptoms seen in FMS (hypersensitivity to multiple sensory stimuli, cognitive dysfunction, and sleep problems) could only be due to CNS abnormalities, and nearly all of the effective pharmacologic and nonpharmacologic therapies for FMS are thought to work primarily in the CNS. In fact, the neural signature of FMS on functional, chemical, and structural neuroimaging is becoming increasingly well understood. We certainly have much to learn about how these CNS symptoms originate, and how they interact with many other peripheral or systemic factors to cause symptoms.

REFERENCES

1. Craig AD. Human feelings: why are some more aware than others? *Trends Cogn Sci (Regul Ed)*. 2004;**8**(6):239–241.
2. Foerster BR, Petrou M, Edden RA, et al. Reduced insular γ-aminobutyric acid in fibromyalgia. *Arthritis Rheum*. 2012;**64**(2):579–583.
3. Geisser ME, Glass JM, Rajcevska LD, et al. A psychophysical study of auditory and pressure sensitivity in patients with fibromyalgia and healthy controls. *J Pain*. 2008;**9**(5):417–422.
4. Gerster JC, Hadj-Djilani A. Hearing and vestibular abnormalities in primary fibrositis syndrome. *J Rheumatol*. 1984;**11**(5):678–680.
5. Giesecke T, Gracely RH, Williams DA, et al. The relationship between depression, clinical pain, and experimental pain in a chronic pain cohort. *Arthritis Rheum*. 2005;**52**(5):1577–1584.
6. Gracely RH, Geisser ME, Giesecke T, et al. Pain catastrophizing and neural responses to pain among persons with fibromyalgia. *Brain*. 2004;**127**(Pt 4):835–843.
7. Gracely RH, Petzke F, Wolf JM, et al. Functional magnetic resonance imaging evidence of augmented pain processing in fibromyalgia. *Arthritis Rheum*. 2002;**46**(5):1333–1343.
8. Harris RE, Clauw DJ, Scott DJ, et al. Decreased central mu-opioid receptor availability in fibromyalgia. *J Neurosci*. 2007;**27**(37):10000–10006.
9. Harris RE, Clauw DJ. How do we know that the pain in fibromyalgia is "real"? *Curr Pain Headache Rep*. 2006;**10**(6):403–407.
10. Harris RE, Napadow V, Huggins JP, et al. Pregabalin rectifies aberrant brain chemistry, connectivity, and functional response in chronic pain patients. *Anesthesiology*. 2013;**119**(6):1453–1464.
11. Harris RE. Elevated excitatory neurotransmitter levels in the fibromyalgia brain. *Arthritis Res Ther*. 2010;**12**(5):141.
12. Harte SE, Ichesco E, Hampson JP, et al. Pharmacologic attenuation of cross-modal sensory augmentation within the chronic pain insula. *Pain*. 2016;**157**(9):1933–1945.
13. Jensen KB, Loitoile R, Kosek E, et al. Patients with fibromyalgia display less functional connectivity in the brain's pain inhibitory network. *Mol Pain*. 2012;**8**:32.
14. Julien N, Goffaux P, Arsenault P, et al. Widespread pain in fibromyalgia is related to a deficit of endogenous pain inhibition. *Pain*. 2005;**114**(1–2):295–302.

15. Kim CH, Vincent A, Clauw DJ, et al. Association between alcohol consumption and symptom severity and quality of life in patients with fibromyalgia. *Arthritis Res Ther*. 2013;**15**(2):R42.
16. López-Solà M, Woo CW, Pujol J, et al. Towards a neurophysiological signature for fibromyalgia. *Pain*. 2017;**158**(1):34–47.
17. Napadow V, LaCount L, Park K, et al. Intrinsic brain connectivity in fibromyalgia is associated with chronic pain intensity. *Arthritis Rheum*. 2010;**62**(8):2545–2555.
18. Petzke F, Gracely RH, Park KM, et al. What do tender points measure? Influence of distress on 4 measures of tenderness. *J Rheumatol*. 2003;**30**(3):567–574.
19. Sluka KA, Clauw DJ. Neurobiology of fibromyalgia and chronic widespread pain. *Neuroscience*. 2016;**338**:114–129.
20. Tracey I. Neuroimaging of pain mechanisms. *Curr Opin Support Palliat Care*. 2007;**1**(2):109–116.
21. Wood PB, Schweinhardt P, Jaeger E, et al. Fibromyalgia patients show an abnormal dopamine response to pain. *Eur J Neurosci*. 2007;**25**(12):3576–3582.

CHAPTER 20

Endogenous Pain Modulation: Effects of Physical Exercise, Cognitive Behavior Therapy, and Pharmacologic Treatments

Eva Kosek

Summary Points

- Fibromyalgia syndrome (FMS) is associated with increased pain sensitivity and reduced ability to recruit endogenous descending pain-inhibitory mechanisms.
- There are overlapping functional and structural changes in the brain of FMS patients, with longer pain duration associated with more severe changes.
- Ratings of depression/anxiety were not related to pain intensity, pain sensitivity, or cerebral pain processing indicating segregated mechanisms of mood and pain processing.
- The genetic polymorphism of the translocator protein (TSPO) gene (*rs6971*) was associated with pain severity and the affective–motivational components of cerebral pain processing.
- Exercise reduced pain, pain sensitivity, and normalized functional resting-state connectivity, but did not affect top-down pain modulation.
- Cognitive behavioral therapy (CBT) improved mood and increased the ability to activate cortical control mechanisms during pain stimulation in FMS patients, thus likely reducing the impact of pain experience.
- Milnacipran reduced pain, pain sensitivity, and increased cerebral pain-related activation within posterior cingulate/precuneus, that is, structures within the default mode network (DMN) in FMS responders.
- Pregabalin reduced pain, pain sensitivity as well as insular glutaminergic activity, and altered resting-state functional connectivity. Neuroimaging markers could predict subsequent analgesic response to pregabalin.

Despite evidence of peripheral aberrations such as muscle and peripheral nerve fiber pathology, FMS is generally regarded as a chronic pain syndrome characterized by dysfunctional endogenous pain modulation. Initial support for central nervous system (CNS) pathology came from behavioral studies demonstrating generalized, multimodal, increase in pain sensitivity, and enhanced temporal as well as spatial summation of nociceptive input when FMS patients were compared to healthy controls. Furthermore, dysfunctional descending pain inhibition affecting conditioning pain modulation (CPM) as well as exercise-induced hypoalgesia (EIH) has been documented in FMS. EIH is particularly interesting, as FMS patients typically report exacerbation of pain during and following physical activity. In accordance with clinical symptoms, FMS patients not only exhibited dysfunctional EIH, but actually reported a paradoxical increase in pain sensitivity during exercise, suggesting that descending pain facilitatory, possibly serotonergic, mechanisms were recruited.[14] However, despite reports of antagonistic interactions between serotonergic and opioid mechanisms, a recent study did not support altered interaction between serotonergic and opioid mechanisms as the basis for dysfunction of EIH in FMS patients.[20]

The behavior studies have been complemented with studies using imaging to assess cerebral pain processing. A recent meta-analysis of brain imaging validated the dysfunction of pain modulation in FMS, showing hypoactivity in the subgenual anterior cingulate cortex (sgACC) and the amygdala, together with hyperactivation of the insula during painful stimuli.[1] Furthermore, FMS patients had lower mu opioid receptor-binding potential (MOR BP) in brain areas implicated in pain-inhibitory networks and placebo analgesia, including rostral ACC (rACC).[3] Recently, Schrepf et al.[19] observed strong associations within-FMS patients between MOR BP and cerebral pain-related activations in rACC, posterior cingulate cortex (PCC), and medial frontal gyrus, which were related to pain intensity. More specifically, lower MOR BP was associated with weaker pain-related brain activations and higher ratings of pain affect. Based on these and previous data, showing high levels of endogenous opioids in the cerebrospinal fluid (CSF) of FMS patients, the authors suggested a model of affective pain dysregulation in FMS whereby initially high levels of tonic endogenous opioids lead to downregulation of MOR on GABAergic interneurons. Because the physiologic effect of MOR is to disinhibit GABAergic inhibitory neurons in rACC and periaqueductal gray (PAG)/brainstem thus activating descending pain-inhibitory mechanisms, the net effect would be a failure to activate descending pain inhibition during painful stimuli.

CEREBRAL PAIN PROCESSING IN FIBROMYALGIA SYNDROME

Given the importance of central mechanisms in FMS, a series of studies using functional magnetic resonance imaging (fMRI) to assess cerebral pain processing and to entangle the effects of genetics and several common treatment modalities on pain modulation were performed. Care was taken to consistently use the same protocol across these studies to enable comparisons (see Table 20.1 for summary). In addition, individually calibrated pain stimuli were used in the scanner to compare pain processing during the same relative pain intensity across subjects and studies. Thumb pressure pain stimuli, carefully calibrated to correspond with every subject's pain intensity rated as 50 mm on a 100-mm visual analog scale (P50), were used and contrasted with non-painful pressure (50 kPa) to assess pain-related brain activations. The stimuli were randomly applied during the fMRI scanning, thus preventing subjects from anticipating the onset time or type of stimuli. As FMS patients have increased pain sensitivity, this meant that on average lower absolute pressure stimuli were used in FMS patients compared to healthy controls.[5] Despite the lower pressure applied in patients, no group differences were found regarding pain-related activations in brain regions associated with sensory-discriminative or affective/motivational aspects of pain processing, revealing amplification of nociceptive input. However, during painful stimulation, FMS patients failed to activate the primary link in the descending pain regulatory system, that is, the rACC, as well as other structures implicated in pain regulation such as thalamus and brainstem.[5] Furthermore, FMS patients had reduced coherent activation among pain-related brain regions. More specifically, reduced pain-related functional connectivity between rACC and PAG/brainstem, rACC and amygdala, rACC and hippocampus as well as between thalamus and orbitofrontal cortex (OBFC) was found in FMS patients.[7] Finally, also structural cerebral abnormalities such as reduced volumes of rACC, OBFC, and amygdala were found,[10] in agreement with previous studies. The cerebral findings were thus in accordance with the results from previous behavior studies revealing a dysfunction of descending pain modulation in FMS patients.

TABLE 20.1 **Summary of FMS treatment studies using the same evoked pressure pain fMRI protocol**

	Clinical improvement	Pain	Pain sensitivity	Peripheral effects	Cerebral effects
Exercise	✓	✓	✓	✓	✓
CBT	✓	**No**	**No**	—	✓
Milnacipran	✓	✓	✓	—	✓

Strengthening exercise twice/week for 15 weeks resulted in clinical improvement; reduced pain and pain sensitivity (n = 130);[15] had beneficial effects on muscle metabolism, which was related to reduced pain (n = 29); normalized cerebral resting-state activity (n = 14);[2] and improved cognitive functioning (n = 19),[17] but did not affect cerebral pain processing (n = 19). CBT for 12 weeks resulted in clinical improvement and activation of cortical control mechanisms likely involved in the reappraisal of pain, but did not affect pain intensity or pain sensitivity (n = 43).[6] Responders to 12 weeks of milnacipran treatment reported clinical improvement, reduced pain intensity and sensitivity, as well as positive effects on top-down pain inhibitory networks or the default mode network during evoked pain (n = 21).[8] Peripheral muscle effects were not assessed following CBT or milnacipran treatment. Note that a responder/nonresponder analysis was only performed in the Milnacipran study and that the results of the exercise and CBT study might have been different if several subjects would allow for a similar responder/nonresponder analysis. CBT, cognitive behavioral therapy; FMS, fibromyalgia syndrome; fMRI, functional magnetic resonance imaging.

Disturbed mood is frequently found in FMS patients and therefore it is of interest to study if psychologic symptoms influence cerebral pain processing. A large cohort of FMS patients ($n = 83$) was used to assess the effects of depressive symptoms, anxiety, and catastrophizing on pain symptoms and general health status as well as on pressure pain sensitivity (P50) and cerebral processing of pressure pain using the fMRI.[9] A large variability was found in the ratings of depressive symptoms on the Beck Depression Inventory (BDI), ranging from what is generally regarded as no depression (BDI ≤ 0 to 9) to severe depression (BDI ≥ 29). Ratings of depression, anxiety, and catastrophizing scores were highly intercorrelated and patients with high ratings of depression or anxiety rated worse general health. However, no correlation was found between the ratings of depression or anxiety and clinical pain or pain sensitivity (P50). Furthermore, pain-related cerebral activation was not modulated by depressive symptoms, anxiety, or catastrophizing indicating partially segregated mechanisms for the processing of nociceptive stimuli and negative affect.[9]

Effects of Pain Duration

FMS is often regarded as an extreme end in a continuum of chronic pain characterized by central sensitization. This view is supported by the fact that more than 80% of FMS patients suffer from localized/regional pain for many years before developing the generalized pain of FMS. Furthermore, regional pain was identified as the main risk factor for the development of widespread pain in prospective studies. Hypothetically, long-term activation of endogenous pain inhibitory mechanisms, as a consequence of living with intractable pain for many years, would lead to a progressive dysfunction of these systems in susceptible individuals. If this hypothesis was true, then more pronounced pain symptoms as well as changes in structure and function in pain-related brain regions would be expected in individuals with long pain duration. Supporting the hypothesis of disease progression, increased pain intensity as well as pressure pain sensitivity was found to be associated with longer duration of FMS.[10] In addition, longer FMS duration was related to widespread reductions in cerebral gray and white matter volumes, as well as significantly smaller rACC and OBFC volumes with the same trend seen for amygdala (although not statistically significant). In the rACC, a distinct overlap was found among decreased cortical thickness, decreased brain volume, and a decrease in functional regional coherence.[10] The findings that pain, pain sensitivity, and rACC atrophy were all associated with FMS duration suggesting that disruptions in endogenous pain modulation were central for the development and maintenance of pain in FMS. The rACC is rich in MOR and the net result of MOR activation in rACC is descending pain inhibition (by inhibiting GABAergic inhibitory neurons). Therefore, the results would be in accordance with a gradual downregulation of MOR in rACC as a consequence of initially high levels of tonic endogenous opioids, as suggested.[19] Thus, an activation of endogenous opioidergic pain inhibitory mechanisms in response to pain, although beneficial short term, could hypothetically have detrimental long-term effects aggravating the painful condition in susceptible individuals.

Effects of Genetics

Although more than 80% of FMS patients initially suffer from regional pain, it must be remembered that only a minority of patients suffering from localized/regional pain eventually develop FMS. Therefore, it is important to investigate factors that could potentially explain the differences in individual susceptibility to FMS and affect the severity of FMS symptoms. An overview of genetic factors affecting individual susceptibility is described in Chapter 16. Recently, a genetic polymorphism of the TSPO (*rs6971*) was associated with pain and other FMS symptoms, as well as cerebral pain processing.[12] TSPO expression is normally low in the brain, but is upregulated during glia activation. TSPO controls expression of interleukin (IL)-8 as well as its receptor, thus affecting IL-8-mediated glia-to-neuron signaling and thereby central sensitization. The latter is underscored by findings of elevated IL-8 in the CSF of patients suffering from FMS, but not rheumatoid arthritis,[11] a condition where descending pain inhibitory mechanisms are normal. The *rs6971* polymorphism regulates binding affinity to the TSPO. FMS patients with genetically inferred TSPO high-affinity binding (HAB) had more pain and more pronounced FMS symptoms compared to intermediate- and low-affinity binders (ILAB).[12] Furthermore, HAB binders had a greater pain-related functional connectivity within the frontoparietal network, a network mainly implicated in the anticipation and appraisal of pain. The data indicated that TSPO-related mechanisms were relevant for anticipatory and affective–motivational components of cerebral pain processing in FMS, rather than the sensory aspects, as no effect on pain sensitivity was seen.

In addition to the IL-8-related mechanisms, TSPO is also implicated in pain modulation by acting as a rate-limiting step for neurosteroid synthesis. Neurosteroids affect synaptic transmission through GABAergic mechanisms acting either as agonists, having analgesic effects, or as antagonists with algesic effects. Serotonergic mechanisms affect the proportions of analgesic/algesic neurosteroids produced. When investigating gene-to-gene interactions between the TSPO polymorphism and the functional polymorphism of the gene-regulating expression of the serotonin transporter (SERT; *5-HTTLPR/rs25531*) and thus serotonin metabolism, a significant gene-to-gene interaction was found.[12] In FMS patients with genetically inferred TSPO HAB, high or intermediate SERT expression (approximately 75% of the population) conferred higher pain intensities, whereas TSPO HAB with genetically inferred low SERT expression had lower pain intensities compared to low/intermediate TSPO affinity binders. The data thus indirectly support the role of neurosteroids in FMS pathology.[12] As neurosteroid regulation has been proposed to be a mechanism of action of antidepressants and because new neurosteroid-acting compounds are currently under development for the treatment of pain and anxiety, a better understanding of these mechanisms regarding the regulation of mood and pain, respectively, is needed, as these rely on segregated mechanisms in FMS.[9]

Implications for Treatment Strategies

Individualized medicine is desirable, but rests on the so far unattainable goal of reliable pretreatment identification of responders. However, with increasing efforts within this research area, certain factors related to pain processing have been identified as predicting treatment outcome. As mentioned earlier, longer pain duration was associated with increased pain, hyperalgesia as well as structural and functional brain pathology, such as deterioration of endogenous pain inhibition.[10] Therefore, it would be expected that shorter pain duration would be favorable for positive treatment outcomes. In support of this notion, short pain duration was the only predictor for a positive response to milnacipran treatment.[8] In addition, short pain duration as well as large variability in pain intensity and low ratings of depression/anxiety predicted positive placebo response in the same randomized controlled trial (RCT).[13] A conjunction analysis of the milnacipran and placebo responders following treatment revealed increased overlapping pain-related activity in amygdala, a pain-defensive region implicated in the motivational/affective aspects of pain inhibition. Unfortunately, the association between pain duration and amygdala activation was not specifically investigated. High variability in pain ratings, that is, a large difference between maximal and minimal ratings of pain intensity on a visual analogue scale (VASmax–VASmin), would suggest better functioning endogenous pain modulation, which could potentially explain the better placebo response.[13] Patients with less negative affect at baseline would also be more likely to expect a positive treatment outcome, thus promoting placebo response, but in accordance with previous research, pretreatment mood did not affect the response to milnacipran.[8] In addition, there is evidence that baseline resting-state functional connectivity measures, fMRI blood oxygenation level dependent testing, and MR spectroscopy can be potentially useful tools to predict FMS treatment response to milnacipran[18] and pregabalin[4] (see the following section). Finally, genotyping could become a valuable tool for individualized medicine in the future. Based on the data regarding gene-to-gene interactions between TSPO and SERT, the most likely responders to selective serotonin reuptake inhibitor/serotonin-noradrenalin reuptake inhibitor (SSRI/SNRI) treatment regarding pain relief would hypothetically be found among FMS patients with the TSPO HAB genotype.[12]

TREATMENT EFFECTS

Exercise

Exercise is the only treatment that received a "strong for" recommendation in the new European FMS treatment guidelines.[16] Good effects have been shown for aerobic as well as strengthening exercise, although the mechanisms of action are not well understood. In a multicenter study where FMS patients were randomized to a 15-week strengthening exercise program or relaxation exercise (controls) both interventions supervised by a physiotherapist twice per week, we found a positive effect of the strengthening exercise on pain, function, and strength.[15] As expected, FMS patients exhibited reduced EIH compared to controls before the intervention, that is, they did not have a normal inhibition of pain sensitivity during static muscular contractions. Contrary to the hypothesis, that exercise can reduce pain in FMS by improving the function of EIH, no improvement of EIH was seen following the intervention (Martinsen et al., in manuscript[17]). These results were in accordance with the fMRI data, showing that when patients were compared before and after the 15-week exercise intervention, no differences in the cerebral processing of painful pressure stimuli were found, although reduced sensitivity to pressure pain was seen following the intervention (Martinsen et al., in manuscript[17]).

Although the strengthening exercise intervention did not affect cerebral pain processing, beneficial cognitive effects as well as a normalization of resting-state activity were seen following the intervention. More specifically, improved executive function reflected as increased processing speed and reduced inference inhibition during the Stroop color-word test was seen, leading to a normalization of the initially impaired cognitive performance in the FMS cohort following the intervention.[17] When cerebral activations during the Stroop paradigm were investigated with fMRI (BOLD), increased bilateral amygdala activations were found following exercise compared to baseline.[17] Regarding resting state, a decreased connectivity between pain-related and sensorimotor brain areas, such as the insula and primary sensorimotor cortex was seen in FMS patients compared to healthy controls at baseline, but this had normalized following the exercise intervention.[2] However, because the changes in resting-state activity did not correlate with any behavior parameters, these results need to be interpreted with caution. In conclusion, the findings indicated that the 15-week strengthening exercise intervention reduced pain and pain sensitivity, but this was not mediated by improved function of descending pain inhibitory mechanisms. Rather, the reduced pain and also the indirectly improved cognitive function could be secondary to the beneficial effects of exercise on peripheral mechanisms, such as muscle pathology (see Chapter 22).

Cognitive Behavior Therapy

Cognitive behavior therapy in general and acceptance commitment therapy (ACT) in particular is currently used in isolation, or as part of multimodal programs to treat chronic pain. The aim of ACT is to encourage patients to pursue valued activities and long-term goals, despite pain and distress, by encouraging acceptance of negative thoughts, emotions, and pain rather than trying to avoid them. The goal is to improve function and quality of life by encouraging exposure to valued activities in life and thus reduce the mental focus on the pain experience. Previous studies, mostly in psychiatric cohorts suffering from depression/anxiety, demonstrated that CBT modifies dysfunctional cognitive and emotional processing by increasing executive control. However, a previous study revealed segregated mechanism of mood and pain modulation in FMS, that is, the degree of rated anxiety and depression was not associated with the degree of clinical pain, pain sensitivity, and cerebral pain processing.[9] Therefore, a mechanistic fMRI study was performed to disentangle the actions of CBT on mood and pain and to assess the effect of CBT on cerebral pain processing in FMS patients. Patients were randomized to a group-based, 12-week ACT program or waiting list controls and cerebral processing (fMRI) of evoked pain was assessed before and following treatment.[6] Compared to waiting list controls, ACT-treated patients reported larger clinical improvement on the patient global impression of change (PGIC) as well as larger reductions of rated depression and anxiety, but no effect was seen regarding pain or pain sensitivity. Increased pain-related activation of brain structures implicated in executive cognitive control, that is, the ventrolateral prefrontal cortex (vlPFC) and OBFC was seen in the ACT-treated patients, but not in controls. Furthermore, the increase in pain-related vlPFC activation following ACT correlated with reduced anxiety. Finally, ACT-treated patients also displayed an increased pain-evoked functional connectivity between the vlPFC and thalamus after treatment, indicating that the connectivity between crucial nodes in the pain modulatory network was significantly changed, despite the fact that ACT had no effects on clinical pain or pain sensitivity.[6] The data indicated that in response to ACT treatment, FMS patients activated cortical control mechanisms leading to an altered cerebral loop among pain signals, emotions, and cognitions with increased access to executive regions for reappraisal of pain. The treatment-related changes correlated with reductions in anxiety, but not with reduced pain or pain sensitivity, thus consolidating the findings of segregated modulation of mood and pain in FMS.[9]

Serotonin–Noradrenalin Reuptake Inhibitors

Serotonin–noradrenalin reuptake inhibitors, that is, milnacipran and duloxetine, constitute one category of drugs that are indicated for the treatment of FMS, the other being anticonvulsants (pregabalin). SNRIs have been shown to reduce pain in FMS independently of their antidepressive and anxiolytic effects, which is in accordance with our finding of segregated mechanisms for the modulation of pain and mood in FMS.[9] Several mechanisms have been proposed to explain the analgesic effects of antidepressants, such as peripheral antinociceptive effects and altered central pain modulation. The elevated concentrations of proinflammatory substances in the CSF of FMS patients suggest glia activation, which would lead to an upregulation of TSPO resulting in increased neurosteroid synthesis. As antidepressants have anti-inflammatory effects and through their effect on serotonin metabolism also regulate the balance between the synthesis of analgesic and algesic neurosteroids, favoring the former, these central mechanisms could also be of importance. In patients with neuropathic pain, duloxetin was associated with improved function of conditioned pain modulation (CPM) and poor CPM at baseline was predictive of a positive treatment response. Furthermore, better pain relief in FMS patients following milnacipran, but not placebo treatment for 6 weeks was associated with lower baseline resting-state functional connectivity between insular cortex and rACC as well as insular cortex and PAG.[18] Hypothetically, patients with reduced resting-state connectivity between brain regions involved in pro- and antinociceptive actions, could be those with reduced CPM, and thus benefit more from a treatment improving the function of CPM.

In order to study the mechanistic effects of SNRIs in FMS, we set out to study the cerebral effects of milnacipran, one of the two SNRI drugs currently indicated for FMS treatment, using the fMRI methodology described earlier. A multicenter, randomized, double-blind, placebo-controlled study of the effects of 12 weeks of milnacipran 100 mg b.i.d. was performed.[8] Patients were randomized to placebo or milnacipran treatment and examined regarding clinical parameters, pressure pain sensitivity, and cerebral pain processing (fMRI BOLD) before and following the treatment. In order to disentangle the mechanisms of action related to pain relief following SNRI treatment in FMS responder, nonresponder analysis was performed. Milnacipran responders had reduced pressure pain sensitivity and increased activation of PCC and precuneus following treatment, which was not seen in placebo responders or milnacipran nonresponders (Fig. 20.1). Furthermore, the increased pain-related activation of PCC/precuneus following milnacipran treatment was associated with the degree of favorable clinical response, such as pain relief and reduced pressure pain intensity. Thus, our results revealed a graded effect of milnacipran response and PCC/precuneus activity, with strong treatment effects corresponding to large increases in PCC activity, moderate effects to moderate increases in PCC activity, and so on (Fig. 20.1). Furthermore, we found a correlation between the antihyperalgesic effect of milnacipran and increased PCC activity specifically in milnacipran responders. The PCC is a core hub in the DMN, a set of brain regions forming an intrinsic network characterized by synchronized spontaneous signal fluctuations related to self-referential mental processes. DMN activity has been shown to decrease during goal-directed behaviors, such as focusing on specific tasks or processing painful stimuli. Disruptions in the DMN have been reported in acute as well as chronic pain and recurrent episodes of acute pain might induce long-term changes in the function of the DMN. Therefore, pain relief resulting in less-directed focus on pain would be expected to result in enhanced DMN activity, as has been shown previously in FMS patients. Further support for the involvement of structures forming part of the DMN in milnacipran treatment effects come from results showing that higher baseline resting-state connectivity between PCC/precuneus and amygdala predicted pain relief following 6-week milnacipran treatment in FMS patients.[18]

The positive drug effect was specifically related to the increase in PCC/precuneus activity, as this was not found in milnacipran nonresponders thus offsetting a nonspecific drug-related effect of milnacipran, nor in placebo responders, thus not related to improvement as such. Contrary to our expectations, the fMRI data did not support that the effects of milnacipran were mediated by normalized pain-related activations in

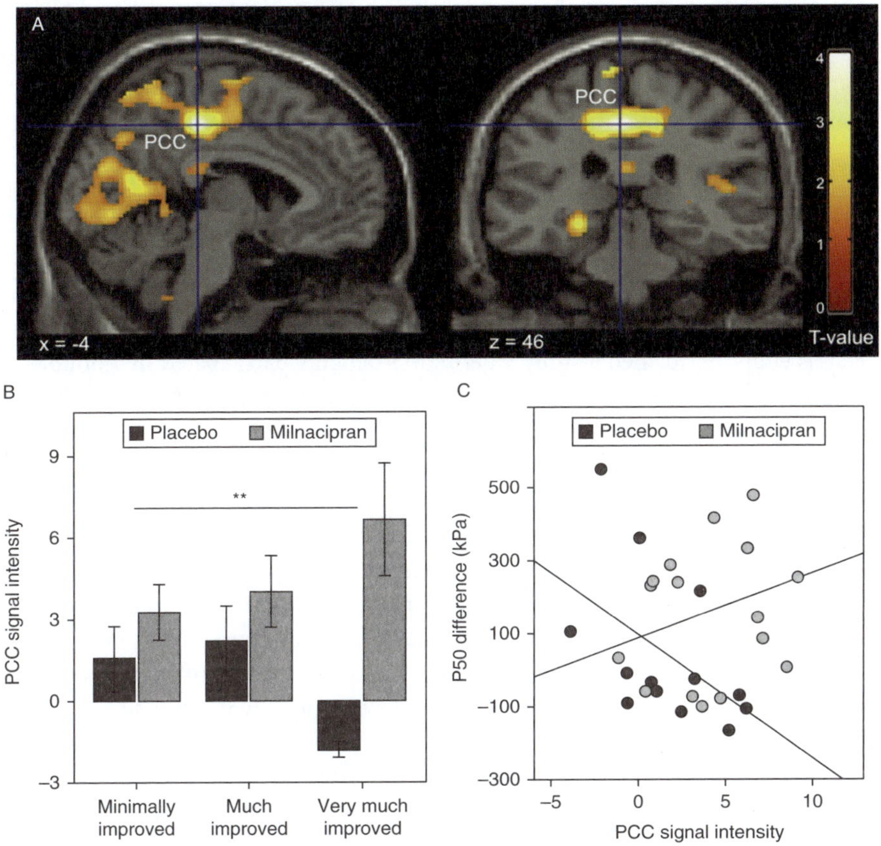

FIGURE 20.1 Posttreatment fMRI and brain activations for different degrees of treatment response. **A**: The anatomic region where pain-evoked brain activity was higher in milnacipran responders, compared to placebo responders, after treatment. The cluster is located in the posterior cingulum. **B**: Pain-evoked signal intensity in the posterior cingulum after treatment in milnacipran responders and placebo responders, clustered according to the magnitude of clinical improvement, rated by PGIC. **Significant main effect of treatment on posterior cingulum activity. **C**: Correlation between pain-evoked signal intensity in the posterior cingulum after treatment and the difference in experimental pain tolerance, calculated as post- minus pre-P50 values. fMRI, functional magnetic resonance imaging; PCC, posterior cingulate cortex; PGIC, patient global impression of change. (From Jensen KB, Petzke F, Carville S, et al. Segregating the cerebral mechanisms of antidepressants and placebo in fibromyalgia. *J Pain*. 2014;15[12]:1328–1337.)

brain regions pertaining to the pain-inhibitory network, that is, rACC, thalamus, and PAG, previously shown to be dysfunctional in FMS. Using the same method of pain stimuli as in our studies, Schrepf et al.[19] demonstrated a positive association between pain-related activation (fMRI BOLD) and MOR BP (PET) in the PCC of FMS subjects. Furthermore, these measures were inversely related to affective/sensory pain ratios of the pressure stimuli, indicating a role of PCC in pain processing related to opioidergic mechanisms in FMS. However, as milnacipran treatment did not affect other areas with high MOR concentrations, such as the rACC, the effect of milnacipran seen in our study was not likely mediated by generalized MOR-dependent mechanisms.

Pregabalin

The second category of drugs indicated for FMS treatment are the anticonvulsants, that is, pregabalin and gabapentin. These drugs bind to the α2δ-subunit of voltage-gated calcium channels and the proposed mode of action is that they reduce synaptic release of glutamate through inhibition of calcium influx into presynaptic neurons. Harris et al.[4] performed a study where FMS patients participated in a double-blind, crossover, placebo-controlled study assessing the effects of 14 days of pregabalin treatment (450 mg/day) on symptoms and cerebral mechanisms. The patients were assessed by fMRI (BOLD and functional connectivity) and proton magnetic resonance spectroscopy (MRS) before and following each treatment. In a previous MRS study, elevated insular glutaminergic activity was reported in FMS patients compared to healthy controls. In the present study, pregabalin treatment reduced insular glutaminergic activity and this was related to reduced pressure pain sensitivity. Furthermore, reduced resting-state functional connectivity between insula and parts of the DMN were seen following pregabalin treatment and were associated with reduced clinical pain ratings. Interestingly, greater pressure pain-related deactivations (BOLD) were seen in the inferior parietal lobule and the PCC following pregabalin treatment. Finally, the baseline values for all three neuroimaging markers predicted subsequent analgesic response to pregabalin but not placebo.

CONCLUSIONS

There is convincing evidence of a generalized increase in pain sensitivity as well as aberrant endogenous pain modulation in FMS. Our treatment studies using the same imaging protocol (see Table 20.1) support the rationale of using a combination of therapies in severe cases of FMS, thereby activating different and complementary pain-relieving mechanisms. There is a need for further studies regarding individualized treatment of FMS, that is, matching each patient with the most beneficial combination of treatments for that particular patient.

REFERENCES

1. Dehghan M, Schmidt-Wilcke T, Pfleiderer B, et al. Coordinate-based (ALE) meta-analysis of brain activation in patients with fibromyalgia. *Hum Brain Mapp*. 2016;**37**(5):1749–1758.
2. Flodin P, Martinsen S, Mannerkorpi K, et al. Normalization of aberrant resting state functional connectivity in fibromyalgia patients following a three month physical exercise therapy. *Neuroimage Clin*. 2015;**9**:134–139.

3. Harris RE, Clauw DJ, Scott DJ, McLean SA, Gracely RH, Zubieta JK. Decreased central mu-opioid receptor availability in fibromyalgia. *J Neurosci*. 2007;**27**(37):10000–10006.
4. Harris RE, Napadow V, Huggins JP, et al. Pregabalin rectifies aberrant brain chemistry, connectivity, and functional response in chronic pain patients. *Anesthesiology*. 2013;**119**(6):1453–1464.
5. Jensen KB, Kosek E, Petzke F, et al. Evidence of dysfunctional pain inhibition in Fibromyalgia reflected in rACC during provoked pain. *Pain*. 2009;**144**(1–2):95–100.
6. Jensen KB, Kosek E, Wicksell R, et al. Cognitive Behavioral Therapy increases pain-evoked activation of the prefrontal cortex in patients with fibromyalgia. *Pain*. 2012;**153**(7):1495–1503.
7. Jensen KB, Loitoile R, Kosek E, et al. Patients with fibromyalgia display less functional connectivity in the brain's pain inhibitory network. *Mol Pain*. 2012;**8**:32.
8. Jensen KB, Petzke F, Carville S, et al. Segregating the cerebral mechanisms of antidepressants and placebo in fibromyalgia. *J Pain*. 2014;**15**(12):1328–1337.
9. Jensen KB, Petzke F, Carville S, et al. Anxiety and depressive symptoms in fibromyalgia are related to poor perception of health but not to pain sensitivity or cerebral processing of pain. *Arthritis Rheum*. 2010;**62**(11):3488–3495.
10. Jensen KB, Srinivasan P, Spaeth R, et al. Overlapping structural and functional brain changes in patients with long-term exposure to fibromyalgia pain. *Arthritis Rheum*. 2013;**65**(12):3293–3303.
11. Kosek E, Altawil R, Kadetoff D, et al. Evidence of different mediators of central inflammation in dysfunctional and inflammatory pain–interleukin-8 in fibromyalgia and interleukin-1 β in rheumatoid arthritis. *J Neuroimmunol*. 2015;**280**:49–55.
12. Kosek E, Martinsen S, Gerdle B, et al. The translocator protein gene is associated with symptom severity and cerebral pain processing in fibromyalgia. *Brain Behav Immun*. 2016;**58**:218–227.
13. Kosek E, Rosen A, Carville S, et al. Lower placebo responses after long-term exposure to fibromyalgia pain. *J Pain*. 2017;**18**(7):835–843.
14. Lannersten L, Kosek E. Dysfunction of endogenous pain inhibition during exercise with painful muscles in patients with shoulder myalgia and fibromyalgia. *Pain*. 2010;**151**(1):77–86.
15. Larsson A, Palstam A, Löfgren M, et al. Resistance exercise improves muscle strength, health status and pain intensity in fibromyalgia—a randomized controlled trial. *Arthritis Res Ther*. 2015;**17**:161.
16. Macfarlane GJ, Kronisch C, Dean LE, et al. EULAR revised recommendations for the management of fibromyalgia. *Ann Rheum Dis*. 2017;**76**(2):318–328.
17. Martinsen S, Flodin P, Berrebi J, et al. The role of long-term physical exercise on performance and brain activation during the Stroop Color Word Task in fibromyalgia patients. *Clin Physiol Function Imag*. 2017. doi:10.1111/cpf.12449.
18. Schmidt-Wilcke T, Ichesco E, Hampson JP, et al. Resting state connectivity correlates with drug and placebo response in fibromyalgia patients. *Neuroimage Clin*. 2014;**6**:252–261.
19. Schrepf A, Harper DE, Harte SE, et al. Endogenous opioidergic dysregulation of pain in fibromyalgia: a PET and fMRI study. *Pain*. 2016;**157**(10):2217–2225.
20. Tour J, Löfgren M, Mannerkorpi K, et al. Gene-to-gene interactions regulate endogenous pain modulation in fibromyalgia patients and healthy controls-antagonistic effects between opioid and serotonin-related genes. *Pain*. 2017;**158**(7):1194–1203.

CHAPTER 21

Small Nerve Fiber Pathology

Nurcan Üçeyler and Claudia Sommer

Summary Points

- Small nerve fibers comprise A-delta and C-nerve fibers with distinct subpopulations.
- Small fiber assessment requires investigations at multiple levels using special small fiber tests.
- Currently, there is no gold standard for the diagnosis of small fiber pathology.
- Small fiber impairment and pathology of so far unknown pathophysiologic impact on pain has been found in subgroups of patients with fibromyalgia syndrome (FMS).
- Future studies are needed and ongoing to decipher the underlying mechanisms.

SMALL NERVE FIBERS AND THEIR ASSESSMENT

Peripheral nerves are classified according to their myelination, diameter, and conduction velocity. The thinly myelinated A-delta fibers and the unmyelinated C-fibers are collectively named "small fibers." Among these, there are subtypes with various functions.[23] In the skin, they conduct sensations such as temperature, pain, itch, and pleasant touch.[33] The autonomic innervation of sweat glands and blood vessels is also provided by small nerve fibers. Their neurons are located in the dorsal root ganglia (DRG), the central axons terminate in lamina I and II of the spinal cord dorsal horn. In the skin, the peripheral endings can be visualized by immunostaining,[15] intra- and subepidermal nerve fibers as well as sweat gland and blood vessel innervation can be quantified. Skin punch biopsies should be obtained from standardized sites like the lateral lower and upper leg, for which published normative values are available. Mostly, skin punch biopsy specimens are immunoreacted with antibodies to the pan-axonal marker protein gene product 9.5 (PGP9.5).[16,19] Fiber subclasses such as peptidergic, cholinergic, and adrenergic nerve fibers can be differentiated by immunohistochemistry.[25]

Quantitative sensory testing (QST) is a psychophysical method used to investigate the function of different afferent nerve fibers and their central connections. Following the standardized protocol of the German Research Network of Neuropathic Pain (Deutscher Forschungsverbund Neuropathischer Schmerz [DFNS]), a reproducible sensory profile of the subject can be obtained.[30] This protocol consists of 13 individual tests that include the determination of thermal and mechanical perception and pain thresholds. The typical finding in patients with pathologic small fiber function is an increase in thermal perception thresholds.

Autonomic function tests can assess sudomotor, adrenergic, and cardiovagal autonomic functions. For example, the quantitative sudomotor axon reflex test (QSART) allows the quantification of sweating at standardized skin sites after stimulation by iontophoresis. Established tests of adrenergic and cardiovagal dysautonomia are the heat-up tilt test, the assessment of the blood pressure, and the heart rate response to the Valsalva maneuver or the examination of heart rate variation.[22]

Standard neurophysiologic tests target large nerve fibers only.[17] Microneurography can be used to record from cutaneous afferents directly and to determine their electrophysiologic properties.[3] After placing a fine needle electrode into a peripheral nerve (e.g., the peroneal nerve) and thermal or mechanical stimulation in the receptive field, individual action potentials can be recorded and analyzed in vivo from single nerve fibers. Sophisticated software has helped to facilitate the method, but subjects still need to cooperate for several hours.[34]

Evoked potentials can be recorded after selective stimulation of the small nerve fibers, and can thus be used to assess their function and that of their central connections. Stimulation can be performed by laser (laser-evoked potentials [LEP]),[1] contact heat (contact heat-evoked potentials [CHEP]),[13] or electrical current (pain-related evoked potentials [PREP]).[14]

Noninvasive investigation of corneal innervation via corneal confocal microscopy (CCM) is increasingly used in conditions with expected small fiber pathology.[32] CCM allows the in vivo assessment of corneal subbasal innervation[27] by visualizing the Bowman membrane and the A-delta and C-nerve fiber plexus.

Small Nerve Fibers in Fibromyalgia Syndrome: Data From Skin Biopsy Studies

The idea to study skin innervation in patients with FMS was derived from the observation that some FMS patients complain of burning pain, similar to that of patients with small fiber neuropathy (SFN).

So far nine studies have been published reporting on a reduction in distal intraepidermal nerve fiber density (IENFD) on skin punch biopsies of patients with FMS.[4,6,8,11,18,20,35,24,26]

In the first study, 25 FMS patients were compared to patients with major depression but no pain and to healthy controls.[35] On average, patients had a lower density of intraepidermal nerve fibers and dermal unmyelinated nerve fiber bundles compared to controls, while numbers of myelinated nerve fibers were not different between groups. In patients with major depression, skin innervation was not different from controls. Looking at individual patient data, about two-thirds of the FMS patients in this cohort had reduced skin innervation. Oaklander et al.[26] found reduced IENFD in 41% of their cohort of 27 FMS patients, Caro and Winter[5] in approximately two-thirds of their 41 patients. In a cohort of 20 Italian FMS patients, 6 had reduced IENFD and fulfilled the criteria for SFN,[11] similarly 15 of 46 Greek patients had reduced IENFD.[18]

In those studies where distal and proximal skin samples from the leg were compared, there was often a non–length-dependent pattern.[4,35] Our own data from two additional groups of FMS patients confirm that IENFD is reduced in many but not all FMS patients, and that the non–length-dependent injury type is more frequent (Fig. 21.1A–C).[8,21] Further than just revealing epidermal innervation density in FMS, these studies brought some additional insights. For example, in the skin samples from the proximal leg of FMS patients, several nerve fibers immunoreactive for growth-associated portein-43 (GAP43), a marker of nerve regeneration that is normally present in healthy skin nerves, was reduced more than what would have been expected proportionally to the counts of PGP9.5 reactive fibers.[35] This may indicate that the natural regenerative capacity of intraepidermal nerve fibers is reduced in FMS patients. Patients with reduced IENFD also had diminished immunoreactivity for insulin growth factor 1 receptor,[21] which is a trophic factor for C-fibers in skin.[10] Furthermore, C-fibers from FMS patients had smaller diameters than those from SFN patients and controls, as morphometrically determined using electron microscopy.[8] As mentioned earlier, myelinated nerve fibers were not affected, pointing toward a specific pathologic process in the small fibers.[6] However, Meissner corpuscles, the rapidly adapting mechanoreceptors in the skin,[12] were markedly reduced in FMS patients.[6] FMS patients had a more rapid reduction of IENFD with aging,[4] potentially pointing toward a neurodegenerative process. Involvement of autonomic skin fibers was also observed[11] and is in line with the complaint of many FMS patients of autonomic symptoms.

A different approach was taken by Albrecht et al.[2] who studied peptidergic innervation of cutaneous arteriole–venule shunts (AVSs) in the palmar glabrous skin of FMS patients. These authors found increased innervation of the AVS in FMS patients compared to controls. This increase was mainly due to vasodilatory sensory fibers, whereas vasoconstrictive sympathetic fibers were not different among the groups. The authors argued that glabrous skin AVS regulate blood flow to the skin in humans for thermoregulation and in other tissues such as skeletal muscle and that they allow increased blood flow during periods of high metabolic demand. They speculated that this increased innervation of the AVS might result in insufficient blood flow in deep tissues like skeletal muscles, which might contribute to the widespread deep pain and fatigue in FMS patients.[2] This is an interesting hypothesis, which would have to be explored in appropriate models.

Small Nerve Fibers in Fibromyalgia Syndrome: Corneal Confocal Microscopy

Corneal innervation has been investigated in two studies so far. In one study, 17 patients with FMS were included and data were compared with 17 healthy controls.[29] The authors describe a smaller diameter of stromal corneal nerves and a diminished subbasal plexus in the FMS group compared to controls. Although the necessary extent of resolution achieved to allow the assessment of corneal nerve fiber thickness is remarkable, the reason and biologic meaning of this finding remain to be determined. In a second study, Oudejans et al.[28] found reduced nerve fiber length, branching, and/or density in 51% of the 39 patients with FSM investigated with CCM when comparing data with published normative values. The pathophysiologic meaning of this finding needs further clarification, but underscores the concept of widespread small fiber pathology in subgroups of patients with FMS (see Fig. 21.1D–F as examples).

Small Nerve Fibers and Their Connections to the Brain: Quantitative Sensory Testing and Evoked Potentials

If a C-fiber or A-delta fiber stimulus is applied in the periphery, and what is received in the central nervous system (CNS) is measured either by asking the participant or by recording of evoked potentials over the skull, not only the peripheral receptors and nerve fibers, but the whole tract from the receptor to the brain is assessed. This has advantages—investigating the complete physiologic tract—and disadvantages, for example not knowing at which level the pathology is, if one is detected.

QST is a psychophysical method that assesses the function of different afferent nerve fibers and their central connections (mentioned earlier). Using QST, functional impairment of the small nerve fibers in FMS was detected in several studies.[8,20,35,29] Detection thresholds for warm and cold stimuli are elevated in FMS, very similar to those in SFN.[35] Also, detection threshold for non-noxious mechanical stimuli is elevated, which seems to have its correspondence in the marked reduction in Meissner corpuscules.[6]

LEP and PREP are both evoked potentials on A-delta fiber stimulation. Although the methods and the stimuli are different, there was an amazing congruence of the findings from two groups of researchers: In our hands, peak-to-peak amplitudes of PREP were reduced in FMS patients, and the same was true in the laboratory of de Tommaso et al. using LEP.[6,35] This was true at proximal and distal stimulation sites, even stimulating at the face (Fig. 21.1G–I). Although we cannot know at present what causes this reduction in amplitude, the pathology of the peripheral receptors

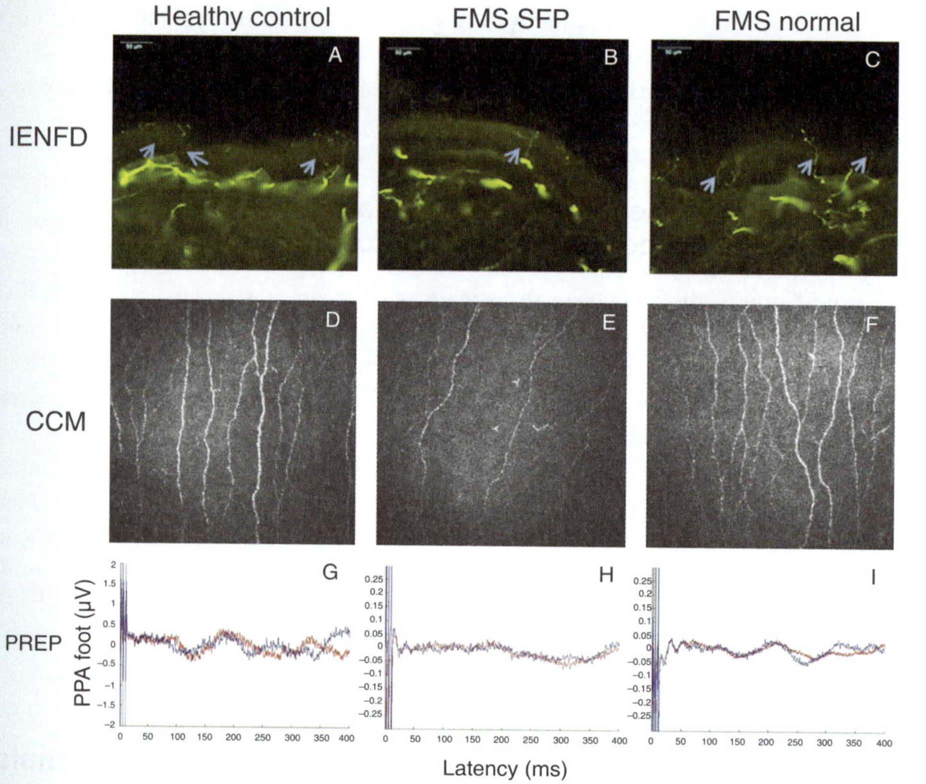

FIGURE 21.1 Examples of intraepidermal nerve fibers on skin punch biopsies (IENFD) (**A–C**), corneal innervation using corneal confocal microscopy (CCM) (**D–F**), and pain-related evoked potential (PREP) obtained from healthy controls, patients with fibromyalgia syndrome (FMS) and small fiber pathology (SFP), and patients with FMS and no SFP (**G–I**). **A–C**: Photomicrographs show intraepidermal nerve fibers (*arrows*) visualized using the pan-axonal marker protein gene product 9.5 (PGP9.5) in skin samples obtained from the lower leg. Fiber density is normal in the healthy control and the FMS patient without SFP, while it is reduced in the patient with FMS SFP. Scale bars: 50 μm. **D–F**: Examples of CCM showing corneal subbasal innervation. Fiber density is normal in the healthy control and the FMS patient without SFP, while it is reduced in the patient with FMS SFP. **G–I**: The graphs show PREP recordings obtained after stimulation at the foot. Peak-to-peak amplitude is normal in the healthy control, while no potential was obtained in the patient with FMS SFP. A normal PREP potential can be seen in the FMS patient without SFP.

described in skin biopsies makes it likely that the reduced amplitudes reflect this deficit in peripheral signal transduction, and not a central conduction deficit.

Microneurography

Microneurography is so far the only method by which the activity of a given C- or A-delta fiber can be directly recorded in humans. In FMS, C-fibers from the peroneal nerve had increased spontaneous activity,[31] a direct correlate of nociceptive signals.

Also, more of the "silent nociceptors" (those normally not responsive to mechanical stimuli) were sensitized to mechanical stimuli. Both the findings of spontaneous activity and of mechanical sensitization were very similar to those in patients with SFN. However, abnormal high slowing of conduction velocity was found in FMS, but neither in SFN nor in controls. Factors discussed as a reason for this slowing were ion channel densities, axon diameter, and environment,[31] Intriguingly, skin axons of FMS patients are indeed thinner than those of SFN patients and of controls.[8] Whether this is a developmental or a neurodegenerative process is as yet unknown.

Relevance of Small Fiber Findings in Fibromyalgia Syndrome

Table 21.1 gives a summary of the findings so far. It is of note that these findings were not present in all FMS patients investigated in the respective study cohorts, but in patient subgroups. For instance, the confidence intervals of the IENFD of FMS patients showed overlap with that of patients with unipolar depression but without pain and also with healthy controls, however, when comparing the entire groups, data of FMS patients differed from both groups.[35] Furthermore, IENFD, QST data, and the result of the neurologic examination of patients with FMS differed from that of patients with idiopathic SFN,[8] which was also true for microneurography results.[31] Thus, small fiber pathology in FMS should not be equaled with idiopathic SFN.[36,7] Small fiber pathology as reflected by reduced IENFD may be present in other chronic pain syndromes, such as postherpetic neuralgia and also in non-painful disorders like Parkinson`s disease. The so far reported findings on small fiber impairment in FMS are thus not specific. Furthermore, future studies need to clarify if and how small nerve fiber pathology may contribute to FMS and which pathomechanisms underlie the small nerve fiber impairment.

Currently, it is not possible to confirm or to exclude the diagnosis of FMS using small nerve fiber tests or any other test. The international American College of Rheumatology (ACR) criteria[37,38] and national criteria (e.g., symptom-based diagnostic criteria of the German S3 FMS guideline[9]) are used, and the diagnosis can be assumed if alternative diagnoses are excluded. The major relevance of the small fiber findings is that for the first time objectively measurable alterations have been detected on multiple levels in the peripheral nervous system of patients diagnosed with FMS. This has changed the view of patients, physicians, and scientists on the syndrome and has initiated the research field of small fiber impairment in FMS. Further research is urgent to now understand potential pathophysiologic connections that may contribute to FMS symptoms.

Pathophysiologic Concept

It is unclear if the mechanisms described for small nerve fiber impairment contribute to the pathophysiology of FMS or if they are sequelae or comorbidities of the syndrome. Current knowledge only allows the assumption that alterations in the central and peripheral nervous system do play a pathophysiologic role in subgroups of

TABLE 21.1 **Summary of results obtained in case–control studies on small fiber impairment in FMS patients**

Reference	Number of FMS patients/controls	Methods used	Main result
23	25/10 healthy controls and 10 patients with unipolar depression without pain	Skin biopsy (distal, proximal) QST PREP	In FMS patients: 6/24: reduced distal IENFD 25/25: elevated thermal perception thresholds 13/20: reduced distal PREP amplitudes
25	27/30 healthy controls	Skin biopsy (distal, proximal) Autonomous tests	Reduced distal IENFD in 41% of patients versus 3% in controls
33	30/9 healthy controls and 17 patients with idiopathic small fiber neuropathy	Microneurography	Distinct pathologic C-Nociceptor activity in subgroups of patients with FMS
17	41/47 healthy controls	Skin biopsy (distal, proximal) cytokines, circulating immune complexes, and complement in serum	In 24/41 cases reduced distal IENFD
21	46/34 healthy controls	Skin biopsy (distal)	Reduced IENFD in 32.6% of FMS patients
18	199/109 healthy controls	LEP (right dorsal hand, right chest, right knee) Skin biopsy (distal) (21/60)	N2–P2-amplitude reduced in FMS patients. Reduced N2–P2 habituation. IENFD reduced in FMS patients and correlates with LEP amplitudes.
20	20/0	Skin biopsy (distal)	In 6/20 cases, reduced IENFD.
19	32/12 small fiber neuropathy/24 healthy controls	Skin biopsy QST	Mean axon diameter of thin myelinated fibers FMS < small fiber neuropathy < healthy controls. Impaired small fiber function in QST. Reduced IENFD in FMS patients. Distinction between FMS and small-fiber neuropathy in both tests
31	17/17 healthy controls	CCM Thickness of stroma nerves in the cornea	Smaller diameter of stromal corneal nerves in FMS patients

TABLE 21.1 **Summary of results obtained in case–control studies on small fiber impairment in FMS patients (*Continued*)**

Reference	Number of FMS patients/controls	Methods used	Main result
33	39/0	CCM QST	Pathologic corneal innervation in 51% of FMS patients (reduced nerve fiber length, branching, and density) Four phenotypes assumed when assessing QST and FMS phenotypes.
22	30/34 healthy controls	Skin biopsy (distal, proximal) QST	In 14/28 cases reduced IENFD. In 12/30 cases elevated thermal perception thresholds in QST

CCM, corneal confocal microscopy; FMS, fibromyalgia syndrome; IENFD, intraepidermal nerve fiber density; LEP, laser-evoked potentials; PREP, pain-related evoked potentials; QST, quantitative sensory testing.

patients with FMS. However, when assessing study results, several caveats need to be taken into account. It is obvious that small nerve fiber impairment cannot account for all FMS symptoms; however, it may underlie peripheral sensitization contributing to FMS pain. It is of note that FMS pain is mostly reported to be localized in muscle tissue and the conceptual gap between impaired superficial skin innervation and deeply situated pain needs to be closed.

Limitations

So far mostly small numbers of patients have been investigated in the different laboratories, so that statistically robust subgroup analysis was hampered, and the heterogeneity of the FMS patient population was only poorly reflected. Also, the scope of investigations was mostly limited to few tests, so that it is unclear in how far the results of different small fiber tests correlate. Longitudinal studies are missing, and the cross-sectional study design does not allow conclusions about causality. It is unclear if the alterations found are epiphenomena of other processes, if they are confounded by other factors, or if they represent an adaptive reaction of the organism, for example, on stress. Furthermore, it is difficult to define a “pure” FMS group because most of the patients with FMS suffer from several comorbidities with functional and psychological impairments. The potential influence of such comorbidities is hardly ever controlled in clinical studies. One key aspect is the lack of specificity of the reported findings. In most studies on FMS pathophysiology, patients’ data are compared with that of age- and gender-matched healthy controls, but not with data of patients with other chronic pain syndromes or psychiatric disorders. It is therefore unclear if the described alterations in the central and peripheral nervous system are specific for FMS. Moreover, the heterogeneity of the methods used hinders direct comparison of the obtained results.

Clinical Implications

Despite the many caveats that need to be considered when interpreting small fiber data in FMS patients, characterization of small nerve fiber impairment in FMS may help to identify subgroups with a neuropathic component of pain, with a specific pathophysiology, and a distinct response to therapy.

Conclusion

Large-scale studies are needed to properly identify FMS subgroups regarding phenotyping and pathophysiology. Longitudinal observations reveal the temporal course of small fiber pathology. The mechanisms underlying nerve fiber degeneration in FMS need to be uncovered, such that they can potentially be used as targets for treatment.

REFERENCES

1. Agostino R, Cruccu G, Romaniello A, et al. Dysfunction of small myelinated afferents in diabetic polyneuropathy, as assessed by laser evoked potentials. *Clin Neurophysiol.* 2000;**111**(2):270–276.
2. Albrecht PJ, Hou Q, Argoff CE, et al. Excessive peptidergic sensory innervation of cutaneous arteriole-venule shunts (AVS) in the palmar glabrous skin of fibromyalgia patients: implications for widespread deep tissue pain and fatigue. *Pain Med.* 2013;**14**(6):895–915.
3. Bennett DL, Woods CG. Painful and painless channelopathies. *Lancet Neurol.* 2014;**13**(6):587–599.
4. Caro XJ, Winter EF. Evidence of abnormal epidermal nerve fiber density in fibromyalgia: clinical and immunologic implications. *Arthritis Rheumatol.* 2014;**66**(7):1945–1954.
5. Caro XJ, Winter EF. The role and importance of small fiber neuropathy in fibromyalgia pain. *Curr Pain Headache Rep.* 2015;**19**(12):55.
6. de Tommaso M, Nolano M, Iannone F, et al. Update on laser-evoked potential findings in fibromyalgia patients in light of clinical and skin biopsy features. *J Neurol.* 2014;**261**(3):461–472.
7. Devigili G, Tugnoli V, Penza P, et al. The diagnostic criteria for small fibre neuropathy: from symptoms to neuropathology. *Brain.* 2008;**131**(Pt 7):1912–1925.
8. Doppler K, Rittner HL, Deckart M, et al. Reduced dermal nerve fiber diameter in skin biopsies of patients with fibromyalgia. *Pain.* 2015;**156**(11):2319–2325.
9. Eich W, Bär KJ, Bernateck M, et al. Definition, classification, clinical diagnosis and prognosis of fibromyalgia syndrome: updated guidelines 2017 and overview of systematic review articles. *Schmerz.* 2017;**31**(3):231–238.
10. Gao WQ, Shinsky N, Ingle G, et al. IGF-I deficient mice show reduced peripheral nerve conduction velocities and decreased axonal diameters and respond to exogenous IGF-I treatment. *J Neurobiol.* 1999;**39**(1):142–152.
11. Giannoccaro MP, Donadio V, Incensi A, et al. Small nerve fiber involvement in patients referred for fibromyalgia. *Muscle Nerve.* 2014;**49**(5):757–759.
12. Hoffmann JN, Montag AG, Dominy NJ. Meissner corpuscles and somatosensory acuity: the prehensile appendages of primates and elephants. *Anat Rec A Discov Mol Cell Evol Biol.* 2004;**281**(1):1138–1147.

13. Jamal GA, Hansen S, Weir AI, et al. Cerebral cortical potentials to pure non-painful temperature stimulation: an objective technique for the assessment of small fibre pathway in man. *J Neurol Neurosurg Psychiatry*. 1989;**52**(1):99–105.
14. Kaube H, Katsarava Z, Käufer T, et al. A new method to increase nociception specificity of the human blink reflex. *Clin Neurophysiol*. 2000;**111**(3):413–416.
15. Kennedy WR, Wendelschafer-Crabb G, Polydefkis M, et al. Pathology and quantitation of cutaneous nerves. In: Dyck PJ, Thomas PK, eds. *Peripheral Neuropathy*. Philadelphia: Elsevier Saunders; 2005:869–896.
16. Kennedy WR, Wendelschafer-Crabb G, Walk D. Use of skin biopsy and skin blister in neurologic practice. *J Clin Neuromuscul Dis*. 2000;**1**(4):196–204.
17. Kimura J. *Electrodiagnosis in Diseases of Nerve and Muscle: Principles and Practice*. New York: Oxford University Press;2001.
18. Kosmidis ML, Koutsogeorgopoulou L, Alexopoulos H, et al. Reduction of intraepidermal nerve fiber density (IENFD) in the skin biopsies of patients with fibromyalgia: a controlled study. *J Neurol Sci*. 2014;**347**(1–2):143–147.
19. Lauria G, Cornblath DR, Johansson O, et al.; European Federation of Neurological Societies. EFNS guidelines on the use of skin biopsy in the diagnosis of peripheral neuropathy. *Eur J Neurol*. 2005;**12**(10):747–758.
20. Leinders M, Doppler K, Klein T, et al. Increased cutaneous miR-let-7d expression correlates with small nerve fiber pathology in patients with fibromyalgia syndrome. *Pain*. 2016;**157**(11):2493–2503.
21. Leinders M, Doppler K, Klein T, et al. Increased cutaneous miR-let-7d expression correlates with small nerve fiber pathology in patients with fibromyalgia syndrome. *Pain*. 2016;**157**(11):2493–2503.
22. Low PA, Tomalia VA, Park KJ. Autonomic function tests: some clinical applications. *J Clin Neurol*. 2013;**9**(1):1–8.
23. Lumpkin EA, Caterina MJ. Mechanisms of sensory transduction in the skin. *Nature*. 2007; **445**(7130):858–865.
24. Martínez-Martínez LA, Mora T, Vargas A, et al. Sympathetic nervous system dysfunction in fibromyalgia, chronic fatigue syndrome, irritable bowel syndrome, and interstitial cystitis: a review of case-control studies. *J Clin Rheumatol*. 2014;**20**(3):146–150.
25. Mellgren SI, Nolano M, Sommer C. The cutaneous nerve biopsy: technical aspects, indications, and contribution. *Handb Clin Neurol*. 2013;**115**:171–188.
26. Oaklander AL, Herzog ZD, Downs HM, et al. Objective evidence that small-fiber polyneuropathy underlies some illnesses currently labeled as fibromyalgia. *Pain*. 2013;**154**(11):2310–2316.
27. Oliveira-Soto L, Efron N. Morphology of corneal nerves using confocal microscopy. *Cornea*. 2001;**20**(4):374–384.
28. Oudejans L, He X, Niesters M, et al. Cornea nerve fiber quantification and construction of phenotypes in patients with fibromyalgia. *Sci Rep*. 2016;**6**:23573.
29. Ramírez M, Martínez-Martínez LA, Hernández-Quintela E, et al. Small fiber neuropathy in women with fibromyalgia. An *in vivo* assessment using corneal confocal bio-microscopy. *Semin Arthritis Rheum*. 2015;**45**(2):214–219.
30. Rolke R, Baron R, Maier C, et al. Quantitative sensory testing in the German Research Network on Neuropathic Pain (DFNS): standardized protocol and reference values. *Pain*. 2006; **123**(3):231–243.
31. Serra J, Collado A, Solà R, et al. Hyperexcitable C nociceptors in fibromyalgia. *Ann Neurol*. 2014;**75**(2):196–208.
32. Tavakoli M, Marshall A, Banka S, et al. Corneal confocal microscopy detects small-fiber neuropathy in Charcot-Marie-Tooth disease type 1A patients. *Muscle Nerve*. 2012;**46**(5):698–704.
33. Themistocleous AC, Ramirez JD, Serra J, et al. The clinical approach to small fibre neuropathy and painful channelopathy. *Pract Neurol*. 2014;**14**(6):368–379.

34. Tomlinson SE, Howells J, Burke D. In vivo assessment of neurological channelopathies: application of peripheral nerve excitability studies. *Neuropharmacology.* 2017;pii:S0028-3908(17)30195-8. doi: 10.1016/j.neuropharm.2017.04.045.
35. Üçeyler N, Zeller D, Kahn AK, et al. Small fibre pathology in patients with fibromyalgia syndrome. *Brain.* 2013;**136**(Pt 6):1857–1867.
36. Üçeyler N. Small fiber pathology—a culprit for many painful disorders? *Pain.* 2016;**157 Suppl 1**:S60–S66.
37. Wolfe F, Clauw DJ, Fitzcharles MA, et al. The American College of Rheumatology preliminary diagnostic criteria for fibromyalgia and measurement of symptom severity. *Arthritis Care Res.* 2010;**62**(5):600–610.
38. Wolfe F, Smythe HA, Yunus MB, et al. The American College of Rheumatology 1990 Criteria for the classification of fibromyalgia. Report of the Multicenter Criteria Committee. *Arthritis Rheum.* 1990;**33**(2):160–172.

CHAPTER 22

Muscle

Björn Gerdle and Britt Larsson

Summary Points

- Historically, several approaches have been used to investigate the presence of muscle engagement, and recent omics methods have produced promising results.
- Although there are clearly central alterations in fibromyalgia syndrome (FMS), it cannot be ruled out that primary nociceptive processes are also present in the periphery (e.g., muscles and nociceptors) in a complex interaction with the immune system.
- Primary muscle alterations (e.g., low-grade inflammation) are indicated by mitochondrial changes, lowered levels of intramuscular adenosine triphosphate (ATP) and phosphocreatine (PCr) concentrations and increased levels of lactate/pyruvate and endogenous lipid mediators together with marked differences in protein patterns between FMS and controls.
- Treatment studies indicate that muscle processes impact pain aspects in FMS.
- Larger proteomic studies that consider comorbidities and fitness level are needed.

EPIDEMIOLOGY AND CLINICAL CONSEQUENCES OF FIBROMYALGIA SYNDROME

FMS has a prevalence of approximately 2% in the population with markedly higher prevalence among females.[66] The American College of Rheumatology classifies FMS as chronic widespread pain (CWP) with simultaneous hyperalgesia/allodynia for mechanical pressure.[157] Hence, FMS is a subgroup of CWP. Spreading of pain is associated with high pain intensity[62,113] and increased prevalence of psychological comorbidities such as anxiety and depression.[113,100] The pain per se or in combination with fear that movements worsen pain can lead to deconditioning and low fitness level. FMS impairs one's ability to work, especially in strenuous occupations, as well as one's quality of life.[66] As clinical syndromes, CWP and FMS could be viewed as heterogeneous conditions based on the process of debut, clinical presentation, activated nociceptive mechanisms, or other circumstances. Presently, there is no standard way to identify robust subgroups based on clinical phenotypes. One-fifth of subjects with regional pain transit to CWP.[143] The risk factors for this transition to CWP/FMS are largely unknown.[89]

CENTRALLY OR PERIPHERALLY DRIVEN PAIN CONDITION?

Without doubt, there are central nervous system (CNS) alterations associated with FMS and other prevalent chronic pain conditions.[15,114,135,74,75] There are different opinions about if and how peripheral and central factors determine the clinical presentation in FMS (i.e., if the drive is mainly peripheral or central). Similar controversies exist for localized/regional chronic pain conditions.[117,118] Understanding these controversies has clear implications for possible treatment strategies.

Some researchers consider FMS as a pain condition associated with central hyperexcitability, whereas others consider FMS as a pain condition associated with peripheral factors in combination with central mechanisms, including hyperexcitability.[15,135,115,92,11,142] It has recently been suggested that FMS is a heterogeneous condition with "a complicated pathobiology with patients falling along a continuum with one end a purely peripherally driven painful condition and the other end of the continuum is when pain is purely centrally driven."[134] According to Sluka and Clauw,[134] most of the evidence suggests CNS mechanisms as the true pathogenesis. The hyperalgesia in FMS is widespread but clinically it cannot be determined whether it is of peripheral and/or central origin. However, FMS is found in increased prevalence in subjects with peripheral pain generators such as rheumatoid arthritis and ankylosing spondyloarthritis.[64] According to animal models, nociceptive inputs from muscle tissues are more effective in inducing changes in the behavior of dorsal horn neurons than inputs from cutaneous nociceptors.[67] CNS alterations in chronic low back pain or chronic hip osteoarthritis were normalized after effective peripheral treatment (surgery or facet joint injections).[130,124,125] Treatment studies of FMS also indicate that localized muscle/joint pain impacts aspects of FMS such as hyperalgesia.[1,58,140,141] The first attempts to understand the pathogenesis of FMS focused on peripheral alterations, a strategy that may have been used because most patients report that their pain condition was initiated as a localized pain condition.

Human skeletal muscle is a heterogeneous and dynamic tissue characterized by the capacity to adjust size and functionality due to both endogenous and exogenous influences. In this chapter, we briefly describe how muscles interact with other tissues and systems, review studies of muscle alterations, synthesize previous knowledge, and identify what is required in future studies. We primarily review studies investigating muscle alterations. Blood (plasma/serum) can also capture the way muscles react; when appropriate, results from such studies should be reported.

POSSIBLE INTERPLAYS BETWEEN MUSCLE, NOCICEPTORS, AND THE IMMUNE SYSTEM

After tissue injury, tissue substances (e.g., bradykinin, prostaglandins, H+, ATP, and nerve growth factor) are released and can stimulate and sensitize nociceptors. Nociceptors cannot be viewed as a pipeline or a conduit as they are heterogenous and highly complex in their expression of ligands, neurotransmitters, and receptors.[19,61] Immune cells, platelets, and other cells are recruited to or activated within the injured area and these cells can release additional substances such as histamine, serotonin, and bradykinin.[96] Nociceptors not only express receptors for and respond to cytokines and chemokines but also produce these substances.[76] Nociceptors (C-fibers) not only transmit action potentials to the spinal cord from the muscle but also transmit action potentials antidromically from junction points back to the muscle. That is, nociceptors can transmit information both from the periphery to the CNS and from the CNS to the periphery.[19] Substances released locally after antidromic firing include substance P, calcitonin gene-related peptide (CGRP), glutamate, and neurokinin A,[92] all contribute to neurogenic inflammation. In other words, the nociceptors influence the surrounding tissue by release of cytokines, chemokines, and neuropeptides.[19] Nonneuronal cells in the periphery such as immune and glial cells can influence these peripheral interactions by releasing neuromodulatory substances in near nociceptors.[76] Nociceptors can also inhibit signals to the CNS (nociceptor-initiated inhibition) from an affected tissue.[15] The excitability of nociceptors can increase (i.e., sensitize), which clinically is noted as primary hyperalgesia with lowered pain thresholds for mechanical pressure. The tissue reactions after injury can range from mild homeostatic reactions to full-scale inflammation.[158] The question arises if and to what extent muscle alterations persist in chronic pain conditions including FMS?

Several research groups have reported alterations of the peripheral nociceptors in FMS and/or FMS subgroups.[107,150,131,31] These modified nociceptors are possible peripheral factors responsible for CNS alterations. Such alterations can be primary nociceptor conditions and/or secondary consequences of tissue alterations. Whatever the cause, it is reasonable that they interact with surrounding tissues such as muscle.

MUSCLE MORPHOLOGIC STUDIES

The proportions of different fiber types were similar in FMS and healthy controls, but FMS patients exhibited greater variability in fiber size and altered fiber size distribution.[139] Several studies have reported atrophy of type II muscle fibers in patients with FMS.[78,121,159] Trapezius muscle fibers with alterations in mitochondrial content (moth-eaten fibers and ragged red fibers) have been reported,[10,8] changes that indicate uneven distribution and proliferation of mitochondria.[10] Also in the quadriceps, different types of muscle alterations have been reported.[91,33,71] However, the literature is not in agreement with respect to such muscle alterations.[129]

Microcirculation

The literature concerning muscle blood flow and oxygen consumption has reported conflicting results.[132,37,99,127] Shang et al.[132] reported that FMS had less oxygen extraction in the muscle during fatiguing exercise and muscle ischemia. Compared to healthy controls, FMS had lowered capillary density.[139,91] Microdialysis (MD) studies (see the following text) have not found alterations in blood flow in the trapezius or vastus lateralis muscles in FMS patients.[47,52]

Electrical Activation

Electromyographic (EMG) techniques—for example, bipolar or multichannel surface EMG—have been used to investigate activations and properties of skeletal muscles in FMS. The electrical activation reflect central (i.e., motor) and peripheral factors (i.e., muscle membrane properties, fiber composition, and fiber diameter).

FMS has a relative inability to relax the antagonists during dynamic muscle contractions[35,36] and another activation pattern of the aching trapezius muscle has been found.[40,51] A significant association existed between the degree of altered neuromuscular control in the trapezius and pain intensity.[69]

Higher conduction velocity (CV) of the muscle fibers in upper body muscles have been reported in most FMS studies,[85,54,84,20] findings that indicate functional abnormalities of the muscle fiber membranes.

Phosphorus Metabolism

The phosphorus metabolism of muscles in patients with FMS has been investigated using ^{96}P magnetic resonance spectroscopy (^{96}P-MRS). The FMS literature is not in agreement: Some studies have found significant muscle alterations[77,137,112,152,97] and other studies have not found any differences.[28,72,133] For example, contradictory findings concerning ATP and PCr concentrations may be because the studies investigated different muscles[77,137,152,97,28,72,133] with different predilections for metabolic alterations. For example, type I muscle fibers have a two- to three-fold higher mitochondrial density and lower capacity for non-oxidative ATP synthesis compared to type II fibers.[119] In addition, the diverse results may be due to the fact that the studies used different types of measures—absolute and relative. From a biochemical point of view, absolute measures are preferred.[104,81] However, the literature is in agreement with respect to absolute measures; the absolute concentrations of ATP and PCr were significantly lower in the quadriceps muscle of FMS patients.[112,48] Similar results have been reported in a study using another technique.[9] The lower absolute concentrations of ATP and PCr might be due to generalized altered mitochondrial function in FMS.

Lactate, Pyruvate, and Glutamate

MD is an in vivo technique for sampling biochemical substances in a tissue, for example, in the muscle where nociceptor-free nerve endings terminate (i.e., extracellular fluid/muscle interstitium), providing information on the local biochemical milieu. In regional chronic neck pain conditions, increased concentrations of glutamate, serotonin, lactate, and/or pyruvate in the trapezius muscle have been found.[53,49] The first MD study of FMS reported an increased concentration of serotonin in the myalgic masseter muscle.[39] Two studies found that FMS patients had higher concentrations of lactate and/or pyruvate in the trapezius[52,55] and one study found similar results for the vastus lateralis.[47] Hence, most studies of FMS, except for one small study,[101] show significant alterations in these substances. Lactate is produced during anaerobic and aerobic conditions and can be metabolized in the same cell or transported to other cells for metabolic use.[16,60,116,32,122,59,3] Increased concentrations of lactate and pyruvate cannot be explained by insufficient oxygen supply because no group difference in blood flow was measured simultaneously with the two metabolites existed.[47,52] A combination of metabolites is needed to activate human nociceptors.[120] Lactic acid is dissociated at body pH.[14] Lactate together with ATP facilitate the response of acid-sensing ion channel 3 (ASIC-3) to low pH.[13,70,83,30] Other receptors for low pH are transient receptor potential (vanilloid-1) receptors (TRPV1),[90] TRPV4,[128] TRPC4, and TRPC5.[34]

Increased levels of glutamate have been found both in trapezius and vastus lateralis of FMS patients[47,52] and in muscles of local/regional pain conditions.[52,53,17] Glutamate can induce experimental pain,[17] and hypertonic saline infusion into muscles releases glutamate.[94,147] Glutamate can be released from peripheral afferent neurons, resulting in excitation and sensitization of the same or adjacent neurons.[17,103,86] Glutamate acts via *N*-methyl-D-aspartate (NMDA), α-amino-3-hydroxy-5-methy-4-isoxazole propionate (AMPA), and possibly TRPV1 receptors.[128,2,23] When NMDA receptors are activated by glutamate, nitric oxide (NO)—a reactive oxygen species (ROS)—is generated[41] and can contribute to peripheral hyperalgesia.[25,7]

The concentrations of lactate, pyruvate, and glutamate correlated to a certain degree with clinical aspects. In one of the MD studies concerning the trapezius muscle, glutamate and lactate levels correlated with pressure pain thresholds (PPTs) and pain intensity in the FMS/CWP group (i.e., 15 out of the 17 CWP patients).[52] In the study of the vastus lateralis muscle, pain intensity decreased, while strength and endurance increased as a consequence of an exercise intervention.[47] The FMS group exhibited significant decreases in mean muscle concentrations of pyruvate, glutamate, and glucose after the exercise intervention[47]; that is, the concentrations were normalized in FMS. The decrease in pain intensity in FMS correlated significantly with the decreases in concentrations of pyruvate and glucose.

N-Acylethanolamines (NAEs)

NAEs belong to a group of endogenous lipid mediators that have a diversity of actions including the regulation of inflammation and pain.[111] Their levels are influenced by diet and associated with energy metabolism.[4,63] NAEs include *N*-palmitoylethanolamide (PEA), *N*-stearoylethanolamine (SEA), *N*-oleoylethanolamine (OEA), and *N*-arachidonoylethanolamine (anandamide, AEA).

An MD study of the trapezius muscle in patients with chronic neck-shoulder pain reported significantly higher concentrations of PEA and SEA than in controls.[57] Another study found that an FMS/CWP cohort mobilized certain NAEs (i.e., PEA and SEA) in the trapezius muscle differently than controls and patients with chronic regional neck-shoulder pain.[56] Increases in pain intensities during a light brief dynamic work (20 minutes) correlated negatively with the levels of PEA and SEA.[56] In addition, acute minor muscle trauma in the same cohort of subjects was associated with significantly higher levels of SEA and OEA during the 120 minutes after the tissue trauma in CWP/FMS,[145] and pain intensity correlated significantly with SEA.

Significantly increased levels of plasma AEA were reported in FMS.[80] Hellstrom et al.[65] found no significant group differences in plasma levels of OEA, PEA, SEA, and other related lipids in CWP compared to healthy controls. In contrast, Stensson et al. found that plasma levels of PEA, OEA, and SEA were significantly higher in CWP/FMS patients than in healthy controls.[144] A possible explanation for the different findings in the two latter studies could be that Stensson et al.'s[144] study had more FMS patients and higher pain intensities.

AEA interacts with cannabinoid receptors and TRPV1 and has antinociceptive actions.[18] According to different pain models, PEA has both anti-inflammatory and antinociceptive effects.[73,26,42,93] PEA acts mainly via peroxisome proliferator-activated receptor type-α (PPAR-α) activation.[93,136,82,95] OEA is also a ligand for this receptor[44] and related to both analgesic properties (independently of PPAR-α activation)[146] and induction of visceral pain (via $TRPV_1$ activation).[155] In addition, SEA has been described as having anti-inflammatory activity[27] not modulated via PPAR-α. Recently, it was shown that SEA influences signaling pathways by inhibition of nuclear factor (NF)-κβ translocation and downregulation of pro-inflammatory cytokines expression.[12]

Cytokines and Chemokines

Proteins can act as signal substances, activate the formation of analgesics, and control nociceptive processes. Cytokines are proteins and act as messengers of the immune system.[123] Chemokines are a special type of proinflammatory cytokines that guide mononuclear cells and participate in synaptic transmission and in the formation of second messenger systems in neurons and glial cells.[123] As mentioned earlier, activated nociceptors (polymodal c-fibers) can secrete cytokines.[21] Different substances such as substance P, glutamate, and brain-derived neurotrophic factor (BDNF) can activate glial cells to release pro-inflammatory cytokines and neuropeptides.

Two studies have investigated cytokines in the muscle of FMS patients. Pro-inflammatory cytokines (i.e., interleukin-1 beta [IL-1β], IL-6, IL-8, and tumor necrosis factor [TNF]) were collected from vastus lateralis using MD.[22] No significant group differences in muscle cytokine levels were found between FMS and controls. Furthermore, no correlation existed between pain or fatigue and the levels of cytokines.[22] Subjects who participated in a 15-week resistance exercise intervention experienced a decrease in pain although no changes occurred in muscle cytokine levels.[38]

Plasma/serum levels of cytokines may reflect peripheral production by C-fibers or neuropeptide stimulation of immune cells in peripheral tissues or from activated glial cells in the CNS.[92] Several studies report that some pro-inflammatory cytokines (IL-1RA, IL-6, and IL-8) are increased in the blood (plasma or serum) of FMS patie nts.[123,149,102,148,154] Also increases in the pro-inflammatory TNF have been reported, but the literature for this substance is not in agreement.[148] There are also reports that inflammatory chemokines are elevated in FMS.[45] In contrast, the two studies investigating cytokines in muscle also investigated plasma levels of pro-inflammatory cytokines but found neither group differences nor changes after an exercise intervention.[22,38] The latter results concerning exercise contrast with a review from 2015 that concluded that exercise interventions may reduce IL-6 and IL-8 levels.[126]

According to two large studies, C-reactive protein (CRP) in serum appears to be associated with FMS and thus indicates the inflammation in FMS.[43,98] A large study of CWP found elevated levels of CRP, IL-6, and TNF when compared to controls,[46] but the significant differences did not remain after controlling for lifestyle and disease factors.

Proteomic Studies of Muscle

Generally, only a few proteins have been investigated simultaneously in each study mentioned earlier. There is growing consensus that a panel of multiple biomarkers, reflecting a so-called molecular signature, will perform better than a single biomarker with respect to understanding activated nociceptive and pain mechanisms. Because omics methods require large-scale data analysis for characterization and quantification of pools of biological molecules, many substances are analyzed simultaneously. Omics have been used to identify potential biomarkers in several neurodegenerative conditions. Omics analyses require powerful and appropriate statistical tools (i.e., multivariate data analysis [MVDA]) to avoid violating traditional classical statistical assumptions. The genome tells us what is possible, whereas the proteome tells us what is functionally present and happening. The proteome is much larger than the genome due to factors such as alternatively spliced RNA, posttranslational modifications of proteins, temporal regulation of protein synthesis, and varying protein–protein interactions.

In a first study—using pooled dialysate—30 out of 97 identified proteins from the interstitium of the trapezius muscle were at least two-fold up- or downregulated in CWP (mainly FMS patients).[108] Marked muscle proteomic differences were found in another cohort of patients with CWP (mainly FMS patients): 17 proteins out of 216 were clearly and highly significantly discriminate between CWP/FMS and healthy controls ($R^2 = 0.81$; CV-analysis of variance [ANOVA]: $p < 0.001$).[109] Using the same CWP/FMS patients, a second study found a highly significant multivariate correlation between pain intensity and a group of 12 proteins ($R^2 = 0.99$; CV-ANOVA: $p < 0.001$).[110] There was also a significant multivariate correlation between pressure pain threshold (PPT) and a group of 16 proteins.[110] The identified proteins in these muscle studies are involved in different processes such as inflammation and stress, muscle damage/recovery, and enzymes involved in metabolic pathways. The proteins of importance for group separation were not identical to those correlating with pain intensity and PPT. The altered expression of these proteins reasonably reflects both direct and indirect nociceptive/inflammatory processes as well as secondary changes.

Proteomics has also been used to investigate plasma. Using the same cohorts of CWP/FMS patients and controls as Olausson et al.,[109] another study found that 22 plasma proteins (out of >300 identified proteins) were important for the significant group separation ($R^2 = 0.84$; CV-ANOVA: $p < 0.001$).[153] The important proteins belonged to inflammatory, immunity, and metabolic processes. Using a special panel of 92 inflammation-related proteins including cytokines and chemokines to investigate the same group of subjects, another study found that 11 of these proteins significantly differentiated the two groups of subjects ($R^2 = 0.58$; CV-ANOVA: $p = 0.006$).[50] These 11 substances consisted of three chemokines, one cytokine, and two growth factors. Interestingly, there was a high degree of overlap with the results presented somewhat later from another FMS cohort using the same panel of 92 proteins.[5] The group of important proteins ($n = 21$) showed good ability to discriminate FMS and controls ($R^2 = 0.97$; CV-ANOVA: $p > 0.001$).[5] In conclusion, proteomic studies indicate systemic inflammation and other alterations in FMS.

CONCLUSION

Human skeletal muscle is a heterogeneous tissue characterized by a large capacity to adjust size and functionality due to both endogenous and exogenous influences. These circumstances contribute to difficulties in detangling possible primary nociceptive and inflammatory processes and secondary consequences of the pain condition per se. Contributing to these difficulties is the fact that muscle is in a bidirectional relationship with nociceptors and the immune system. For example, nociceptors (C-fibers) not only transmit action potentials to the spinal cord from the muscle but also transmit antidromically—from junction points back to the muscle.[92] The studies reviewed indicate that peripheral factors in the muscle are present and may contribute to maintaining central alterations. Alterations in mitochondrial distribution, shape, volume, and orientation have been reported[159,138] as well as a mitochondrial dysfunction in blood mononuclear cells of FMS.[24] Both the alterations in lactate/pyruvate metabolism and the lowered concentrations of ATP and PCr can be due to mitochondrial alterations/insufficiency.

Altered activation patterns of the fibromyalgic muscle[35,40,51,6] may indicate muscular overactivity and thereby higher lactate and possibly pyruvate levels.[29,151] Increased concentrations of lactate and pyruvate cannot be explained by insufficient oxygen supply because no group difference in blood flow measured simultaneously with the two metabolites existed.[47,52] Furthermore, other studies of blood flow and oxygenation are conflicting with respect to the possible role of relative ischemia in the muscle.

In FMS/CWP, muscular fitness is reduced.[10,47,106] The content and function of mitochondria depend on physical activity level[87,88]; the mitochondrial density increases as a result of exercise.[68,105] The aerobic capacity of the muscle is largely governed by several mitochondria and their enzymes.[156] Lower capillary density and enzymes associated with aerobic metabolism in vastus lateralis muscle of FMS have been reported.[91] However, the capillary density depends on physical activity level. That is, inactivity and deconditioning may alter phosphorus metabolism (ATP and PCr) and lactate/pyruvate metabolism in FMS patients.[87]

The increased levels of glutamate found both in muscles of FMS[47,52] and as a result of local/regional pain conditions[52,53,17] can have either have a nociceptor origin or be the result of intramuscular processes. A combination of metabolites is needed to activate human nociceptors.[120] Glutamate in combination with increased lactate and pyruvate levels may contribute to nociceptor activation in FMS. However, there is a need to investigate other substances (e.g., serotonin, bradykinin, nerve growth factor, and substance P) using MD. MD studies of cytokines are few and the studies of pro-inflammatory cytokines do not indicate prominent ongoing cytokine signaling in muscle. The few studies of NAEs indicate activation of anti-inflammatory and analgesic substances. In addition, MD studies of FMS need to include other anti-inflammatory and analgesic substances such as endorphins; a recent MD study of chronic neck-shoulder pain reported elevated levels of beta-endorphin and glutamate in the trapezius muscle.[79] Studies of cytokines in plasma of mainly pro-inflammatory cytokines in FMS have yielded conflicting results, although one study has reported increased levels of certain NAEs.

Generally, few substances have been investigated in each biochemical study using a hypothesis-driven approach. In omics studies, a more explorative approach is chosen and many substances are analyzed simultaneously. Proteomics has not been extensively used in human studies of chronic pain conditions in contrast to the field of neurodegenerative disorders. Both the studies of muscles and plasma in FMS report prominent and highly significant multivariate differences in protein patterns between FMS and controls. In these studies, the identified significant proteins were involved in different processes such as inflammation and stress, muscle damage/recovery, and enzymes involved metabolic pathways. It was also obvious that certain proteins correlated with pain intensity and pain sensitivity aspects. Furthermore, studies using the broader panel of inflammatory substances (i.e., 92 proteins) reported significant alterations in FMS compared to controls, and several of the important proteins are replicated in different FMS cohorts.

The proteomic studies may indicate low-grade inflammation in FMS. Although the results are promising, several studies and subjects are relatively few. In larger cohorts of patients with FMS and healthy controls, it is necessary in the MVDA analyses to also consider the presence of comorbidities such as anxiety and depression and overweight/obesity, because these conditions also have been associated with low-grade inflammation. Another factor to consider is the activity level and muscle fitness level because several of the alterations reported earlier may be activity dependent (e.g., capillary density and mitochondrial density). Most studies reviewed have been cross-sectional and there is a need for different longitudinal studies, for example, investigations of interventions, and studies of transitions from local to generalized pain conditions. Future proteomic studies should include more detailed bioinformatic analyses. In addition, future studies should investigate whether the found alterations in muscle and proteins are specific for FMS/CWP or common across chronic pain conditions. Investigations of rheumatoid arthritis patients with and without FMS may shed light on the specificity of proteomic findings.

In conclusion, although the few studies that have been conducted indicate activations of anti-inflammatory and antinociceptive mechanisms in muscle tissue and plasma in patients with FMS/CWP, more research is needed to confirm these results.

FUNDING

This chapter was sponsored by research grants from the Swedish Research Council and AFA Insurance. The sponsors had no role in study design, selection of articles, data interpretation, writing of the chapter, or the decision to submit for publication.

REFERENCES

1. Affaitati G, Costantini R, Fabrizio A, Lapenna D, Tafuri E, Giamberardino M. Effects of treatment of peripheral pain generators in fibromyalgia patients. *Eur J Pain*. 2011;**15**(1):61–69.
2. Alfredson H, Forsgren S, Thorsen K, Lorentzon R. In vivo microdialysis and immunohistochemical analyses of tendon tissue demonstrated high amounts of free glutamate and glutamate NMDAR1 receptors, but no signs of inflammation, in Jumper's knee. *J Orthop Res*. 2001;**19**(5):881–886.
3. Allen M. Lactate and acid base as a hemodynamic monitor and markers of cellular perfusion. *Pediatr Crit Care Med*. 2011;**12**(4 Suppl):S43–S49.
4. Artmann A, Petersen G, Hellgren LI, Boberg J, Skonberg C, Nellemann C. Influence of dietary fatty acids on endocannabinoid and N-acylethanolamine levels in rat brain, liver and small intestine. *Biochim Biophys Acta*. 2008;**1781**(4):200–212.
5. Bäckryd E, Tanum L, Lind A, Larsson A, Gordh T. Evidence of both systemic inflammation and neuroinflammation in fibromyalgia patients, as assessed by a multiplex protein panel applied to the cerebrospinal fluid and to plasma. *J Pain Res*. 2017;**10**:515–525.
6. Bazzichi L, Dini M, Rossi A, Corbianco S, De Feo F, Giacomelli C. Muscle modifications in fibromyalgic patients revealed by surface electromyography (SEMG) analysis. *BMC Musculoskelet Disord*. 2009;**10**:36.
7. Benarroch EE. Nitric oxide: a pleiotropic signal in the nervous system. *Neurology*. 2011;**77**(16):1568–1576.
8. Bengtsson A, Henriksson KG, Larsson J. Muscle biopsy in primary fibromyalgia. Light-microscopical and histochemical findings. *Scand J Rheumatol*. 1986;**15**(1):1–6.
9. Bengtsson A, Henriksson KG, Larsson J. Reduced high-energy phosphate levels in the painful muscles of patients with primary fibromyalgia. *Arthritis Rheum*. 1986;**29**(7):817–821.
10. Bengtsson A. Editorial, the muscle in fibromyalgia. *Rheumatology*. 2002;**41**:721–724.
11. Bennett RM. Emerging concepts in the neurobiology of chronic pain: evidence of abnormal sensory processing in fibromyalgia. *Mayo Clin Proc*. 1999;**74**:385–398.
12. Berdyshev AG, Kosiakova HV, Onopchenko OV, Panchuk RR, Stoika RS, Hula NM. N-stearoylethanolamine suppresses the pro-inflammatory cytokines production by inhibition of NF-kappaB translocation. *Prostagland Other Lipid Mediat*. 2015;121(Pt A):91–96.

13. Birdsong WT, Fierro L, Williams FG, Spelta V, Naves LA, Knowles M. Sensing muscle ischemia: coincident detection of acid and ATP via interplay of two ion channels. *Neuron.* 2010;**68**(4):739–749.
14. Birklein F, Weber M, Neundorfer B. Increased skin lactate in complex regional pain syndrome: evidence for tissue hypoxia? *Neurology.* 2000;**55**(8):1213–1215.
15. Bradley LA. Pathophysiology of fibromyalgia. *Am J Med.* 2009;**122**(12 Suppl):S22–S30.
16. Brooks GA. Cell-cell and intracellular lactate shuttles. *J Physiol.* 2009;**587**(Pt 23):5591–5600.
17. Cairns BE, Dong X. The role of peripheral glutamate and glutamate receptors in muscle pain. *J Musculoskelet Pain.* 2008;**16**(1–2):85–91.
18. Calignano A, La Rana G, Giuffrida A, Piomelli D. Control of pain initiation by endogenous cannabinoids. *Nature.* 1998;**394**:277–281.
19. Carlton SM. Nociceptive primary afferents: they have a mind of their own. *J Physiol.* 2014;**592**(16): 3403–3411.
20. Casale R, Sarzi-Puttini P, Atzeni F, Gazzoni M, Buskila D, Rainoldi A. Central motor control failure in fibromyalgia: a surface electromyography study. *BMC Musculoskelet Disord.* 2009;**10**:78.
21. Chiu IM, von Hehn CA, Woolf CJ. Neurogenic inflammation and the peripheral nervous system in host defense and immunopathology. *Nat Neurosci.* 2012;**15**(8):1063–1067.
22. Christidis N, Ghafouri B, Larsson A, Palstam A, Mannerkorpi K, Bileviciute-Ljungar I. Comparison of the levels of pro-inflammatory cytokines released in the vastus lateralis muscle of patients with fibromyalgia and healthy controls during contractions of the quadriceps muscle—a microdialysis study. *PLoS One.* 2015;**10**(12):e0143856.
23. Coggeshall RE, Carlton SM. Ultrastructural analysis of NMDA, AMPA, and kainate receptors on unmyelinated and myelinated axons in the periphery. *J Comp Neurol.* 1998;**391**(1):78–86.
24. Cordero MD, De Miguel M, Moreno Fernandez AM, Carmona Lopez IM, Garrido Maraver J, Cotan D. Mitochondrial dysfunction and mitophagy activation in blood mononuclear cells of fibromyalgia patients: implications in the pathogenesis of the disease. *Arthritis Res Ther.* 2010;**12**(1):R17.
25. Cury Y, Picolo G, Gutierrez VP, Ferreira SH. Pain and analgesia: the dual effect of nitric oxide in the nociceptive system. *Nitric Oxide.* 2011;**25**(3):243–254.
26. D'Agostino G, La Rana G, Russo R, Sasso O, Iacono A, Esposito E. Central administration of palmitoylethanolamide reduces hyperalgesia in mice via inhibition of NF-κB nuclear signalling in dorsal root ganglia. *Eur J Pharmacol.* 2009;**613**(1–3):54–59.
27. Dalle Carbonare M, Del Giudice E, Stecca A, Colavito D, Fabris M, D'Arrigo A. A saturated N-acylethanolamine other than N-palmitoyl ethanolamine with anti-inflammatory properties: a neglected story. *J Neuroendocrinol.* 2008;20 Suppl 1:26–34.
28. de Blecourt AC, Wolf RF, van Rijswijk MH, Kamman RL, Knipping AA, Mooyaart E. 68In vivo 31P magnetic resonance spectroscopy (MRS) of tender points in patients with primary fibromyalgia syndrome. *Rheumatol Int.* 1991;**11**(2):51–54.
29. de Paoli FV, Ortenblad N, Pedersen TH, Jorgensen R, Nielsen OB. Lactate per se improves the excitability of depolarized rat skeletal muscle by reducing the Cl-conductance. *J Physiol.* 2010;588(Pt 23):4785–4794.
30. Deval E, Gasull X, Noel J, Salinas M, Baron A, Diochot S. Acid-sensing ion channels (ASICs): pharmacology and implication in pain. *Pharmacol Ther.* 2010;**128**(3):549–558.
31. Doppler K, Rittner HL, Deckart M, Sommer C. Reduced dermal nerve fiber diameter in skin biopsies of patients with fibromyalgia. *Pain.* 2015;**156**(11):2319–2325.
32. Draoui N, Feron O. Lactate shuttles at a glance: from physiological paradigms to anti-cancer treatments. *Dis Model Mech.* 2011;**4**(6):727–732.
33. Drewes AM, Andreasen A, Schroder HD, Hogsaa B, Jennum P. Pathology of skeletal muscle in fibromyalgia: a histo-immuno-chemical and ultrastructural study. *Br J Rheumatol.* 1993;**32**(6):479–483.
34. Eisenhut M, Wallace H. Ion channels in inflammation. *Pflugers Arch.* 2011;**461**(4):401–421.
35. Elert J, Aspegren Kendall S, Larsson B, Månsson B, Gerdle B. Chronic pain and difficulty in relaxing postural muscles in patients with fibromylgia and chronic whiplash associated disorders. *J Rheumatol.* 2001;**28**:1361–1368.

36. Elert JE, Rantapaa-Dahlqvist SB, Henriksson-Larsen K, Lorentzon R, Gerdle B. Muscle performance, electromyography and fibre type composition in fibromyalgia and work-related myalgia. *Scand J Rheumatol.* 1992;**21**(1):28–34.
37. Elvin A, Siosteen AK, Nilsson A, Kosek E. Decreased muscle blood flow in fibromyalgia patients during standardised muscle exercise: a contrast media enhanced colour Doppler study. *Eur J Pain.* 2006;**10**(2):137–144.
38. Ernberg M, Christidis N, Ghafouri B, Bileviciute-Ljungar I, Lofgren M, Larsson A. Effects of 15 weeks of resistance exercise on pro-inflammatory cytokine levels in the vastus lateralis muscle of patients with fibromyalgia. *Arthritis Res Ther.* 2016;**18**(1):137.
39. Ernberg M, Hedenberg-Magnusson B, Alstergren P, Kopp S. The level of serotonin in the superficial masseter muscle in relation to local pain and allodynia. *Life Sci.* 1999;**65**(3):313–325.
40. Falla D, Andersen H, Danneskiold-Samsøe B, Arendt-Nielsen L, Farina D. Adaptations of upper trapezius muscle activity during sustained contractions in women with fibromyalgia. *J Electromyogr Kinesiol.* 2010;**20**(3):457–464.
41. Fan W, Huang F, Wu Z, Zhu X, Li D, He H. The role of nitric oxide in orofacial pain. *Nitric Oxide.* 2012;**26**(1):32–37.
42. Farquhar-Smith W, Jaggar S, Rice A. Attenuation of nerve growth factor-induced visceral hyperalgesia via cannabinoid CB1 and CB2-like receptors. *Pain.* 2002;**97**:11–21.
43. Feinberg T, Sambamoorthi U, Lilly C, Innes KK. Potential mediators between fibromyalgia and C-reactive protein: results from a large U.S. community survey. *BMC Musculoskelet Disord.* 2017;**18**(1):294.
44. Fu J, Gaetani S, Oveisi F, Lo Verme J, Serrano A, Rodriguez De Fonseca F. Oleylethanolamide regulates feeding and body weight through activation of the nuclear receptor PPAR-alpha. *Nature.* 2003;**425**(6953):90–93.
45. Garcia JJ, Cidoncha A, Bote ME, Hinchado MD, Ortega E. Altered profile of chemokines in fibromyalgia patients. *Ann Clin Biochem.* 2014;**51**(Pt 5):576–581.
46. Generaal E, Vogelzangs N, Macfarlane GJ, Geenen R, Smit JH, Dekker J. Basal inflammation and innate immune response in chronic multisite musculoskeletal pain. *Pain.* 2014;**155**(8):1605–1612.
47. Gerdle B, Ernberg M, Mannerkorpi K, Larsson B, Kosek E, Christidis N. Increased interstitial concentrations of glutamate and pyruvate in vastus lateralis of women with fibromyalgia syndrome are normalized after an exercise intervention—a case-control study. *PLoS One.* 2016;**11**(10):e0162010.
48. Gerdle B, Forsgren MF, Bengtsson A, Leinhard OD, Soren B, Karlsson A. Decreased muscle concentrations of ATP and PCR in the quadriceps muscle of fibromyalgia patients—a 31P-MRS study. *Eur J Pain.* 2013;**17**(8):1205–1215.
49. Gerdle B, Ghafouri B, Ernberg M, Larsson B. Chronic musculoskeletal pain: review of mechanisms and biochemical biomarkers as assessed by the microdialysis technique. *J Pain Res.* 2014;**7**:313–326.
50. Gerdle B, Ghafouri B, Ghafouri N, Backryd E, Gordh T. Signs of ongoing inflammation in female patients with chronic widespread pain: a multivariate, explorative, cross-sectional study of blood samples. *Medicine.* 2017;**96**(9):e6130.
51. Gerdle B, Grönlund C, Karlsson S, Holtermann A, Roeleveld K. Altered neuromuscular control mechanisms of the trapezius muscle in fibromyalgia. *BMC Musculoskelet Disord.* 2010;**11**:42. doi:10.1186/471-2474-11-42v.
52. Gerdle B, Larsson B, Forsberg F, Ghafouri N, Karlsson L, Stensson N. Chronic widespread pain: increased glutamate and lactate concentrations in the trapezius muscle and plasma. *Clin J Pain.* 2014;**30**(5):409–420.
53. Gerdle B, Larsson B. Potential muscle biomarkers of chronic myalgia in humans—a systematic review of microdialysis studies. In: Khan T, ed. *Biomarker in Press.* Rijeka, Croatia: INTECH Open Access Publisher; 2012.
54. Gerdle B, Ostlund N, Gronlund C, Roeleveld K, Karlsson J. Firing rate and conduction velocity of single motor units in the trapezius muscle in fibromyalgia patients and healthy controls. *J Electromyogr Kinesiol.* 2008;**18**(5):707–716.

55. Gerdle B, Soderberg K, Salvador Puigvert L, Rosendal L, Larsson B. Increased interstitial concentrations of pyruvate and lactate in the trapezius muscle of patients with fibromyalgia: a microdialysis study. *J Rehabil Med.* 2010;**42**(7):679–687.
56. Ghafouri N, Ghafouri B, Larsson B, Stensson N, Fowler CJ, Gerdle B. Palmitoylethanolamide and stearoylethanolamide levels in the interstitium of the trapezius muscle of women with chronic widespread pain and chronic neck-shoulder pain correlate with pain intensity and sensitivity. *Pain.* 2013;**154**(9):1649–1658.
57. Ghafouri N, Ghafouri B, Larsson B, Turkina MV, Karlsson L, Fowler C. High levels of N-palmitoylethanolamide and N-stearoylethanolamide in microdialysate samples from myalgic trapezius muscle in women. *PLoS One.* 2011;**6**(11):e27257.
58. Giamberardino MA, Affaitati G, Fabrizio A, Costantini R. Effects of treatment of myofascial trigger points on the pain of fibromyalgia. *Curr Pain Headache Rep.* 2011;**15**(5):393–399.
59. Gjedsted J, Buhl M, Nielsen S, Schmitz O, Vestergaard ET, Tonnesen E. Effects of adrenaline on lactate, glucose, lipid and protein metabolism in the placebo controlled bilaterally perfused human leg. *Acta Physiol.* 2011;**202**(4):641–648.
60. Gladden LB. Lactate metabolism: a new paradigm for the third millenium. *J Physiol.* 2004;**558**(1): 5–30.
61. Gold MS, Gebhart GF. Nociceptor sensitization in pain pathogenesis. *Nat Med.* 2010;**16**(11):1248–1257.
62. Grimby-Ekman A, Gerdle B, Bjork J, Larsson B. Comorbidities, intensity, frequency and duration of pain, daily functioning and health care seeking in local, regional, and widespread pain—a descriptive population-based survey (SwePain). *BMC Musculoskelet Disord.* 2015;**16**:165.
63. Hansen HS. Role of anorectic N-acylethanolamines in intestinal physiology and satiety control with respect to dietary fat. *Pharmacol Res.* 2014;**86**:18–25.
64. Hauser W, Ablin J, Fitzcharles MA, Littlejohn G, Luciano JV, Usui C. Fibromyalgia. *Nat Rev Dis Primers.* 2015;**1**:15022.
65. Hellstrom F, Gouveia-Figueira S, Nording ML, Bjorklund M, Fowler CJ. Association between plasma concentrations of linoleic acid-derived oxylipins and the perceived pain scores in an exploratory study in women with chronic neck pain. *BMC Musculoskelet Disord.* 2016;**17**:103.
66. Henriksson CM, Liedberg GM, Gerdle B. 1.Women with fibromyalgia: work and rehabilitation. *Disabil Rehabil.* 2005;**27**(12):685–695.
67. Hoheisel U, Mense S. Response behaviour of cat dorsal horn neurons receiving input from skeletal muscle and other deep somatic tissues. *J Physiol.* 1990;**426**:265–280.
68. Holloszy JO. Biochemical adaptations in muscle. Effects of exercise on mitochondrial oxygen uptake and respiratory enzyme activity in skeletal muscle. *J Biol Chem.* 1967;**242**(9):2278–2282.
69. Holtermann A, Gronlund C, Roeleveld K, Gerdle B. The relation between neuromuscular control and pain intensity in fibromyalgia. *J Electromyogr Kinesiol.* 2011;**21**(3):519–524.
70. Immke DC, McCleskey EW. ASIC3: a lactic acid sensor for cardiac pain. *Scient World J.* 2001;**1**:510–512.
71. Jacobsen S, Bartels EM, Danneskiold-Samsoe B. Single cell morphology of muscle in patients with chronic muscle pain. *Scand J Rheumatol.* 1991;**20**(5):336–343.
72. Jacobsen S, Jensen KE, Thomsen C, Danneskiold-Samsoe B, Henriksen O. 31P magnetic resonance spectroscopy of skeletal muscle in patients with fibromyalgia. *J Rheumatol.* 1992;**19**(10):1600–1603.
73. Jaggar SI, Hasnie FS, Sellaturay S, Rice AS. The anti-hyperalgesic actions of the cannabinoid anandamide and the putative CB2 receptor agonist palmitoylethanolamide in visceral and somatic inflammatory pain. *Pain.* 1998;**76**(1–2):189–199.
74. Jensen K, Kosek E, Petzke F, Carville S, Fransson P, Marcus H. Evidence of dysfunctional pain inhibition in fibromyalgia reflected in rACC during provoked pain. *Pain.* 2009;**144**(1–2):95–100.
75. Jensen KB, Srinivasan P, Spaeth R, Tan Y, Kosek E, Petzke F. Overlapping structural and functional brain changes in patients with long-term exposure to fibromyalgia pain. *Arthritis Rheum.* 2013;**65**(12):3293–3303.
76. Ji RR, Chamessian A, Zhang YQ. Pain regulation by non-neuronal cells and inflammation. *Science.* 2016;**354**(6312):572–577.

77. Jubrias SA, Bennett RM, Klug GA. Increased incidence of a resonance in the phosphodiester region of 31P nuclear magnetic resonance spectra in the skeletal muscle of fibromyalgia patients. *Arthritis Rheum.* 1994;**37**(6):801–807.
78. Kalyan-Raman UP, Kalyan-Raman K, Yunus MB, Masi A. Muscle pathology in primary fibromyalgia syndrome: a light microscopic, histochemical and ultrastructural study. *J Rheumatol.* 1984;**11**(6):808–813.
79. Karlsson L, Gerdle B, Ghafouri B, Backryd E, Olausson P, Ghafouri N. Intramuscular pain modulatory substances before and after exercise in women with chronic neck pain. *Eur J Pain.* 2015;**19**(8):1075–1085.
80. Kaufmann I, Schelling G, Eisner C, Richter HP, Krauseneck T, Vogeser M. Anandamide and neutrophil function in patients with fibromyalgia. *Psychoneuroendocrinology.* 2008;**33**(5):676–685.
81. Kemp GJ, Meyerspeer M, Moser E. Absolute quantification of phosphorus metabolite concentrations in human muscle in vivo by 31P MRS: a quantitative review. *NMR Biomed.* 2007;**20**(6):555–565.
82. Khasabova IA, Xiong Y, Coicou LG, Piomelli D, Seybold V. Peroxisome proliferator-activated receptor alpha mediates acute effects of palmitoylethanolamide on sensory neurons. *J Neurosci.* 2012;**32**(37):12735–12743.
83. Kim TJ, Freml L, Park SS, Brennan T. Lactate concentrations in incisions indicate ischemic-like conditions may contribute to postoperative pain. *J Pain.* 2007;**8**(1):59–66.
84. Klaver-Krol EG, Rasker JJ, Henriquez NR, Verheijen WG, Zwarts M. Muscle fiber velocity and electromyographic signs of fatigue in fibromyalgia. *Muscle Nerve.* 2012;**46**(5):738–745.
85. Klaver-Krol EG, Zwarts MJ, Ten Klooster PM, Rasker J. Abnormal muscle membrane function in fibromyalgia patients and its relationship to the number of tender points. *Clin Exp Rheumatol.* 2012;**30**(6 Suppl 74):44–50.
86. Lam D, Hu J, Sessle B, Cairns B. Neural mechanisms of temporomandibular joint and masticatory muscle pain: a possible role for peripheral glutamate receptor mechanisms. *Pain Res Manag.* 2005;**10**:145–152.
87. Lanza IR, Nair KS. Muscle mitochondrial changes with aging and exercise. *Am J Clin Nutr.* 2009;**89**(1):467S–71S.
88. Lanza IR, Short DK, Short KR, Raghavakaimal S, Basu R, Joyner MJ. Endurance exercise as a countermeasure for aging. *Diabetes.* 2008;**57**(11):2933–2942.
89. Larsson B, Björk J, Börsbo B, Gerdle B. A systematic review of risk factors associated with transitioning from regional musculoskeletal pain to chronic widespread pain. *Eur J Pain.* 2012;**16**(8):1084–1093.
90. Lee Y, Lee CH, Oh U. Painful channels in sensory neurons. *Mol Cells.* 2005;**20**(3):315–324.
91. Lindh M, Johansson G, Hedberg M, Henning GB, Grimby G. Muscle fiber characteristics, capillaries and enzymes in patients with fibromyalgia and controls. *Scand J Rheumatol.* 1995;**24**(1):34–37.
92. Littlejohn G. Neurogenic neuroinflammation in fibromyalgia and complex regional pain syndrome. *Nat Rev Rheumatol.* 2015;**11**(11):639–648.
93. Lo Verme J, Fu J, Astarita G, La Rana G, Russo R, Calignano A. The nuclear receptor peroxisome proliferator-activated receptor alpha mediates the anti-inflammatory actions of palmitoylethanolamide. *Mol Pharmacol.* 2005;**67**:15–19.
94. Louca S, Christidis N, Ghafouri B, Gerdle B, Svensson P, List T. Serotonin, glutamate and glycerol are released after the injection of hypertonic saline into human masseter muscles—a microdialysis study. *J Headache Pain.* 2014;**15**(1):89.
95. LoVerme J, Russo R, La Rana G, Fu J, Farthing J, Mattace-Raso G. Rapid broad-spectrum analgesia through activation of peroxisome proliferator-activated receptor-alpha. *J Pharmacol Exp Ther.* 2006;**319**(3):1051–1061.
96. Loyd DR, Henry MA, Hargreaves KM. Serotonergic neuromodulation of peripheral nociceptors. *Semin Cell Dev Biol.* 2013;**24**(1):51–57.
97. Lund E, Kendall SA, Janerot-Sjoberg B, Bengtsson A. Muscle metabolism in fibromyalgia studied by P-31 magnetic resonance spectroscopy during aerobic and anaerobic exercise. *Scand J Rheumatol.* 2003;**32**(3):138–145.

98. Lund Haheim L, Nafstad P, Olsen I, Schwarze P, Ronningen KS. C-reactive protein variations for different chronic somatic disorders. *Scand J Public Health.* 2009;**37**(6):640–646.

99. Lund N, Bengtsson A, Thorborg P. Muscle tissue oxygen pressure in primary fibromyalgia. *Scand J Rheumatol.* 1986;**15**(2):165–173.

100. Mayer TG, Towns BL, Neblett R, Theodore BR, Gatchel R. Chronic widespread pain in patients with occupational spinal disorders: prevalence, psychiatric comorbidity, and association with outcomes. *Spine.* 2008;**33**(17):1889–1897.

101. McIver KL, Evans C, Kraus RM, Ispas L, Sciotti VM, Hickner R. NO-mediated alterations in skeletal muscle nutritive blood flow and lactate metabolism in fibromyalgia. *Pain.* 2006;**120**(1–2):161–169.

102. Mendieta D, De la Cruz-Aguilera DL, Barrera-Villalpando MI, Becerril-Villanueva E, Arreola R, Hernandez-Ferreira E. IL-8 and IL-6 primarily mediate the inflammatory response in fibromyalgia patients. *J Neuroimmunol.* 2016;**290**:22–25.

103. Miller KE, Hoffman EM, Sutharshan M, Schechter R. Glutamate pharmacology and metabolism in peripheral primary afferents: physiological and pathophysiological mechanisms. *Pharmacol Ther.* 2011;**130**(3):283–309.

104. Noren B, Lundberg P, Ressner M, Wirell S, Almer S, Smedby O. Absolute quantification of human liver metabolite concentrations by localized in vivo 31P NMR spectroscopy in diffuse liver disease. *Eur Radiol.* 2005;**15**(1):148–157.

105. Norrbom J. *Exercise and Regulation of Mithochondrial Biogenesis Factors in Human Skeletal Muscle.* Stockholm: Karolinska Institute; 2008.

106. Norregaard J, Bulow PM, Danneskiold-Samsoe B. Muscle strength, voluntary activation, twitch properties, and endurance in patients with fibromyalgia. *J Neurol Neurosurg Psychiat.* 1994;**57**(9):1106–1111.

107. Oaklander AL, Herzog ZD, Downs HM, Klein M. Objective evidence that small-fiber polyneuropathy underlies some illnesses currently labeled as fibromyalgia. *Pain.* 2013;**154**(11):2310–2316.

108. Olausson P, Gerdle B, Ghafouri N, Larsson B, Ghafouri B. Identification of proteins from interstitium of trapezius muscle in women with chronic myalgia using microdialysis in combination with proteomics. *PLoS One.* 2012;**7**(12):e52560.

109. Olausson P, Gerdle B, Ghafouri N, Sjostrom D, Blixt E, Ghafouri B. Protein alterations in women with chronic widespread pain—an explorative proteomic study of the trapezius muscle. *Sci Rep.* 2015;**5**:11894.

110. Olausson P, Ghafouri B, Ghafouri N, Gerdle B. Specific proteins of the trapezius muscle correlate with pain intensity and sensitivity—an explorative multivariate proteomic study of the trapezius muscle in women with chronic widespread pain. *J Pain Res.* 2016;**9**:345–356.

111. Pacher P, Batkai S, Kunos G. The endocannabinoid system as an emerging target of pharmacotherapy. *Pharmacol Rev.* 2006;**58**(3):389–462.

112. Park JH, Phothimat P, Oates CT, Hernanz-Schulman M, Olsen N. Use of P-31 magnetic resonance spectroscopy to detect metabolic abnormalities in muscles of patients with fibromyalgia. *Arthritis Rheum.* 1998;**41**(3):406–413.

113. Peolsson M, Borsbo B, Gerdle B. Generalized pain is associated with more negative consequences than local or regional pain: a study of chronic whiplash-associated disorders. *J Rehabil Med.* 2007;**39**(3):260–268.

114. Petersel D, Dror V, Cheung R. Central amplification and fibromyalgia: disorder of pain processing. *J Neurosci Res.* 2011;**89**(1):29–34.

115. Petersel DL, Dror V, Cheung R. Central amplification and fibromyalgia: disorder of pain processing. *J Neurosci Res.* 2011;**89**(1):29–34.

116. Philip A, Macdonald AL, Watt PW. Lactate—a signal coordnating cell and systemic function. *Exp Biol.* 2005;**208**:4561–4575.

117. Phillips K, Clauw DJ. Central pain mechanisms in chronic pain states—maybe it is all in their head. *Best Pract Res Clin Rheumatol.* 2011;**25**(2):141–154.

118. Phillips K, Clauw DJ. Central pain mechanisms in the rheumatic diseases: future directions. *Arthritis Rheum.* 2013;**65**(2):291–302.

119. Picard M, Hepple RT, Burelle Y. Mitochondrial functional specialization in glycolytic and oxidative muscle fibers: tailoring the organelle for optimal function. *Am J Physiol Cell Physiol.* 2012;**302**(4):C629–C641.
120. Pollak KA, Swenson JD, Vanhaitsma TA, Hughen RW, Jo D, White AT. Exogenously applied muscle metabolites synergistically evoke sensations of muscle fatigue and pain in human subjects. *Exp Physiol.* 2014;**99**(2):368–380.
121. Pongratz DE, Spath M. Morphologic aspects of fibromyalgia. *Z Rheumatol.* 1998;**57** Suppl 2:47–51.
122. Robergs RA, Ghiasvand F, Parker D. Biochemistry of exercise-induced metabolic acidosis. *Am J Physiol Regulat Integrat Comparat Physiol.* 2004;**287**:R502–R516.
123. Rodriguez-Pinto I, Agmon-Levin N, Howard A, Shoenfeld Y. Fibromyalgia and cytokines. *Immunol Lett.* 2014;**161**(2):200–203.
124. Rodriguez-Raecke R, Niemeier A, Ihle K, Ruether W, May A. Brain gray matter decrease in chronic pain is the consequence and not the cause of pain. *J Neurosci.* 2009;**29**(44):13746–13750.
125. Rodriguez-Raecke R, Niemeier A, Ihle K, Ruether W, May A. Structural brain changes in chronic pain reflect probably neither damage nor atrophy. *PLoS One.* 2013;**8**(2):e54475.
126. Sanada K, Diez MA, Valero MS, Perez-Yus MC, Demarzo MM, Garcia-Toro M. Effects of non-pharmacological interventions on inflammatory biomarker expression in patients with fibromyalgia: a systematic review. *Arthritis Res Ther.* 2015;**17**:272.
127. Sandberg M, Lindberg LG, Gerdle B. Peripheral effects of needle stimulation (acupuncture) on skin and muscle blood flow in fibromyalgia. *Eur J Pain.* 2004;**8**(2):163–171.
128. Schaible HG, Ebersberger A, Natura G. Update on peripheral mechanisms of pain: beyond prostaglandins and cytokines. *Arthritis Res Ther.* 2011;**13**(2):210.
129. Schmidt-Wilcke T, Clauw DJ. Fibromyalgia: from pathophysiology to therapy. *Nat Rev Rheumatol.* 2011;**7**(9):518–527.
130. Seminowicz DA, Wideman TH, Naso L, Hatami-Khoroushahi Z, Fallatah S, Ware MA. Effective treatment of chronic low back pain in humans reverses abnormal brain anatomy and function. *J Neurosci.* 2011;**31**(20):7540–7550.
131. Serra J, Collado A, Sola R, Antonelli F, Torres X, Salgueiro M. Hyperexcitable C nociceptors in fibromyalgia. *Ann Neurol.* 2014;**75**(2):196–208.
132. Shang Y, Gurley K, Symons B, Long D, Srikuea R, Crofford LJ. Noninvasive optical characterization of muscle blood flow, oxygenation, and metabolism in women with fibromyalgia. *Arthritis Res Ther.* 2012;**14**(6):R236.
133. Simms RW, Roy SH, Hrovat M, Anderson JJ, Skrinar G, LePoole SR. Lack of association between fibromyalgia syndrome and abnormalities in muscle energy metabolism. *Arthritis Rheum.* 1994;**37**(6):794–800.
134. Sluka KA, Clauw DJ. Neurobiology of fibromyalgia and chronic widespread pain. *Neuroscience.* 2016;**338**:114–129.
135. Smith H, Harris R, Clauw D. Fibromyalgia: an afferent processing disorder leading to a complex pain generalized syndrome. *Pain Phys.* 2011;**14**(2):E217–E245.
136. Solorzano C, Zhu C, Battista N, Astarita G, Lodola A, Rivara S. Selective N-acylethanolamine-hydrolyzing acid amidase inhibition reveals a key role for endogenous palmitoylethanolamide in inflammation. *Proc Natl Acad Sci USA.* 2009;**106**(49):20966–20971.
137. Sprott H, Rzanny R, Reichenbach JR, Kaiser WA, Hein G, Stein G. 31P magnetic resonance spectroscopy in fibromyalgic muscle. *Rheumatology.* 2000;**39**(10):1121–1125.
138. Sprott H, Salemi S, Gay RE, Bradley LA, Alarcon GS, Oh SJ. Increased DNA fragmentation and ultrastructural changes in fibromyalgic muscle fibres. *Ann Rheumat Dis.* 2004;**63**(3):245–251.
139. Srikuea R, Symons TB, Long DE, Lee JD, Shang Y, Chomentowski PJ. Association of fibromyalgia with altered skeletal muscle characteristics which may contribute to postexertional fatigue in postmenopausal women. *Arthritis Rheum.* 2013;**65**(2):519–528.

140. Staud R, Nagel S, Robinson ME, Price D. Enhanced central pain processing of fibromyalgia patients is maintained by muscle afferent input: a randomized, double-blind, placebo-controlled study. *Pain.* 2009;**145**(1–2):96–104.
141. Staud R, Weyl EE, Bartley E, Price DD, Robinson M. Analgesic and anti-hyperalgesic effects of muscle injections with lidocaine or saline in patients with fibromyalgia syndrome. *Eur J Pain.* 2014;**18**(6):803–812.
142. Staud R. The role of peripheral input for chronic pain syndromes like fibromyalgia syndrome. *J Musculoskelet Pain.* 2008;**16**(1–2):67–74.
143. Staud R. Is it all central sensitization? Role of peripheral tissue nociception in chronic musculoskeletal pain. *Curr Rheumatol Rep.* 2010;**12**(6):448–454.
144. Stensson N, Ghafouri B, Gerdle B, Ghafouri N. Alterations of anti-inflammatory lipids in plasma from women with chronic widespread pain—a case control study. *Lipids Health Dis.* 2017;**16**(1):112.
145. Stensson N, Ghafouri B, Ghafouri N, Gerdle B. High levels of endogenous lipid mediators (N-acylethanolamines) in women with chronic widespread pain during acute tissue trauma. *Mol Pain.* 2016;12:1–11.
146. Suardiaz M, Estivill-Torrus G, Goicoechea C, Bilbao A, Rodriguez de Fonseca F. Analgesic properties of oleoylethanolamide (OEA) in visceral and inflammatory pain. *Pain.* 2007;**133**(1–3):99–110.
147. Tegeder L, Zimmermann J, Meller S, Geisslinger G. Release of algesic substances in human experimental muscle pain. *Inflamm Res.* 2002 **51**(8):393–402.
148. Tsilioni I, Russell IJ, Stewart JM, Gleason RM, Theoharides TC. Neuropeptides CRH, SP, HK-1, and inflammatory cytokines IL-6 and TNF are increased in serum of patients with fibromyalgia syndrome, implicating mast cells. *J Pharmacol Exp Ther.* 2016;**356**(3):664–672.
149. Uceyler N, Hauser W, Sommer C. Systematic review with meta-analysis: cytokines in fibromyalgia syndrome. *BMC Musculoskelet Disord.* 2011;**12**:245.
150. Uceyler N, Zeller D, Kahn AK, Kewenig S, Kittel-Schneider S, Schmid A. Small fibre pathology in patients with fibromyalgia syndrome. *Brain.* 2013;**136**(Pt 6):1857–1867.
151. van Hall G. Lactate kinetics in human tissues at rest and during exercise. *Acta Physiol.* 2010;**199**(4):499–508.
152. Vestergaard-Poulsen P, Thomsen C, Nørregaard J, Bülow P, Sinkjaer T, Henriksen O. 31P NMR spectroscopy and electromyography during exercise and recovery in patients with fibromyalgia. *J Rheumatol.* 1995;**22**(8):1544–1551.
153. Wahlen K, Olausson P, Carlsson A, Ghafouri N, Gerdle B, Ghafouri B. Systemic alterations in plasma proteins from women with chronic widespread pain compared to healthy controls: a proteomic study. *J Pain Res.* 2017;**10**:797–809.
154. Wang H, Moser M, Schiltenwolf M, Buchner M. Circulating cytokine levels compared to pain in patients with fibromyalgia—a prospective longitudinal study over 6 months. *J Rheumatol.* 2008;**35**(7):1366–1370.
155. Wang X, Miyares RL, Ahern GP. Oleoylethanolamide excites vagal sensory neurones, induces visceral pain and reduces short-term food intake in mice via capsaicin receptor TRPV1. *J Physiol.* 2005;**564**(Pt 2):541–547.
156. Weibel ER, Hoppeler H. Exercise-induced maximal metabolic rate scales with muscle aerobic capacity. *J Exp Biol.* 2005;**208**:1635–1644.
157. Wolfe F, Smythe HA, Yunus MB, Bennett RM, Bombardier C, Goldenberg DL. The American College of Rheumatology 1990 criteria for the classification of fibromyalgia. Report of the multicenter criteria committee. *Arthritis Rheum.* 1990;**33**(2):160–172.
158. Xanthos DN, Sandkuhler J. Neurogenic neuroinflammation: inflammatory CNS reactions in response to neuronal activity. *Nat Rev Neurosci.* 2014;**15**(1):43–53.
159. Yunus MB, Kalyan-Raman UP, Kalyan-Raman K, Masi A. Pathologic changes in muscle in primary fibromyalgia syndrome. *Am J Med.* 1986;**81**(3A):38–42.

CHAPTER 23

Autoimmunity

Fabiola Atzeni, Rossella Talotta, and Piercarlo Sarzi-Puttini

Fibromyalgia syndrome (FMS) is a heterogeneous syndrome that is characterized by chronic pain, fatigue, and hyperalgesia, which may be associated with a wide range of symptoms including memory, sleep, and mood disorders. The etiology of the disease is still debated: It is far from being considered an autoimmune or auto-inflammatory disease, but it may develop after the activation of the innate or adaptive immune system (although data are still controversial),[7] and it is associated with other autoimmune diseases such as Sjögren's syndrome (SS), systemic lupus erythematosus (SLE), other connective tissue diseases, and rheumatoid arthritis (RA).[22,20,6,3] An association has been found between FMS and celiac disease or autoimmune thyroiditis, especially in the antibodies against thyroid-stimulating hormone (TSH).[17,16] However, aberrant immune response, increased C-reactive protein (CRP) levels, and increased erythrocyte sedimentation rate (ESR) have rarely been described in primary FMS, and perhaps characterize a distinct phenotype of the disease.[15]

An activated auto-inflammatory response has recently been found in FMS. Experiments on human peripheral blood mononuclear cells (PBMCs) and animal models have demonstrated the activation of the NACHT, LRR, and PYD domain-containing protein 3 (NALP3)/caspase-1 inflammasome, which may be related to mitochondrial dysfunction. Polymorphic variants of cytochrome b and a deficit in the Q10 coenzyme may favor oxidative stress and consequently trigger the NALP3/caspase-1 inflammasome.[29] Moreover, oxidative stress and a deficit in the Q10 coenzyme may synergistically favor the activation of innate immunity and the production of interleukin (IL)-1β and IL-18, which are typically increased in hyperalgesia.[8] Other authors have demonstrated that the activation of the NALP3 inflammasome in the PBMCs of FMS patients may be mediated by a deficit in protein kinase induced by adenosine monophosphate (AMPK).[4]

The activation of the adaptive immune response is less clearly characterized in FMS than in chronic fatigue syndrome (CFS). Although it belongs to the spectrum of algo-dysfunctional syndromes, CFS seems to develop after a viral, protozoan, or bacterial infection and the subsequent activation of B memory cells and $CD8^+$ T cells, and the production of IL-10, IL-8, and IL-1β, and tumor necrosis factor-α (TNF-α) and anti-serotonin antibodies.[21,13,12]

On the contrary, FMS does not seem to have a proper "infectious" pathogenesis, but is more related to chronic neuromuscular damage with and subsequent activation of innate immunity. Chronic neuronal damage inducing the release of substance P (SP) may favor the activation of PBMCs and the production of cytokines such as IL-10, IL-18, and TNF-α that may tune nociception.[14] The overexpression of SP, corticotropin-releasing hormone (CRH), and SP-structurally related hemokinin-1 (HK-1) that has been reported in FMS patients may favor the synthesis of proinflammatory cytokines (TNF-α and IL-6) by mast cells, thus sensitizing central and peripheral nervous cells to pain.[23]

A recent study of 114 post-vaccinated hepatitis B virus (HBV) patients found 19 cases of CFS and FMS due to vaccination. These patients satisfied the criteria for autoimmune/inflammatory syndrome induced by adjuvants (ASIA), and some of them also had detectable antinuclear antibodies (ANAs), rheumatoid factor (RF), and antibodies directed against Ro and La or ribonucleoprotein antigens.[1] Similarly, cases of FMS related to metal allergy have been described and attributed to an immune-mediated response.[19] Therefore, although the immune system seems to be more markedly involved in the pathogenesis of CFS, an external stimulus (including microbial antigens) may sometimes determine the onset of FMS as a result of the development of an immune-mediated response possibly in genetically susceptible subjects.

A recent genomic and proteogenomic study of FMS patients has demonstrated the overexpression of genes coding for glucocorticoid signaling molecules and the mediators involved in the development and proliferation of B cells even though no clear activation of this immune pathway was observed in these patients.[11] Another study found that the amount of IL-6, IL-8, macrophage inflammatory protein-1α (MIP-1α) and MIP-1β produced in vitro by stimulated PBMCs was significantly lower in the case of PBMCs from FMS patients than in those from SLE and RA patients.[25] The significant difference in IL-6 levels between FMS PBMCs and the RA/SLE controls may explain the reduced B cell responses observed in FMS patients in comparison with patients affected by inflammatory autoimmune diseases,[9] although other authors have reported higher serum IL-6 levels in FMS patients than in healthy controls.[23] A systematic review showed that FMS patients had higher serum levels of IL-1 receptor antagonist, IL-6, and IL-8, and higher plasma levels of IL-8. Moreover, the meta-analysis of eligible studies revealed that FMS patients had higher plasma IL-6 levels compared to controls (standard mean difference [SMD] = −0.34 to 0.64; −0.03 95% CI; $P = .03$).[24]

Obesity may aggravate the production of proinflammatory cytokines. One recent study has reported higher serum CRP, IL-6, and IL-8 levels in obese FMS patients than in body mass index (BMI)-matched controls.[26] However, increased CRP levels are uncommon in FMS and may depend on the presence of single-nucleotide polymorphism (SNP) in the gene of brain-derived neurotrophic factor.[27] A meta-analysis of 82 studies showed that levels of IL-6, TNF-α, IL-10, the soluble IL-2 receptor, C–C chemokine ligand 2, IL-13, IL-18, IL-12, the IL-1 receptor antagonist, and the soluble

TNF receptor 2 were elevated in patients with major depressive disturbance (MDD) compared to healthy controls, whereas interferon-γ levels were lower suggesting a typical cytokine/chemokine profile associated with MDD.[10] However, there are no studies assessing whether depression, anxiety, and stress could be responsible for the association between FMS and proinflammatory cytokines.

Anti-68/48 kD and anti-45 kD protein antibodies have been described in primary FMS (the former are associated with sleep disturbances and cognitive impairment),[5] but other autoantibodies such as ANAs that may sometimes be detected with speckled and diffuse patterns are not diagnostic or prognostic in FMS, although some authors have described an association with a separate inflammatory form of FMS.[28, 2, 18]

CONCLUSION

In conclusion, the contribution of autoimmunity or autoinflammation to the pathogenesis of FMS is still unclear, and it is not known whether primary nervous system damage may trigger an immune-mediated response. Infections and exposure to external antigens have been considered in the first steps of the pathogenesis of the disease, but no evidence is available. In genetically predisposed patients, the production of cytokines and the activation of some cell subsets (albeit in a less pronounced manner than in the case of inflammatory immune-mediated diseases) may favor the generation of a systemic *micro-inflammatory* substrate that accounts for the multifaceted disease expression of FMS. However, as immunosuppressive therapies and anti-inflammatory drugs are generally unhelpful in improving FMS symptoms, pathogenetic mechanisms other than the activation of the immune system may play a more crucial role in establishing and maintaining the disease.

REFERENCES

1. Agmon-Levin N, Zafrir Y, Kivity S, et al. Chronic fatigue syndrome and fibromyalgia following immunization with the hepatitis B vaccine: another angle of the 'autoimmune (auto-inflammatory) syndrome induced by adjuvants' (ASIA). *Immunol Res.* 2014;**60**(2–3):376–383.
2. Al-Allaf AW, Ottewell L, Pullar T. The prevalence and significance of positive antinuclear antibodies in patients with fibromyalgia syndrome: 2-4 years' follow-up. *Clin Rheumatol.* 2002;**21**(6):472–477.
3. Atzeni F, Masala IF, Salaffi F, et al. Pain in systemic inflammatory rheumatic diseases. *Best Pract Res Clin Rheumatol.* 2015;**29**(1):42–52.
4. Bullón P, Alcocer-Gómez E, Carrión AM, et al. AMPK phosphorylation modulates pain by activation of NLRP3 inflammasome. *Antioxid Redox Signal.* 2016;**24**(3):157–170.
5. Buskila D, Sarzi-Puttini P. Fibromyalgia and autoimmune diseases: the pain behind autoimmunity. *Isr Med Assoc J.* 2008;**10**(1):77–78.
6. Choi BY, Oh HJ, Lee YJ, et al. Prevalence and clinical impact of fibromyalgia in patients with primary Sjögren's syndrome. *Clin Exp Rheumatol.* 2016;**34**(2 Suppl 96):S9–S13.
7. Clauw DJ. Fibromyalgia and related conditions. *Mayo Clin Proc.* 2015;**90**(5):680–692.
8. Cordero MD, Alcocer-Gómez E, Culic O, et al. NLRP3 inflammasome is activated in fibromyalgia: the effect of coenzyme Q10. *Antioxid Redox Signal.* 2014;**20**(8):1169–1180.

9. Jego G, Pascual V, Palucka AK, et al. Dendritic cells control B cell growth and differentiation. *Curr Dir Autoimmun.* 2005;**8**:124–139.
10. Köhler CA, Freitas TH, Maes M, et al. Peripheral cytokine and chemokine alterations in depression: a meta-analysis of 82 studies. *Acta Psychiatr Scand.* 2017;**135**(5):373–387.
11. Lukkahatai N, Walitt B, Espina A, et al. Comparing genomic profiles of women with and without fibromyalgia. *Biol Res Nurs.* 2015;**17**(4):373–383.
12. Maes M, Bosmans E, Kubera M. Increased expression of activation antigens on CD8+ T lymphocytes in myalgic encephalomyelitis/chronic fatigue syndrome: inverse associations with lowered CD19+ expression and CD4+/CD8+ ratio, but no associations with (auto)immune, leaky gut, oxidative and nitrosative stress biomarkers. *Neuro Endocrinol Lett.* 2015;**36**(5):439–446.
13. Maes M, Ringel K, Kubera M, et al. In myalgic encephalomyelitis/chronic fatigue syndrome, increased autoimmune activity against 5-HT is associated with immuno-inflammatory pathways and bacterial translocation. *J Affect Disord.* 2013;**150**(2):223–230.
14. Mashaghi A, Marmalidou A, Tehrani M, et al. Neuropeptide substance P and the immune response. *Cell Mol Life Sci.* 2016;**73**(22):4249–4264.
15. Metyas SK, Solyman JS, Arkfeld DG. Inflammatory fibromyalgia: is it real? *Curr Rheumatol Rev.* 2015;**11**(1):15–17.
16. Nishioka K, Uchida T, Usui C, et al. High prevalence of anti-TSH receptor antibody in fibromyalgia syndrome. *Int J Rheum Dis.* 2017;**20**(6):685–690.
17. Rubio-Tapia A, Jansson-Knodell CL, Rahim MW, et al. Influence of gender on the clinical presentation and associated diseases in adults with celiac disease. *Gac Med Mex.* 2016;**152**(Suppl 2):38–46.
18. Smart PA, Waylonis GW, Hackshaw KV. Immunologic profile of patients with fibromyalgia. *Am J Phys Med Rehabil.* 1997;**76**(3):231–234.
19. Stejskal V. Metals as a common trigger of inflammation resulting in non-specific symptoms: diagnosis and treatment. *Isr Med Assoc J.* 2014;**16**(12):753–758.
20. Stisi S, Sarzi-Puttini P, Benucci M, et al. Pain in systemic sclerosis. *Reumatismo.* 2014;**66**(1):44–47.
21. Talotta R, Atzeni F, Bazzichi L, et al. Algo-dysfunctional syndromes: a critical digest of the recent literature. *Clin Exp Rheumatol.* 2015;**33**(1 Suppl 88):S102–S108.
22. Torrente-Segarra V, Salman-Monte TC, Rúa-Figueroa Í, et al.; RELESSER Study Group of the Spanish Society of Rheumatology (SER); Study Group of Systemic Autoimmune Diseases of the SER (EAS-SER). Fibromyalgia prevalence and related factors in a large registry of patients with systemic lupus erythematosus. *Clin Exp Rheumatol.* 2016;**34**(2 Suppl 96):S40–S47.
23. Tsilioni I, Russell IJ, Stewart JM, et al. Neuropeptides CRH, SP, HK-1, and inflammatory cytokines IL-6 and TNF are increased in serum of patients with fibromyalgia syndrome, implicating mast cells. *J Pharmacol Exp Ther.* 2016;**356**(3):664–672.
24. Uçeyler N, Häuser W, Sommer C. Systematic review with meta-analysis: cytokines in fibromyalgia syndrome. *BMC Musculoskelet Disord.* 2011;**12**:245.
25. Wallace DJ, Gavin IM, Karpenko O, et al. Cytokine and chemokine profiles in fibromyalgia, rheumatoid arthritis and systemic lupus erythematosus: a potentially useful tool in differential diagnosis. *Rheumatol Int.* 2015;**35**(6):991–996.
26. Xiao Y, Haynes WL, Michalek JE, et al. Elevated serum high-sensitivity C-reactive protein levels in fibromyalgia syndrome patients correlate with body mass index, interleukin-6, interleukin-8, erythrocyte sedimentation rate. *Rheumatol Int.* 2013;**33**(5):1259–1264.
27. Xiao Y, Russell IJ, Liu YG. A brain-derived neurotrophic factor polymorphism Val66Met identifies fibromyalgia syndrome subgroup with higher body mass index and C-reactive protein. *Rheumatol Int.* 2012;**32**(8):2479–2485.
28. Yunus MB, Hussey FX, Aldag JC. Antinuclear antibodies and connective tissue disease features in fibromyalgia syndrome: a controlled study. *J Rheumatol.* 1993;**20**(9):1557–1560.
29. Zhang H, Li F, Li WW, et al. The inflammasome as a target for pain therapy. *Br J Anaesth.* 2016;**117**(6):693–707.

CHAPTER 24

Stress-Induced Hyperalgesia

Winfried Häuser

Summary Points

- Many patients with fibromyalgia syndrome (FMS) report childhood adversities and prolonged stress during their life span.
- The model of stress-induced hyperalgesia (SIH) postulates that chronic stress can lead to maladaptive neurobiologic changes in pathways associated with pain processing.
- The model of SIH is compatible with current pathophysiologic concepts of central sensitization and sympathetic nervous system dysfunction in FMS.
- SIH might apply to many, but not to all FMS patients.

FIBROMYALGIA SYNDROME—A STRESS DISORDER

Since the 1990s, mental health care specialists were impressed by the amount of psychological suffering during the life span (childhood adversities such as physical and sexual abuse and emotional neglect, major life and traumatic events, prolonged daily hassles) of FMS patients. The term "pain-prone patient" created by Engel[12,2] seems to ring true for many patients with FMS: "Some of them seem to have suffered the most and extraordinary number of defeats, humiliations and unpleasant experiences."[12] These concepts described by G. Engel led to the creation of the category "psychogenic pain" in the *Diagnostic and Statistical Manual of Psychiatric Diseases Version III* and later to the category "somatoform pain disorder" in the *Diagnostic and Statistical Manual of Psychiatric Diseases Version IV*.[4,5] However, FMS is still regarded to be a somatoform pain disorder by many European mental health care specialists, especially for those in psychosomatic medicine.[11,16] The association of retrospective self-reports of childhood adversities and adult FMS has been confirmed by systematic reviews of case–control studies.[18,3] Traumatic events in childhood and adulthood for a considerable number of FMS patients have been described by case-controlled studies in Germany[15] and by case series in Germany,[17,26] Israel,[20] and the United States.[17] In 2004, Van Houdenhove and

Egle[25] synthesized the findings of adverse life experiences with stress regulation and pain-processing mechanisms and postulated that FMS is a stress disorder.

FIBROMYALGIA SYNDROME AND STRESS-INDUCED HYPERALGESIA

A wealth of research over the past two decades has expanded our understanding of the impact of early-life adversity on physiologic function. Early-life adversity increases the risk of developing a number of so-called functional somatic pain syndromes or central hypersensitivity syndromes such as FMS and irritable bowel syndrome.[22] Evidence supports the notion that exposure to chronic or repeated stress can produce maladaptive neurobiologic changes in pathways associated with pain processing, resulting in SIH.[21] There are certain key neurobiologic substrates for SIH, including the hypothalamic–pituitary–adrenal axis, monoaminergic, opioidergic, endocannabinoid, and immune systems.[6] SIH can be demonstrated in animals, as well as healthy persons and persons with FMS.[8]

The concept of SIH is compatible with current pathophysiologic models of FMS. The best-established pathophysiologic features are those of central sensitization (i.e., augmented pain and sensory processing in the brain, with increased functional connectivity to pronociceptive brain regions and decreased connectivity to antinociceptive regions) and accompanying changes in central nervous system (CNS) neurotransmitters as well as the size and shape of brain regions.[7] Enhancement of central sensitization was detected in persons with high levels of childhood adversities and may provide a mechanism underlying the pain hypersensitivity.[27]

Studies in animals have described a chronic stress-related sensitization of muscle nociceptors that may relate to stress-related cytokine release.[9] Furthermore, increased prostaglandin E2 expression in stressed newborn rats causes hyperalgesia in these animals throughout their life span.[13] Because patients with FMS display a correlation of muscle pain with levels of prostaglandin E2,[19] hyperalgesic/allodynic reactions could be based on stress-related alterations of their muscle nociceptors.[8]

Sympathetic nervous system dysfunction is another pathophysiologic model of FMS. The sympathetic nervous system is a key element of the stress response system and might be altered by traumatic and or prolonged stress.[23]

LIMITATIONS

Most of the studies in this field have been cross-sectional or retrospective in design, and caution is advised when interpreting results. It is possible that some findings may be subjected to recall bias, and reverse causation is also a potential concern, but several prospective studies that provide more robust evidence are reassuring.[22] In addition, retrospective reports are known to rather underestimate than overestimate the rates of childhood adversities.[10]

The association of childhood adversities and traumatic events in FMS patients is likely mediated by depression and might therefore be only valid for FMS patients with comorbid affective disorders.[14]

FMS is a heterogenous condition from a clinical and pathophysiologic point of view. The biopsychosocial model postulates the interaction of biological, psychological, and social factors in the predisposition, triggering, and maintenance of FMS.[24] Prolonged stress by major life and traumatic events during the whole life span and the consequence of SIH might be a pathway to FMS in many, but not all FMS patients. Although characterization of patient populations facilitates the classification, strengthens the search for common underlying mechanisms, and helps to design treatment plans, it is important that providers not fall victim to the "patient uniformity" or "patient-homogeneity" myth.[1]

REFERENCES

1. Adams LM, Turk DC. Psychosocial factors and central sensitivity syndromes. *Curr Rheumatol Rev.* 2015;**11**(2):96–108.
2. Adler RH, Zlot S, Hürny C, Minder C. Engel's "Psychogenic Pain and the Pain-Prone Patient": a retrospective, controlled clinical study. *Psychosom Med.* 1989;**51**(1):87–101.
3. Afari N, Ahumada SM, Wright LJ, et al. Psychological trauma and functional somatic syndromes: a systematic review and meta-analysis. *Psychosom Med.* 2014;**76**(1):2–11.
4. American Psychiatric Association Task Force on DSM-IV. *Diagnostic and Statistical Manual of Mental Disorders: DSM-III-TR.* Arlington, VA: American Psychiatric Publishing; 1987.
5. American Psychiatric Association Task Force on DSM-IV. *Diagnostic and Statistical Manual of Mental Disorders: DSM-IV-TR.* Arlington, VA: American Psychiatric Publishing; 2000.
6. Burke NN, Finn DP, McGuire BE, Roche M. Psychological stress in early life as a predisposing factor for the development of chronic pain: clinical and preclinical evidence and neurobiological mechanisms. *J Neurosci Res.* 2017;**95**(6):1257–1270.
7. Clauw DJ. Fibromyalgia: a clinical review. *JAMA.* 2014;**311**(15):1547–1555.
8. Crettaz B, Marziniak M, Willeke P, et al. Stress-induced allodynia—evidence of increased pain sensitivity in healthy humans and patients with chronic pain after experimentally induced psychosocial stress. *PLoS ONE.* 2013;**8**(8):e69460.
9. Dina OA, Levine JD, Green PG. Enhanced cytokine-induced mechanical hyperalgesia in skeletal muscle produced by a novel mechanism in rats exposed to unpredictable sound stress. *Eur J Pain.* 2011;**15**(8):796–800.
10. Egle UT, Egloff N, von Känel R. Stress-induced hyperalgesia (SIH) as a consequence of emotional deprivation and psychosocial traumatization in childhood: implications for the treatment of chronic pain. *Schmerz.* 2016;**30**(6):526–536.
11. Egle UT, Nickel R, Schwab R, Hoffmann SO. Somatoform pain disorder. *Dtsch Arztebl.* 2000;**97**(21):A-1469/B-1229/C-1149.
12. Engel GL. Psychogenic pain and pain-prone patient. *Am J Med.* 1959;**26**(6):899–918.
13. Green PG, Chen X, Alvarez P, Ferrari LF, Levine JD. Early-life stress produces muscle hyperalgesia and nociceptor sensitization in the adult rat. *Pain.* 2011;**152**(11):2549–2556.
14. Häuser W, Bohn D, Kühn-Becker H, Erdkönig R, Brähler E, Glaesmer H. Is the association of self-reported childhood maltreatments and adult fibromyalgia syndrome attributable to depression? A case control study. *Clin Exp Rheumatol.* 2012;**30**(6 Suppl 74):59–64.

15. Häuser W, Galek A, Erbslöh-Möller B, et al. Posttraumatic stress disorder in fibromyalgia syndrome: prevalence, temporal relationship between posttraumatic stress and fibromyalgia symptoms, and impact on clinical outcome. *Pain.* 2013;**154**(8):1216–1223.
16. Häuser W, Henningsen P. Fibromyalgia syndrome: a somatoform disorder? *Eur J Pain.* 2014;**18**(8): 1052–1059.
17. Häuser W, Hoffmann EM, Wolfe F, et al. Self-reported childhood maltreatment, lifelong traumatic events and mental disorders in fibromyalgia syndrome: a comparison of US and German outpatients. *Clin Exp Rheumatol.* 2015;**33**(1 Suppl 88):S86–S92.
18. Häuser W, Kosseva M, Üceyler N, Klose P, Sommer C. Emotional, physical, and sexual abuse in fibromyalgia syndrome: a systematic review with meta-analysis. *Arthritis Care Res.* 2011;**63**(6):808–820.
19. Hedenberg-Magnusson B, Ernberg M, Alstergren P, Kopp S. Pain mediation by prostaglandin E2 and leukotriene B4 in the human masseter muscle. *Acta Odontol Scand.* 2001;**59**(6):348–355.
20. Hellou R, Häuser W, Brenner I, et al. Self-reported childhood maltreatment and traumatic events among Israeli patients suffering from fibromyalgia and rheumatoid arthritis. *Pain Res Manag.* 2017;**2017**:3865249.
21. Jennings EM, Okine BN, Roche M, Finn DP. Stress-induced hyperalgesia. *Prog Neurobiol.* 2014;**121**:1–18.
22. Jones GT. Psychosocial vulnerability and early life adversity as risk factors for central sensitivity syndromes. *Curr Rheumatol Rev.* 2016;**12**(2):140–153.
23. Martínez-Martínez LA, Mora T, Vargas A, Fuentes-Iniestra M, Martínez-Lavín M. Sympathetic nervous system dysfunction in fibromyalgia, chronic fatigue syndrome, irritable bowel syndrome, and interstitial cystitis: a review of case-control studies. *J Clin Rheumatol.* 2014;**20**(3):146–150.
24. Üçeyler N, Burgmer M, Friedel E, et al. Etiology and pathophysiology of fibromyalgia syndrome: updated guidelines 2017, overview of systematic review articles and overview of studies on small fiber neuropathy in FMS subgroups. *Schmerz.* 2017;**31**(3):239–245.
25. Van Houdenhove B, Egle UT. Fibromyalgia: a stress disorder? Piecing the biopsychosocial puzzle together. *Psychother Psychosom.* 2004;**73**(5):267–275.
26. Waller E, Scheidt CE, Endorf K, Hartmann A, Zimmermann P. Unresolved trauma in fibromyalgia: a cross-sectional study. *J Health Psychol.* 2015;pii:1359105315580460. [Epub ahead of print]
27. You DS, Meagher MW. Childhood adversity and pain sensitization. *Psychosom Med.* 2016; **78**(9): 1084–1093.

SECTION 6

Management Approaches in Fibromyalgia Syndrome

CHAPTER 25

Pharmacologic Approaches: From Meta-Analyses and Reviews to Clinical Guidelines

Serge Perrot

Summary Points

- Drugs are not very effective in fibromyalgia syndrome (FMS) and both physicians and patients should have realistic expectations about the efficacy of drugs in FMS.
- Pharmacologic therapy should be considered as an adjunct to non-pharmacologic intervention.
- Pain relief should not be considered as the single aim of the management. An individualized approach to patient care is imperative, adapted to the core set of symptom domains, including pain, fatigue, sleep and mood disturbance, and cognitive dysfunction.
- The choice of pharmaceutical therapies should be guided by the patient's clinical features, side-effect profile, and response: FMS patients who started pharmaceutical therapies should be reviewed frequently and the dose titrated up based on the patient's response.
  - Further research on new therapies with different mechanisms and side-effect profiles is needed.

Despite increased understanding of FMS and numerous clinical trials, there is no gold standard treatment for FMS. Numerous meta-analyses on pharmacologic and non-pharmacologic approaches have been published. Classically, most trials and meta-analyses have evaluated pain and physical function (Fibromyalgia Impact Questionnaire) as the primary outcome measures. To provide a complete assessment of a treatment for FMS, the Outcome Measures in Rheumatology Clinical Trials (OMERACT) group defined core symptomatic domains that should be measured in all FMS randomized controlled trials (RCTs).[22] These core domains included pain, sleep dysfunction, fatigue, depression, and multidimensional function, with second-level outcome domains to be measured in some but not all clinical trials included cognitive dysfunction, anxiety, and tenderness. Literature reviews and meta-analyses on pharmacologic and non-pharmacologic treatments for FMS have concluded that treatments may be effective at managing a few core FMS symptoms, mainly pain and function.[18,6,25] One meta-analysis looked at efficacy profiles of pharmacologic and non-pharmacologic interventions for the management of the six core FMS clinical domains as defined by OMERACT: pain, sleep dysfunction, fatigue, depression, physical dysfunction, and cognitive dysfunction.[28]

Based on literature analyses, recent guidelines for FMS treatment[33,13,12,21] have been proposed, which include both pharmacologic and non-pharmacologic approaches, with a recent increased focus on non-pharmacologic therapies. However, pharmacology remains the basis of therapy, including classical analgesic therapies, but also antidepressants, anticonvulsants, and numerous others drugs, proposed according to various pathophysiologic pathways. The wide range of therapies often leads to confusion both for prescribers and patients, and the evidence supporting pharmacologic therapies is often limited with discrepancies across countries according to their market authorization. As an example, in Europe, no drug is approved particularly for FMS. European Medicine Agency (EMA) refused the approval of duloxetine, milnacipran, and pregabalin—in contrast to Food and Drug Administration (FDA). In this chapter, we review meta-analyses, literature reviews on pharmacologic approaches, and how these pharmacologic approaches have been integrated in the guidelines.

SIMPLE ANALGESICS

Because pain is the major symptom in FMS, simple analgesics are widely used by patients, but their efficacy is poor with very few studies. A recent Cochrane review on nonsteroidal anti-inflammatory drugs (NSAIDs) in FMS does not recommend their use[11] and there is no evidence for the use of acetaminophen except it is used in combination with tramadol.[2]

Tramadol is a weak opioid with combined 5-hydroxytryptamine (5-HT) and norepinephrine reuptake inhibition activity, studied in two trials, one combined with acetaminophen[2] and one as single therapy,[30] demonstrating some efficacy, mainly on the short term, and is being proposed in the guidelines for severe pain.[12,21]

STRONG OPIOIDS

No controlled study with strong opioids in FMS has been conducted.[33] The Cochrane review on oxycodone[14] concluded that there is no randomized trial evidence to support or refute the use of FMS. All FMS guidelines recommend against the use of opioid analgesics and observational studies have found that patients with FMS receiving opioids have poorer outcomes than patients receiving nonopioids.[15]

CANNABINOIDS

Cannabinoid molecules have been shown to have analgesic properties as well as sleep-promoting effects.[18] The Canadian guidelines[13,12] recommend the use of pharmacologic cannabinoids, particularly in the setting of sleep disturbance. Both the European League Against Rheumatism and the German guidelines gave a recommendation not to use cannabis-based drugs in FMS[33,21] and further research should demonstrate their safety in FMS. The Cochrane review on cannabinoids in FMS found no convincing evidence for their use in FMS.[40]

PHARMACOLOGIC APPROACHES BASED ON PAIN PATHWAYS MODULATION: ANTIDEPRESSANTS

Antidepressants have been proposed for years in FMS, independently of their effect on mood disorders and, aside anticonvulsants, represent the first-line treatment for FMS. Patients with FMS have been found to have decreased concentration of 5-HT and its precursor (tryptophan) in serum and cerebrospinal fluid.[32] Descending pain inhibitory pathways dysfunctions have also been found in FMS, with the implication of serotonin and noradrenaline. This could represent the pathophysiologic basis for the use of antidepressants in FMS, independently of their use for concomitant mood disorders. Globally, antidepressants are effective in FMS.[28,24,17,42,37] When looking more precisely on different FMS domains,[28] it can be confirmed that amitriptyline is effective at reducing pain and sleep disturbances and for improving fatigue, whereas citalopram has weak and nonsignificant effects on pain, fatigue, and sleep disturbances. Nishishinya et al.[24] also concluded that amitriptyline 25 mg/day improved pain, sleep, and fatigue at 6 to 8 weeks with no evidence for 50 mg/day. A statistically significant improvement in reducing pain, sleep disturbance, fatigue, affective symptoms, functional deficit, and cognitive impairment has been noted for duloxetine treatment, but with small treatment effects.[28] Fluoxetine treatment demonstrated a medium effect for pain, mainly at high dosages (80 mg/day), small effects on sleep disturbance, affective symptoms, and functional impact.[1] Milnacipran demonstrated a small but significant effect on pain, while there were no effects on sleep disturbance, fatigue, affective symptoms, functional deficit, or cognitive impairment.[10] Finally, cyclobenzaprine, an antidepressant used as a muscle relaxant and only available in few countries has demonstrated some effects[37]: weak on pain, better on sleep, but not on fatigue or allodynia. All FMS guidelines recommend the use of antidepressants in FMS, especially amitriptyline at low doses.

ANTICONVULSANTS

Anticonvulsants are also first-line drug treatment options for FMS. FMS has features in common with neuropathic pain, including changes in the central nervous system (CNS), especially central sensitization,[4] but also in peripheral nerve fibers.[26] In this line, anticonvulsants have been proposed in FMS, and, as in neuropathic pain, mostly pregabalin and gabapentin. Pregabalin and gabapentin are structurally similar to the neurotransmitter gamma-aminobutyric acid (GABA), but their analgesic effect is not related to GABA's neuronal system. Their effect on pain is linked to their affinity to the voltage-gated calcium channels in the CNS.[36]

Pregabalin

In two Cochrane reviews,[38,9] authors concluded that pregabalin produces a major reduction in pain intensity for more than 12 to 26 weeks with tolerable adverse events for a small proportion of people (about 10% more than placebo) with moderate or severe pain due to FMS. The degree of pain relief is known to be accompanied by improvements in other symptoms, quality of life, and function. This effect on pain was confirmed in a review on effects on specific FMS domains,[28] with effects also on function. Due to the unavailability of data, the effects of pregabalin on affective symptoms and cognitive impairment cannot be concluded. Pregabalin is proposed in FMS in all guidelines.

Gabapentin and Other Anticonvulsants

In their Cochrane review, the conclusion of Üçeyler et al.[38] was that amount and quality of evidence were insufficient to draw definite conclusions on the efficacy and safety of gabapentin, lacosamide, and levetiracetam in FMS. The amount of evidence for gabapentin in FMS was also considered very limited in a third Cochrane review and the conclusion was that there is insufficient evidence to support or refute the suggestion that gabapentin reduces pain in FMS.[7]

PHARMACOLOGIC APPROACHES BASED ON EXPERIMENTAL FINDINGS

Because numerous causes have been suggested in FMS, several drugs have proposed based on specific pathophysiologic pathways and experimental findings.

Growth Hormone

Growth hormone was found to be decreased in a subset of FMS patients and daily injections were tested as a treatment of FMS.[8] It induced a substantial reduction in pain and an improvement in functional deficit.

Hypnotics

Sleep disturbances are prevalent in FMS, and some treatments dedicated to sleep disorders have been tested in FMS. Hypnotics did not demonstrate any efficacy on pain or function, only on sleep.[23] However, sodium oxybate reduced sleep disturbance, fatigue, and pain,[34] but FDA and EMA refused the approval of sodium oxybate in FMS due to safety concerns.

Dopamine Agonists

Pramipexole was the first dopamine agonist to be tested in FMS,[19] with important effects that were never confirmed in clinical practice.

Setrons

Russell et al.[32] showed decreased levels of serum serotonin and its metabolite 5-hydroxyindoleacetic acid (5-HIA) in the cerebrospinal fluid and increase of serotonin receptors in platelets of patients with FMS.[31] Among the subtypes of receptors for serotonin, 5-HT3 receptors are located on neurons in the central and peripheral nervous system and several studies have tested setrons (tropisetron, ondansetron, granisetron, and dolasetron) in FMS that are highly selective and competitive receptor 5-HT3 antagonists. Setrons, injected intravenously, demonstrated some effect on pain but not on other symptoms.[35,39]

N-Methyl-D-Aspartate Receptor Antagonists

Central sensitization is an important feature in FMS, suggesting some efficacy of *N*-methyl-D-aspartate (NMDA) receptor antagonists. Only one small single-center study has demonstrated efficacy of memantine[27] on pain and quality of life. Overall, benefits with NMDA receptor antagonists (ketamine, memantine) are not defined and there is a need for better strategy trials to clarify optimal dose schedules and to delineate potential longer term adverse events.[20]

Antipsychotics

The conclusion of the Cochrane review[41] on antipsychotics in FMS was negative, with the exception of comorbid major depression not responding to antidepressants, a condition where antipsychotics are also recommended by the German guidelines.

DISCUSSION AND CONCLUSION

Globally, drugs do not demonstrate important improvement in most of the FMS patients, either on pain or on other dimensions, with important side effects for most of the drugs. This is probably not specific to FMS because it has been observed in other chronic pain conditions, like chronic low back pain.[5] Thus, both physicians and patients should have realistic expectations about the efficacy of drugs in FMS. Although patients may initially experience some symptom relief, the majority will ultimately discontinue therapy because of inadequate response or unacceptable side effects.[29] Non-pharmacologic approaches such as self-management, aerobic and strengthening exercises, psychological therapies have demonstrated higher efficacy on the long term, with reduced side effects.[28] Some strategies have suggested the use of drugs based on FMS symptoms (e.g., pain, sleep disturbances, mood disorders),[3] but, as suggested in the guidelines, drug therapy may be added to non-pharmacologic treatments and not used as a single management strategy.[16] Pharmacologic therapies should be considered for patients with severe FMS involving several domains, with a graded approach, adapted to the severity. The choice of pharmaceutical therapies should be guided by the patient's clinical features, side-effect profile, and response: FMS patients who started pharmaceutical therapies should be reviewed frequently and the dose titrated up based on the patient's response. Where therapy has not demonstrated a positive effect, or where side effects are prominent, treatment should be discontinued. In all cases, as recommended in all guidelines, an individualized approach to patient care is imperative, and both patients and physician should now be aware that pharmacologic therapy should be considered as an adjunct to non-pharmacologic intervention.

REFERENCES

1. Arnold LM, Hess EV, Hudson JI, Welge JA, Berno SE, Keck PE Jr. A randomized, placebo-controlled, double-blind, flexible-dose study of fluoxetine in the treatment of women with fibromyalgia. *Am J Med.* 2002;**112**:191–197.
2. Bennett RM, Kamin M, Karim R, Rosenthal N. Tramadol and acetaminophen combination tablets in the treatment of fibromyalgia pain: a double-blind, randomized, placebo-controlled study. *Am J Med.* 2003;**114**:537–545.
3. Boomershine CS, Crofford LJ. A symptom-based approach to pharmacologic management of fibromyalgia. *Nat Rev Rheumatol.* 2009;**5**:191–199.
4. Boomershine CS. Fibromyalgia: the prototypical central sensitivity syndrome. *Curr Rheumatol Rev.* 2015;**11**:131–145.
5. Chou R. Pharmacological management of low back pain. *Drugs.* 2010;**70**:387–402.
6. Choy E, Marshall D, Gabriel ZL, Mitchell SA, Gylee E, Dakin HA. Systematic review and mixed treatment comparison of the efficacy of pharmacological treatments for fibromyalgia. *Semin Arthritis Rheum.* 2011;**41**:335–345.
7. Cooper TE, Derry S, Wiffen PJ, Moore RA. Gabapentin for fibromyalgia pain in adults. *Cochrane Database Syst Rev.* 2017;(**1**):CD012188.
8. Cuatrecasas G, Alegre C, Fernandez-Solà J, et al. Growth hormone treatment for sustained pain reduction and improvement in quality of life in severe fibromyalgia. *Pain.* 2012;**153**:1382–1389.
9. Derry S, Cording M, Wiffen PJ, Law S, Phillips T, Moore RA. Pregabalin for pain in fibromyalgia in adults. *Cochrane Database Syst Rev.* 2016;(**9**):CD011790.
10. Derry S, Gill D, Phillips T, Moore RA. Milnacipran for neuropathic pain and fibromyalgia in adults. *Cochrane Database Syst Rev.* 2012;(**3**):CD008244.

11. Derry S, Wiffen PJ, Häuser W, et al. Oral nonsteroidal anti-inflammatory drugs for fibromyalgia in adults. *Cochrane Database Syst Rev*. 2017;(**3**):CD012332.
12. Fitzcharles MA, Ste Marie PA, Goldenberg DL, et al. Canadian guidelines for the diagnosis and management of fibromyalgia syndrome. *Pain Res Manag*. 2013;**18**(3):119–126.
13. Fitzcharles MA, Ste-Marie PA, Goldenberg DL, et al. Canadian guidelines for the diagnosis and management of fibromyalgia syndrome: executive summary. *Pain Res Manag*. 2013;**18**:119–126.
14. Gaskell H, Moore RA, Derry S, Stannard C. Oxycodone for pain in fibromyalgia in adults. *Cochrane Database Syst Rev*. 2016;(**9**):CD012329.
15. Goldenberg DL, Clauw DJ, Palmer RE, Clair AG. Opioid use in fibromyalgia: a cautionary tale. *Mayo Clin Proc*. 2016;**91**:640–648.
16. Häuser W, Ablin J, Perrot S, Fitzcharles MA. Management of fibromyalgia: practical guides from recent evidence-based guidelines. *Pol Arch Intern Med*. 2017;**127**:47–56.
17. Hauser W, Urrutia G, Tort S, Uceyler N, Walitt B. Serotonin and noradrenaline reuptake inhibitors (SNRIs) for fibromyalgia syndrome. *Cochrane Database Syst Rev*. 2013;(1):CD010292.
18. Hauser W, Walitt B, Fitzcharles MA, Sommer C. Review of pharmacological therapies in fibromyalgia syndrome. *Arthritis Res Ther*. 2014;**16**:201.
19. Holman AJ, Myers RR. A randomized, double-blind, placebo-controlled trial of pramipexole, a dopamine agonist, in patients with fibromyalgia receiving concomitant medications. *Arthritis Rheum*. 2005;**52**:2495–2505.
20. Littlejohn G, Guymer E. Modulation of NMDA receptor activity in fibromyalgia. *Biomedicines*. 2017;**5**:2.
21. Macfarlane GJ, Kronisch C, Dean LE, et al. EULAR revised recommendations for the management of fibromyalgia. *Ann Rheum Dis*. 2017;**76**:318–328.
22. Mease P, Arnold LM, Choy EH, et al. Fibromyalgia syndrome module at OMERACT 9. *J Rheumatol*. 2009;**36**:2318–2329.
23. Moldofsky H, Lue FA, Mously C, Roth-Schechter B, Reynolds WJ. The effect of zolpidem in patients with fibromyalgia: a dose ranging, double blind, placebo controlled, modified crossover study. *J Rheumatol*. 1996;**23**:529–533.
24. Nishishinya B, Urrútia G, Walitt B, et al. Amitriptyline in the treatment of fibromyalgia: a systematic review of its efficacy. *Rheumatology*. 2008;**47**:1741–1746.
25. Nüesch E, Häuser W, Bernardy K, Barth J, Jüni P. Comparative efficacy of pharmacological and non-pharmacological interventions in fibromyalgia syndrome: network meta-analysis. *Ann Rheum Dis*. 2013;**72**:955–962.
26. Oaklander AL, Herzog ZD, Downs HM, Klein MM. Objective evidence that small-fiber polyneuropathy underlies some illnesses currently labeled as fibromyalgia. *Pain*. 2013;**154**:2310–2316.
27. Olivan-Blázquez B, Herrera-Mercadal P, Puebla-Guedea M, et al. Efficacy of memantine in the treatment of fibromyalgia: a double-blind, randomised, controlled trial with 6-month follow-up. *Pain*. 2014;**155**:2517–2525.
28. Perrot S, Russell IJ. More ubiquitous effects from non-pharmacologic than from pharmacologic treatments for fibromyalgia syndrome: a meta-analysis examining six core symptoms. *Eur J Pain*. 2014;**18**:1067–1080.
29. Robinson RL, Kroenke K, Mease P, et al. Burden of illness and treatment patterns for patients with fibromyalgia. *Pain Med*. 2012;**13**:1366–1376.
30. Russell IJ, Kamin M, Bennett RM, Schnitzer TJ, Green JA, Katz WA. Efficacy of tramadol in treatment of pain in fibromyalgia. *J Clin Rheumatol*. 2000;**6**:250–257.
31. Russell IJ, Michalek JE, Vipraio GA, Fletcher EM, Javors MA, Bowden CA. Platelet 3H-imipramine uptake receptor density and serum serotonin levels in patients with fibromyalgia/fibrositis syndrome. *J Rheumatol*. 1992;**19**:104–109.
32. Russell IJ, Vaeroy H, Javors M, Nyberg F. Cerebrospinal fluid biogenic amine metabolites in fibromyalgia/fibrositis syndrome and rheumatoid arthritis. *Arthritis Rheum*. 1992;**35**:550–556.

33. Sommer C, Alten R, Bär KJ, et al. Drug therapy of fibromyalgia syndrome: updated guidelines 2017 and overview of systematic review articles. *Schmerz.* 2017;**31**(3):274–284.
34. Spaeth M, Bennett RM, Benson BA, Wang YG, Lai C, Choy EH. Sodium oxybate therapy provides multidimensional improvement in fibromyalgia: results of an international phase 3 trial. *Ann Rheum Dis.* 2012;**71**:935–942.
35. Späth M, Stratz T, Neeck G, et al. Efficacy and tolerability of intravenous tropisetron in the treatment of fibromyalgia. *Scand J Rheumatol.* 2004;**33**:267–270.
36. Taylor CP. Mechanisms of analgesia by gabapentin and pregabalin—calcium channel α2-Δ [cavα2-Δ] ligands. *Pain.* 2009;**142**:13–16.
37. Tofferi JK, Jackson JL, O'Malley PG. Treatment of fibromyalgia with cyclobenzaprine: a meta-analysis. *Arthritis Care Res.* 2004;**51**:9–13.
38. Üçeyler N, Sommer C, Walitt B, Häuser W. Anticonvulsants for fibromyalgia. *Cochrane Database Syst Rev.* 2013;(**10**):CD010782.
39. Vergne-Salle P, Dufauret-Lombard C, Bonnet C, et al. A randomised, double-blind, placebo-controlled trial of dolasetron, a 5-hydroxytryptamine 3 receptor antagonist, in patients with fibromyalgia. *Eur J Pain.* 2011;**15**:509–514.
40. Walitt B, Klose P, Fitzcharles MA, Phillips T, Häuser W. Cannabinoids for fibromyalgia. *Cochrane Database Syst Rev.* 2016;(**7**):CD011694.
41. Walitt B, Klose P, Üçeyler N, Phillips T, Häuser W. Antipsychotics for fibromyalgia in adults. *Cochrane Database Syst Rev.* 2016;(**6**):CD011804.
42. Walitt B, Urrútia G, Nishishinya MB, Cantrell SE, Häuser W. Selective serotonin reuptake inhibitors for fibromyalgia syndrome. *Cochrane Database Syst Rev.* 2015;(6):CD011735.

CHAPTER 26

Psychological Approaches

Françoise Laroche

Summary Points

- Patients suffering from fibromyalgia syndrome (FMS) usually present with negative beliefs about pain, dysfunctional coping strategies, and emotional distress. Multidisciplinary approach combining pharmacologic and non-pharmacologic therapies are recommended.
- High stress and physical tension may maintain pain and psychological training may reduce pain and pain-related distress. Interventions proposed should be explained and adapted to the patients' symptoms, comorbidities, preferences, and expectations, in order to increase patients' active engagement and chances of success.
- Different techniques and therapies are available:
  - Structured education may be the first step of psychotherapies, including information on the disease and its self-management.
  - Cognitive behavioral therapy (CBT) is the predominant intervention used. Most of the international guidelines recommend CBT for FMS.
  - Mindfulness-based stress reduction's (MBSR) objectives are to change the state of consciousness during meditation in order to take distance with personal thoughts. International recommendations regarding MBSR are conflicting.
  - Acceptance and commitment therapy (ACT) tries to help patients' acceptance of pain in order to enhance patients' ability to commit to their personal values despite pain. Recommendations for ACT are lacking.
  - Hypnosis and biofeedback are also used in FMS. However, efficacy results and recommendations are conflicting.

Chronic pain including FMS is usually conceptualized as a combination of central and peripheral sensitization in a specific context for each patient. FMS is a chronic pain disorder that often impairs quality of life, day life activities, and socio-professional abilities. It is responsible for heavy economic burdens on society and patients.[2,10] Emotional distress is usually associated with FMS and includes frustration, anger, resentment, helplessness, hostility, and feelings of injustice, but also negative beliefs about pain, generalized negative thinking patterns, and dysfunctional coping strategies.

The evaluation and management of FMS require a full understanding of the biopsychosocial model of chronic pain, and should provide a multidisciplinary approach combining pharmacologic and non-pharmacologic therapies. Psychotherapeutic approaches have to be considered as an adjuvant therapy in this multidisciplinary approach, and psychological interventions should be offered at the same time with physical interventions.[3,8,18] Education in a structured way is the beginning of the process.[3]

Even if the management of psychological factors is a necessity, we do not know exactly what works for whom.[28] The rationale of these psychological interventions should be explained to the patient; emphasizing that high stress and physical tension can maintain pain, and that psychological training may reduce pain and pain-related distress. Interventions provided should be adapted to the patients' symptoms and comorbidities. Different authors have raised the importance of being involved as patient in the decision-making process. Patients' preferences and expectations should also be taken into account to increase patients' active engagement and chances of success. Therefore, motivational interviewing and enhancement therapy should be proposed to help patients' understanding and commitment.[29] Pain therapies discussed in this chapter are CBTs, MBSR, and ACT. Among mind–body therapies, we discuss hypnosis and biofeedback.

STRUCTURED EDUCATION

Model

Education means information in a "structured way." Indeed, it includes information on the disease and its self-management. It emphasizes that pain is real, explaining the psychophysiologic mechanisms of pain amplification (such as muscle tension, insomnia, fatigue, cognitive, emotional, and behavioral pain dysfunction). Moreover, explaining that pain will persist is extremely important (even if a decrease may be possible and control of flares may become an objective). Patients are encouraged to perform new behaviors or skills.

Structured education is one part of CBT for most of the authors. Indeed, CBTs usually include education (information on the etiology of the disease including importance of psychological factors, treatment options, working mechanisms of psychological and drug therapies).[3]

Mechanism of Action

Educational studies have demonstrated reduction in pain and improvement in psychological and disability measures immediately on completion of the program.[26]

Objectives

Understanding the disease and the need to perform personnel skills and adapted coping strategies.

Procedure

Education on FMS is provided to the patients in different ways: groups or individual, once or repetitive, alone or associated to another intervention. Responses to what is FMS are provided. The reason for FMS, the diagnosis, and prognosis are explained. Education emphasizes that the disease is benign (without damage) and that distress, depression, anxiety, sleep disorder, trauma, and an excess of activities may increase symptoms. Strategies for coping are discussed including the need of adaptation to daily activities. The patient is taught to stay active and to learn new skills.[15] In Koçyigit et al.'s[15] study, education session lasted 20 minutes and each session was given face-to-face with the patient by the same doctor. Several sessions vary between studies published.

Efficacy

In literature, few studies evaluated the effectiveness of education alone.[15,14] They usually combine education and physical exercise.

A new study protocol published by Musekamp among 566 inpatients in rehabilitation will give more answers. The objective is to compare two education program. The evaluation is planned at 6 and 12 months by questionnaires. FMS is a complex chronic condition that makes high demands on patients' self-management skills. Thus, patient education is considered an important component of multimodal therapy, although evidence regarding its effectiveness is scarce. The main objective of this study is to assess the effectiveness of an advanced self-management patient education program for patients with FMS as compared to usual care in the context of inpatient rehabilitation. Primary outcomes are patients' disease- and treatment-specific knowledge and self-management skills after 6 months. Other outcomes are also important (satisfaction, attitudes and coping competences, health-promoting behavior, psychological distress, health impairment, and participation).[22]

Recommendations

Patient education is a method recommended in FMS treatment guidelines.[8] The necessity of informing about the natural course of the disease at the moment of the diagnosis and during follow up is reported.[8]

The last guidelines published were developed by 13 scientific societies and 2 patient self-help organizations coordinated by the German Pain Society, including 42 members. Systematic reviews on randomized, controlled trials on patient education and shared decision making were analyzed (December 2010–May 2016). The conclusions are: "The diagnosis of fibromyalgia syndrome should be explicitly communicated to the affected individual. Shared decision-making with the patient on the therapeutic options based on individual preferences of the patient, comorbidities and the success of previous treatment is recommended. A step-wise treatment approach depending on the severity of fibromyalgia syndrome and the response to therapeutic measures is recommended."[23]

PATIENT INSTRUCTIONS BEFORE PAIN PSYCHOTHERAPY

Patients may need exhaustive information on chronic pain and FMS process before entering a psychotherapy approach. The therapy proposed has to be relevant and understandable for the patient. Indeed, a partnership between patient and therapist is needed because patients have to be engaged and motivated in this approach unless failing to succeed. Pain intensity should not be the main objective keeping in mind that the primary focus of these therapies is not symptom reduction. Function and quality of life as goals should be discussed with patients.

USUAL PSYCHOLOGICAL APPROACHES

Different psychotherapies are available, explained by distinct models, mechanisms of action, objectives, and procedures.

"Traditional" Cognitive Behavioral Therapy

Model

CBT is the predominant intervention used for chronic pain–FMS management. This form of psychotherapy is known since the 1950s. It was previously developed for the treatment of mental disorders. The multidimensional conceptualization of pain is suitable for CBT even if the condition seems to be only physical. The CBT model of pain is based on the idea that chronic pain is maintained, because of dysfunctional thinking, emotional distress, and pain behaviors. The goals of the CBTs are to target cognitive, emotional, and behavioral factors:

- The cognitive behavioral model endorses the view that affective, behavioral, cognitive, and sensory or physical aspects are important for understanding the patient's experience of pain. This model emphasizes the influence of the individual's beliefs and (mis)interpretations of the pain experience.
- The operant treatment model (operant conditioning) considers that pain behaviors have been inadequately reinforced, at the cost of healthy behaviors.

Mechanisms of Action

Mechanisms of action of pain CBT include a decrease of pain catastrophizing and an increase in self-efficacy.[27] Improvements in both concepts have shown to be associated with improvement in pain intensity and functioning because of their mediator role.[27,24]

Objectives

Primary goals of CBT include increasing a patient's sense of personal control over his or her pain and decreasing dysfunctional thought patterns. Psychotherapists' objectives are to target beliefs, expectations, emotional distress, and pain behaviors. The objective is to improve functioning and decrease interference of pain.

Procedure

The intervention usually includes education about chronic pain. The relationships among maladaptive thoughts (including pain catastrophizing—exaggerating the significance of a negative event such as pain), beliefs (inability to control pain), emotional and physical reactions are discussed. Patients are trained in identifying maladaptive thoughts, finding behavioral goals, problem solving, relaxation procedure, activity pacing, distraction techniques, and coping with pain flare-ups in the everyday life. Ability to cope with pain such as ignoring pain behaviors and reinforcing well behaviors is also used during the therapy. Sleep problems, relapse prevention, and maintenance of gains are also addressed. Moreover, physical components are included in a broader rehabilitation program with behavioral activation, coping strategies, increased activity level, and modify inappropriate behaviors such as medication consumption. For example, pain catastrophizing is a negative thinking that is associated with altered behaviors. Therapy focuses on its importance and impact with cognitive restructuring techniques and emotional distress management.

Efficacy

One high-quality review including 23 trials (among FMS patients) has been published in 2013.[3] Results showed a reduction of depressed mood and improvement in self-efficacy compared with control arms after treatment. However, the authors concluded no positive effects on the key symptoms of FMS. But the general quality of trial was poor with various control groups. And it is important to stress that efficacy on sleep, depression, catastrophizing were not usually evaluated in these trials. The conclusion can be drawn that the greatest benefit of CBT is observed for improved function and that CBT programs are effective in small groups of patients, including Internet programs (which are more convenient for patients still active in the workforce). No significant side effects have been reported.[6]

Recommendations

Four guidelines on the management of FMS from Europe, Canada, Israel, and Germany have been recently published.[8,18,1,12] German, Canadian, and Israeli guidelines graded at a level of evidence with a strong (A) recommendation, which is similar to the previous American Pain Society recommendation in 2005.[4] However, CBTs are recommended in the EULAR with a weak strength (agreement for 100%).[18] In the EULAR guidelines, five reviews were discussed including up to 30 trials (n = 2,031 participants). The effect of CBT was weak on pain intensity (−0.29; −0.49 to −0.17) and disability (−0.30; −0.51 to −0.08) at the end of treatment. But results were sustained in long term.[21] The differences between the guidelines may partly be explained by using different evidence.

Whatever source, all the guidelines agree with the need for tailored therapy to the individual and the first-line role of non-pharmacologic therapies. Indeed, the EULAR guidelines emphasize: "Fibromyalgia should be recognised as a complex and heterogeneous condition where there is abnormal pain processing and other secondary features. Treatment modalities should be tailored according to pain intensity, function, associated features (such as depression), fatigue, sleep disturbance and patient preferences and comorbidities; by shared decision-making with the patient. Initial management should focus on non-pharmacological therapies."[18]

Mindfulness-Based Stress Reduction

Model

Mindfulness is considered by most psychotherapists as part of the "third wave" of CBT. It is an emotional approach oriented to mindfulness meditation developed in the 1980s. MBSR is defined as "an attention to the present moment without judgment." MBSR psychotherapists define MBSR as a psychological approach of its own. Mindfulness integrated with cognitive therapy is called mindfulness-based cognitive therapy (MBCT). It is also one of the strategies included in the ACT. A mindful person may change his or her perception with mental distance taking. MBSR exercises include different meditation practices, yoga, and training. Mindfulness was primarily used to prevent depressive relapse and studies reported MBSR effects on anxiety, physical functioning, and quality of life.

Mechanism of Action

Mindfulness acts as a central mechanism in order to increase pain acceptance and flexibility.[5]

Objectives

The objectives are to change the state of consciousness during meditation in order to take distance with personal thoughts.

Procedure

Mindful individuals may be attentive to thoughts, emotions, and body consciousness without judging them. Some therapists add meditative movement, and such a combination is also called mind–body therapy.

Efficacy

One recent review, a meta-analysis of six trials ($n = 674$) provided evidence that MBSR resulted in improvements in pain intensity immediately posttreatment compared with usual care but not to active interventions.[16] However, the clinical relevance of the results is weak, and the exact number of participants are unclear.[18] Among several pain diagnoses (FMS, osteoarthritis, rheumatoid arthritis), MBSR changed pain perception, well-being, and quality of life.[21]

Recommendation

The EULAR recommendation is "weak" for mindfulness/mind–body therapy (73% agreement—evidence level III).[18] The German guideline gave a negative recommendation (weak against) for MBSR as a single therapy, while the Canadian guidelines are strong for mindfulness (evidence level I). We may conclude that the international guidelines are not helpful for this therapy, because of conflicting recommendations.

Acceptance and Commitment Therapy

Model

ACT is considered a third-generation psychological therapy derived from CBT. It is increasingly used in the treatment of chronic pain. The six core processes of ACT are Acceptance, Cognitive Defusion, Being Present, Self as Context, Values, and Committed Action (https://contextualscience.org/the_six_core_processes_of_act). ACT focuses on the increase of psychological flexibility.[13,20] ACT encourages patients in accepting pain and being mindful. ACT is not oriented to control-oriented treatments such as CBT.

Mechanism of Action

ACT targets maladaptive coping strategies and avoidance behavior.[13]

Objectives

Patients learn to let go of pain control strategies in favor of acceptance of pain as a part of their daily lives. The objective is to improve functioning and decrease interference of pain. The goal is to enhance patients' ability to commit to their personal values despite pain.

Procedure

ACT focuses on emotion and attention as well as MBSR. Patient's training uses mindfulness procedure, meaning being in contact with unpleasant emotions, sensations, and thoughts. Exposure to negative thoughts is the target. No action to change their content is warranted.[7]

Efficacy

Wicksell et al.[30] included 40 FMS women in a randomized study of 12 weekly group sessions of ACT or a waiting list. The results are to be interpreted with caution, given the absence of active control group, the small sample sizes, and the short follow-up period (3 months). Luciano et al.[17] published a larger study of 156 patients suffering from FMS ($n > 50$ in each study arm) and increased the follow-up period to 6 months. The patients were randomly assigned to ACT versus best pharmacologic treatment (pregabalin and in case of major depression duloxetine) or a waiting list control. ACT was not superior to drug therapy in most outcomes; the number needed to treat (NNT) for 50% improvement was 46, and the NNT to decrease the Fibromyalgia Impact Questionnaire (FIQ) total score (<39) was also 46. McCracken published in 2013 a trial implemented in general practice.[19] A 3-month multidisciplinary program was conducted in 73 chronic pain patients (30 diagnosed with FMS). They were randomized to ACT and physical activity or usual treatment. The effect sizes were 0.46 for depression after treatment and 0.58 at follow-up. There was also a significantly higher increase in pain acceptance in the active group.

Recommendation

ACT is not mentioned in EULAR guidelines.[18]

Multicomponent Therapy

Hauser et al.[11] conducted a review of management involving both educational or psychological therapies and exercise. In his meta-analysis of nine trials (1,119 patients), multicomponent therapy was effective in reducing pain, depressive symptoms, fatigue and increasing quality of life, physical function, and self-efficacy after treatment, compared with waiting list, relaxation, treatment as usual, and education. However, effects were small and short-lived. Two reviews including 27 trials ($n = 2407$) examined the additional benefit of combining therapies, compared to individual therapy in the EULAR recommendation.[18]

The EULAR recommendation is "weak" for these therapies with an evidence level II (*93% agreement*).[18] But the Canadian, Israeli, and German recommendations (level of evidence Ia) as well as the American Pain Society[4] strongly recommend multicomponent therapies.[8,1,12]

HYPNOTHERAPY

Nine randomized controlled trials including 484 FMS patients were included in a meta-analysis.[31] Around nine hypnosis/guided imagery sessions were generally performed. No long-term follow-up was performed (maximum 3 months). The results did not show a clinical benefit compared to controls on pain and psychological distress at the end of the sessions and at 3-month follow-up. EULAR 2016 recommendation for the use of hypnosis in FMS is "weak against" (*86% agreement*).[18] It was also weak for the American Pain Society guidelines in 2005.[4] However, hypnosis/guided imagery received a "weak for" recommendation by the German (IIB) and Israeli guidelines.[1,12] Hypnosis with analgesia suggestion is considered as a psychological intervention in the Canadian recommendation with effect on pain.

BIOFEEDBACK

A review of seven studies ($n = 321$) has been published in 2013.[9] Biofeedback reportedly consisted of 6 to 22 sessions. Controls groups were various; sham biofeedback, attention control, medication, and usual treatment. Pain intensity was slightly reduced, but all trials were of poor quality. There was no evidence of fatigue, sleep, depression, or quality of life. The EULAR recommendation is weak against (100% agreement).[18] The German recommendation is a "weak for."[12] There was no comment in the Israeli recommendation.[1]

DISCUSSION—METHODOLOGIC ISSUES

Thieme et al.[25] just published a comparison of three recent available guidelines: Canadian (2013), German (2012), and EULAR (2016) and the former American Pain Society published in 2005. The methodologic analysis shows a consistency regarding CBT and multicomponent treatments, which are all strongly recommended, except for EULAR guidelines (weak for).[18] Indeed, there is a large number of studies and participants included. The benefits of CBT on different outcomes (pain, function, anxiety) are considered as maintained. However, regarding other therapies, there are clear discrepancies. Methodologic issues may explain the inconsistencies between guidelines (studies included, patient's inclusion criteria, number of patients, outcome measures, etc.). Outcomes Measures in Rheumatology (OMERACT) recommends evaluating different outcomes: pain, sleep, fatigue, affects, function, and cognitive function.

But they are rarely reported among studies.[30] Moreover, we still do not know what minimal outcome effects should be relevant. Pain intensity was the most used outcome measure in the included studies, which is in accordance with The Initiative on Methods, Measurement, and Pain Assessment in Clinical Trials (IMMPACT) recommendations. But pain reduction should not be the primary outcome of these psychotherapies because pain is persistent. FMS is also a heterogeneous syndrome with some patients being more severe and showing less response to treatments. All these factors may explain why guidelines are difficult to compare.

CONCLUSION

FMS is a multi-symptom disorder that is difficult to treat. Different modalities and combination of treatments should be provided. Psychotherapies have shown benefits, especially for CBT. Systematic reviews show methodologic limiting or conflicting conclusion for other therapies. There is a need to harmonize the management guidelines. However, there is a consensus that self-management strategies and multicomponent therapies may help patients to improve function and quality of life. It is important to consider the treatment as individually tailored to the patient's characteristics. Some questions are still remaining: Are combined pharmacologic and non-pharmacologic approaches more effective than single modality management? Are there characteristics of patients with FMS that predict response to specific therapies? Are there "tailored therapies" to specific subgroups such as posttraumatic stress disorder (PTSD), major depression, and so on?

ACKNOWLEDGMENT

I thank Mr Johan Vlaeyen for kindly reviewing the manuscript.

REFERENCES

1. Ablin J, Fitzcharles MA, Buskila D, et al. Treatment of fibromyalgia syndrome: recommendations of recent evidence-based interdisciplinary guidelines with special emphasis on complementary and alternative therapies. *Evid Based Compl Alt Med*. 2013;Article ID 485272:7.
2. Berger A, Dukes E, Martin S, Edelsberg J, Oster G. Characteristics and healthcare costs of patients with fibromyalgia syndrome. *Int J Clin Pract*. 2007;**61**:1498–1508.
3. Bernardy K, Klose P, Busch AJ, et al. Cognitive behavioural therapies for fibromyalgia. *Coch Database Syst Rev*. 2013;(9):CD009796.
4. Buckhardt C, Goldenberg D, Crofford L, Gerwin R, Gowens S. Guidelines for the management of fibromyalgia syndrome pain in adults and children. Glenview, IL: American Pain Society; 2005.
5. Chiesa A, Serretti A. Mindfulness-based interventions for chronic pain: a systematic review of the evidence. *J Alt Compl Med*. 2011;**17**:83–93.
6. Clauw D. Fibromyalgia: a clinical review. *JAMA*. 2014;**311**:1547–1555.

7. Dahl J, Wilson KG, Nilsson A. Acceptance and commitment therapy and the treatment of persons at risk for long-term disability resulting from stress and pain symptoms: a preliminary randomized trial. *Behav Ther*. 2004;**35**:785–801.
8. Fitzcharles MA, Ste Marie P, Goldenberg D, Pereira J, Abbey S. The National Fibromyalgia Guideline Advisory Panel: 2012 Canadian guidelines for the diagnosis and management of fibromyalgia syndrome: executive summary. *Pain Res Manag*. 2013;**18**:119–126.
9. Glombiewski, J, Bernardy, K, Häuser W. Efficacy of EMG-and EEG-biofeedback in fibromyalgia syndrome: a meta-analysis and a systematic review of randomized controlled trials. *Evid Based Compl Alt Med*. 2013;Article ID 962741:11.
10. Goldenberg D, Schaefer C, Ryan K, Chandran A, Slateva G. What is the true cost of fibromyalgia to our society: results from a cross-sectional survey in the United States. Paper presented at American College of Rheumatology, Philadelphia, PA, October 18, 2009.
11. Hauser W, Bernardy K, Arnold B, Offenbacher M. Efficacy of multicomponent treatment in fibromyalgia syndrome: a meta-analysis of randomized controlled clinical trials. *Arthritis Rheum*. 2009;**61**:216–224.
12. Hauser W, Thieme K, Turk DC. Guidelines on the management of fibromyalgia syndrome—a systematic review. *Eur J Pain*. 2010;**14**:5–10.
13. Hayes SC, Strosahl K, Wilson KG. Acceptance and commitment therapy. New York: Guilford Press; 1999.
14. King SJ, Wessel J, Bhambhani Y, Sholter D, Maksymowych W. The effects of exercise and education, individually or combined, in women with fibromyalgia. *J Rheumatol*. 2002;**29**:2620–2627.
15. Koçyigit BF, Gür A, Altindag O, Akyol A, Gürsoy S. Comparison of education and balneotherapy efficacy in patients with fibromyalgia syndrome: a randomized, controlled clinical study Fibromiyalji sendromlu hastalarda eğitim ve balneoterapinin. *Agri*. 2016;**28**(2):72–78.
16. Lauche R, Cramer H, Dobos G, Langhorst J, Schmidt S. A systematic review and meta-analysis of mindfulness-based stress reduction for the fibromyalgia syndrome. *J Psychosomat Res*. 2013;**75**:500–510.
17. Luciano J, Guallar J, Aguado J, López-del-Hoyo Y, Olivan B, Magallón R. Effectiveness of group acceptance and commitment therapy for fibromyalgia: a 6-month randomized controlled trial (EFFIGACT study). *Pain*. 2014;**155**:693–702.
18. Macfarlane G, Kronisch C, Dean LE, Atzeni F, Häuser W. EULAR revised recommendations for the management of fibromyalgia. *Ann Rheum Dis*. 2017;**76**:318–328.
19. McCracken LM, Sato A, Taylor GJ. A trial of a brief group-based form of acceptance and commitment therapy (ACT) for chronic pain in general practice: pilot outcome and process results. *J Pain*. 2013;**14**:1398–1406.
20. Mease P, Arnold L, Choy E, et al. Fibromyalgia symptom module at OMERACT 9: domain construct. *J Rheumatol*. 2009;**36**:2318–2329.
21. Merkes M. Mindfulness-based stress reduction for people with chronic diseases. *Aust J Prim Health*. 2010;**16**:200–210.
22. Musekamp G, Gerlich C, Ehlebracht-König I, Faller H, Reusch A. Evaluation of a self-management patient education program for patients with fibromyalgia syndrome: study protocol of a cluster randomized controlled trial. *BMC Musculoskelet Disord*. 2016;**17**:55.
23. Petzke F, Brückle W, Eidmann U, et al. General treatment principles, coordination of care and patient education in fibromyalgia syndrome: updated guidelines 2017 and overview of systematic review articles. *Schmerz*. 2017;**31**:246–254. doi:10.1007/s00482-017-0201-6.
24. Smeets RJ, Vlaeyen JW, Kester AD, Knottnerus JA. Reduction of pain catastrophizing mediates the outcome of both physical and cognitive-behavioral treatment in chronic low back pain. *J Pain*. 2006;7(4):261–271.
25. Thieme K, Mathys M, Turk D. Evidenced-based guidelines on the treatment of fibromyalgia patients: are they consistent and if not, why not? Have effective psychological treatments been overlooked? *J Pain*. 2017;**18**:747–756.

26. Turk DC, Okifuji A, Sinclair JD, Starz TW. Interdisciplinary treatment for fibromyalgia syndrome: clinical and statistical significance. *Arthritis Care Res.* 1998;**11**:186–195.
27. Turner JA, Holtzman S, Mancl L. Mediators, moderators, and predictors of therapeutic change in cognitive-behavioral therapy for chronic pain. *Pain.* 2007;**127**:276–286.
28. Vlaeyen JW, Morley SC. Cognitive-behavioral treatments for chronic pain: what works for whom? *Clin J Pain.* 2005;**21**:1–8.
29. Vong SK, Cheing GL, Chan F, So EM, Chan CC. Motivational enhancement therapy in addition to physical therapy improves motivational factors and treatment outcomes in people with low back pain: a randomized controlled trial. *Arch Phys Med Rehabil.* 2011;**92**:176–183.
30. Wicksell RK, Kemani M, Jensen K, et al. Acceptance and commitment therapy for fibromyalgia: a randomized controlled trial. *Eur J Pain.* 2013;**17**:599–611.
31. Zech N, Hansen E, Bernardy K, Häuser W. Efficacy, acceptability and safety of guided imagery/hypnosis in fibromyalgia—a systematic review and meta-analysis of randomized controlled trials. *Eur J Pain.* 2017;**21**:217–227.

CHAPTER 27

Physiotherapy and Physical Approaches

Andreas Winkelmann

Summary Points

- There is strong evidence that physical exercise such as aerobic exercise and resistance training leads to positive effects such as improvement of pain, fatigue, physical and cognitive function, other fibromyalgia syndrome (FMS) symptoms, and quality of life.
- That is why physical approaches play a key role in the management of the different potentially disabling FMS symptoms.
- Physical exercise could reduce pain, pain sensitivity, and normalize functional resting-state connectivity, but does not influence top-down pain modulation. The mechanisms of how the effects of physical modalities could be achieved are not yet completely clear.
- Regular and long-term activities are necessary for success (especially best possible function for activities of daily living, quality of life, pain management, energy/reduction of fatigue), adapted to the capacity and preferences of the FMS patients.
- Strong recommendations (suitable for almost all FMS patients) exist for aerobic exercise with light-to-medium intensity, for example, walking, cycling, or swimming, and for resistance, exercise training with at least moderate intensity.
- A recommendation (suitable for a big number of FMS patients) can be given for Spa therapy, balneotherapy, and hydrotherapy.
- FMS management strategies that may be considered (weak evidence, without health risks with FMS patient-tailored intensity, helpful for a smaller number of FMS patients) are physiotherapy (PT) and/or occupational therapy (OT; if limitations in activities in daily living are reported) with temporary use within a guided multicomponent therapy concept, and stretching or whole body vibration therapy (WBV).

- Due to lack of evidence, no recommendations for or against the following FMS management strategies can be given: hydrogalvanic baths (within a guided multidisciplinary therapy concept), manual lymph drainage therapy, osteopathic/craniosacral therapy, and thermotherapy heat.
- Based on lack of evidence or negative results in randomized controlled trials (RCTs), recommendations against the management of FMS include chiropractic/manual therapy, electrotherapy (e.g., transcutaneous electric nerve stimulation [TENS]), hyperbaric oxygen therapy, laser therapy, magnetic field therapy, massage, and transcranial current stimulation.

VALUE OF PHYSIOTHERAPY AND PHYSICAL APPROACHES

The Health Professional Perspective

Although FMS is listed in the International Statistical Classification of Diseases and Related Health Problems–10th Revision (ICD-10) by the World Health Organization (WHO), and characterized and defined by American College of Rheumatology (ACR) 1990, ACR 2010 Criteria and in the different national and European guidelines and recommendations, many health professionals have difficulties following these guidelines and criteria because of the lack of FMS-characteristic pathologic findings. As described in Chapter 20, physical exercise could reduce pain, pain sensitivity, and normalize functional resting-state connectivity, but not influence top-down pain modulation. The mechanisms of how the effects of physical modalities could be achieved are not yet completely clear (Chapter 20).

Even though the mechanisms of exercise and physical approaches are not completely understood, there is no doubt that physical exercise, adapted to capacity and comorbidities, should be recommended for FMS and chronic widespread pain (CWP) patients.

The Fibromyalgia Syndrome Patients' Perspective

Many patients with FMS and CWP feel helpless with their numerous disabling symptoms. Although different guidelines[24,8,1] and recommendations[22] on FMS exist, many of the patients suffering from FMS and CWP argue that due to pain, they cannot begin recommended physical exercise or therapy. Pain relief would be necessary first before starting exercise, such as endurance or resistance training, land or water based (walking, running, cycling, swimming) or stretching. However, sufficient pain relief with pain medication is not possible in many cases. Less-intense physical therapy such as thermotherapy with hot packs (strongly preferred to cold in self-reported strategies used by FMS patients) is best rated by FMS patients.[12,13,2] and could be easily and safely used for short-term pain relief by the patients themselves. Due to lack of evidence, these strategies are less recommended by health professionals. As shown in the German consumer reports,[12,13] the top category or strategy used by almost all German FMS patients (about 95%) was activity-related self-management (e.g., functional training, walking, distraction, muscle stretching, and strengthening) and similar reports were shown in self-care groups in the United States.[2] The biggest difference in self-management use was for aerobic exercise (32% in the United States vs. 58% in Germany).[13] Self-management seems to be very significant and used most frequently.

Most beneficial (0 = no effectiveness, 10 = maximum effectiveness) strategies as shown in Table 27.1 was reported by the German FMS patients for whole-body warmth therapy (7.1), thermal baths (7.0), FMS education (6.8), resting (6.6), local warmth therapy (6.6), lymph drainage (6.4), functional training (6.2), warm baths (6.1), osteopathy (6.0), and dance therapy (6.0).

Most harmful in the top 10 strategies were cold (twice, local, and whole-body cold) and drugs (eight times medication, e.g., the non-recommended strong opioids and also guideline-recommended medication).

TABLE 27.1 Top 10 most effective management/therapy strategies, rated by FMS patients

		Effectiveness	
Order	**Management strategy**	***N*; Mean benefit (*SD*) (0–10)[a]**	**High benefit (8–10) *N* (%)[a]**
1	Whole-body warmth therapy	984; 7.1 (2.6)	507 (51.5)
2	Thermal bathes	699; 7.0 (2.7)	354 (50.6)
3	FMS education	649; 6.8 (2.7)	304 (46.8)
4	Resting	1296; 6.6 (2.5)	519 (40.1)
5	Local warmth therapy	1088; 6.6 (2.5)	452 (41.6)
6	Lymph drainage	481; 6.4 (2.8)	197 (41.0)
7	Functional training[b]	781; 6.2 (2.7)	271 (34.7)
8	Warm bathes	681; 6.1 (2.9)	250 (36.7)
9	Osteopathy	445; 6.0 (3.1)	177 (38.8)
10	Dance therapy	159; 6.0 (2.9)	60 (37 7)

0 = no benefit; 10 = maximum benefit.

[a]The discrepancies between the number of persons in the different rows are due to missing items.

[b]Combination of land- and water-based exercises (stretching, aerobic exercise) guided by a licensed trainer; the costs are covered for years by German health insurance companies if prescribed by a physician. The efficacy ratings of all management strategies are available on request.

From Häuser W, Jung E, Erbslöh-Möller B, et al. The German fibromyalgia consumer reports (Table 3)—a cross-sectional survey. *BMC Musculoskelet Disord*. 2012;13:74. http://www.biomedcentral.com/1471–2474/13/74.

There was a discrepancy between the most effective/useful and most harmful therapy strategies reported by the patients[12,13] and the guideline-based recommended therapy strategies. Some of them were not listed in the top 10 of the self-reported most useful therapy strategies (such as aerobic exercise or resistance training). For almost all of the top 10 most useful therapy strategies rated by patients, we have no sufficient evidence (e.g., whole-body warmth therapy, resting, lymph drainage, or osteopathy).

For FMS patients, it is important to know that the guideline-recommended therapy interventions or strategies are not dangerous and we do not expect risk of tissue damage or risk of death—even if the patients can feel pain or discomfort while practicing the recommended physical exercise or therapy. Therefore, it is crucial to show the patients how to practice the different evidence-based therapy strategies.

In this chapter, we highlight the therapies that could be part of a PT, physical therapy, or other physical exercise training. We emphasize the patient perspective and give information on possibilities of different therapies with various dosages. Guided therapy also for physical therapy can prevent negative/harmful feelings or experiences (cold in the right dosage is not dangerous for patients with FMS alone, for some of the FMS patients, guided therapy, e.g., also with cold packs could be experienced as helpful in self-management, e.g., before stretching, although we have no evidence for cold by the literature).

In the long term, the goal is to inform and guide FMS and CWP patients in order for them to be able to train themselves independently and regularly, using long-term self-management strategies, ultimately increasing function and quality of life.

RECOMMENDATIONS WITH EXPLANATION AND DISCUSSION OF THE DIFFERENT PHYSICAL THERAPIES, PHYSIOTHERAPY, AND EXERCISE THERAPIES

The order of the different physical therapy modalities is listed by the strength of recommendations, strongest recommendation, best evidence first, then listed alphabetically; also see Tables 27.2 and 27.3 with improvements of FMS symptoms with recommended physical approaches/therapies.

Strong Recommendation

Aerobic Exercise—Endurance Training, Low-to-Moderate Intensity (Evidence Level 1a)

Based on the results of systematic reviews,[24,8,1,22,3,5,4,26,25] low-to-moderate intensity aerobic exercise (low intensity with 50% to 70% of maximum heart rate (HR); moderate with 70% to 85% of maximum HR)—endurance training land or water based (e.g., walking, running, cycling or aquatic exercise, swimming, aquatic exercise) is strongly recommended. If performed regularly (at least twice a week with at least

TABLE 27.2 **Strengths of recommendation for physical approaches, physical therapy, and exercise training by FMS guidelines of Canada, Germany, and Israel; EULAR recommendations within the fields**

	Canada	EULAR	Germany	Israel
Aerobic exercise	Strong for (as an example for regular physical activity)	Strong for	Strong for	Strong for
Aquatic exercise	Strong for (as an example for regular physical activity)	Strong for	Strong for	—
Land-based exercise	Strong for (as an example for regular physical activity)	Strong for	Strong for	—
Resistance/strength training	Strong for (as an example for regular physical activity)	Strong for	Weak for	—
Spa-/balneo-/ hydrotherapy	—	Weak for	Weak for	Open/Consider (weak evidence)
Acupuncture in EULAR recommendation as a physical therapy; others as a complementary therapy.	No recommendation (weak evidence)	Weak for	Open/consider (weak evidence)	—
OT within a guided multidisciplinary therapy concept	Weak for multimodal/ multidisciplinary therapy concept	Weak for multimodal/ multidisciplinary therapy concept	Open/consider (weak evidence)	—

(Continued)

TABLE 27.2 Strengths of recommendation for physical approaches, physical therapy, and exercise training by FMS guidelines of Canada, Germany, and Israel; EULAR recommendations within the fields *(Continued)*

	Canada	EULAR	Germany	Israel
PT within a guided multidisciplinary therapy concept	Weak for multimodal/ multidisciplinary therapy concept	Weak for multimodal/ multidisciplinary therapy concept	Open/consider (weak evidence)	—
Stretching	—	—	Open/consider (weak evidence)	—
WBV therapy	—	—	Open/consider (weak evidence)	—
Hydrogalvanic baths within a guided multidisciplinary therapy concept	—	—	No recommendation (weak evidence)	—
Manual lymph drainage therapy	—	—	No recommendation (weak evidence)	—
Osteopathic therapy/craniosacral therapy	—	—	No recommendation (weak evidence)	—
Thermotherapy heat	—	—	No recommendation (weak evidence)	—
Chiropractic/manual therapy	—	Strong against (no evidence)	Weak against (no evidence)	—
Electrotherapy/TENS	—	No recommendation	Weak against (no evidence)	—
Hyperbaric oxygen therapy	—	—	Weak against (no evidence)	—

Laser therapy	—	—	Weak against (no evidence; health risks with high energy laser)	—
Magnetic field therapy	—	No recommendation	Weak against (no evidence)	—
Massage therapy	—	Weak against (no evidence)	Weak against (no evidence)	—
Thermotherapy cold	—	—	Weak against (no evidence)	—
Transcranial current stimulation	—	No recommendation	Weak against (no evidence)	—

—, no statement to this item was given.

OT, occupational therapy; PT, physiotherapy; TENS, transcutan electric nerve stimulation; WBV, whole-body vibration therapy.

From Petzke F, Brückle W, Eidmann U, et al. General treatment principles, coordination of care and patient education in fibromyalgia syndrome: updated guidelines 2017 and overview of systematic review articles. *Schmerz*. 2017;31(3):246–254; Fitzcharles M-A, Ste-Marie PA, Goldenberg DL, et al; the National Fibromyalgia Guideline Advisory Panel. 2012 Canadian guidelines for the diagnosis and management of fibromyalgia syndrome: executive summary. *Pain Res Manag*. 2013;18(3):119–126; Ablin JN, Amital H, Ehrenfeld M, et al. Guidelines for the diagnosis and treatment of the fibromyalgia syndrome. Israeli Rheumatology Association. *Harefuah*. 2013;152(12):742–747, 751, 750. Hebrew; Macfarlane GJ, Kronisch C, Dean LE, et al. EULAR revised recommendations for the management of fibromyalgia. *Ann Rheum Dis*. 2017;76:318–328. doi:10.1136/annrheumdis-2016–209724.

TABLE 27.3 Symptom improvements for recommended physical approaches, physical therapy, and exercise training (FMS guidelines of Canada, Germany, and Israel; EULAR recommendations)

	Improvements
Aerobic exercise	Pain (VAS −3.6/10 vs. controls), multidimensional function (FIQ, −22.2/100 better than. controls), stiffness 8%, quality of life/HRQL 7%
– Aquatic exercise	– In favor to reduce stiffness
– Land-based exercise	– In favor to improve isokinetic strength (knee extension and handgrip) + 37%
Resistance/strength training	Pain (VAS −2.5/10 vs. controls), multidimensional function (FIQ, 16.7/100 better than controls), tender point count −2.5/18 better than controls), fatigue (−14.7/100 better than controls), and muscle strength (lifting +27 kg more in concentric leg extension than controls)
Spa/balneo/hydrotherapy[24,8,1,22,18]	Pain (VAS −2.0/10 vs. controls; SMD −1.36 vs. aerobic exercise −0.40), multidimensional function (FIQ, 24/100 better than controls), quality of life (SMD −1.38 vs. aerobic exercise −0.38), tender point count −2.0/18 better than controls), fatigue (MFIS −8.5)

FMS, fibromyalgia syndrome; FIQ, Fibromyalgia Impact Questionnaire; MFIS, Modified Fatigue Impact Scale; HRQL, health-related quality of life; SMD, standardized mean difference; VAS, Visual Analogue Scale.

From Petzke F, Brückle W, Eidmann U, et al. General treatment principles, coordination of care and patient education in fibromyalgia syndrome: updated guidelines 2017 and overview of systematic review articles. *Schmerz*. 2017;31(3):246–254; Fitzcharles M-A, Ste-Marie PA, Goldenberg DL, et al; the National Fibromyalgia Guideline Advisory Panel. 2012 Canadian guidelines for the diagnosis and management of fibromyalgia syndrome: executive summary. *Pain Res Manag*. 2013;18(3):119–126; Ablin JN, Amital H, Ehrenfeld M, et al. Guidelines for the diagnosis and treatment of the fibromyalgia syndrome. Israeli Rheumatology Association. *Harefuah*. 2013;152(12):742–747, 751, 750. Hebrew; Macfarlane GJ, Kronisch C, Dean LE, et al. EULAR revised recommendations for the management of fibromyalgia. *Ann Rheum Dis*. 2017;76:318–328. doi:10.1136/annrheumdis-2016–209724.

30 minutes training, better with at least 3 hours of training time distributed over the week) and long-term therapeutic effects improve pain 11%, physical function 10% (Fibromyalgia Impact Questionnaire [FIQ]), stiffness 8%, quality of life/health-related quality of life (HRQL) 7%, with low or moderate evidence because of low numbers of participants included in the studies.[26,25] A water-based training (standing in the pool water for guided exercise) is favorable in reducing stiffness; land-based training is in slight favor of improving strength (measured with isokinetic strength of knee extension and handgrip +37%).[3]

Resistance Exercise Training or Strength Training With Devices (Evidence Level 1a)

Improving pain (Visual Analogue Scale [VAS] 2.5/10 better than controls, 8 weeks moderate-intensity resistance training suggests less effects than aerobic exercise for pain [VAS −2.7 vs. −3.57]) and multidimensional function in FIQ (16.7/100 better than controls; improving −15.85 vs. aerobic exercise −21.33 FIQ units), self-reported physical function (5.7/100 better), tenderness (2.5/18 better), and muscle strength (lifting +27 kg more in concentric leg extension than controls) could be demonstrated.[5,26,25] At least moderate-intensity training is recommended. Strength training can be performed within the scope of a PT or self-care after instructions from physiotherapists, occupational therapists, or sports therapists.

Recommendation

Spa Therapy (Evidence Level 2a)

Hydrotherapy (hot water including whirlpool), spa therapy (bathing in mineral water), and thalassotherapy (bathing in seawater) were taken into account in reviews and meta-analysis for the evaluation of spa therapy.

With spa therapy (mud and balneotherapy), a high effect size is confirmed for pain relief at the end of randomized clinical trials, in reviews, and meta-analysis.[26,25,19,23,9,18,17,10,11] Smaller effects are also shown for depression and minor FMS symptoms.[10]

Balneotherapy combined with information seems to increase the effects for pain (VAS [0 to 10] − 2 and tender point count [0 to 18] − 2; compared with controls), multidimensional function (FIQ −24), and fatigue (Modified Fatigue Impact Scale [MFIS] −8.5) shown in one RCT.[18] These results have to be confirmed in further RCTs with larger numbers of participants and optimized study design, but placebo-controlled trials for spa therapy are almost impossible.

Open Recommendation (Consider)

OT (if limitations in activities in daily living are reported) or PT can be used temporarily within a guided multidisciplinary, multicomponent so-called multimodal therapy concept, stretching, WBV.[26,25,21,6,15,14]

No Recommendation and Recommendation Against the Use of the Following Listed Therapies (Because of Lack of Benefit or Lack of Evidence by Randomized Controlled Trials or Negative Side Effects Reported by Fibromyalgia Syndrome Patients)

No recommendation to use or not to use these strategies/therapies, because of insufficient data from RCTs could be given for hydrogalvanic baths (part or in most cases whole-body baths), manual lymph drainage therapy, osteopathic therapy/craniosacral therapy, or thermotherapy—heat (whole body or local).[26,25,16] Recommendation, against the use of the following listed therapies (because of lack of benefit or lack of evidence by RCTs or negative side effects reported by FMS patients): Chiropractic/manual therapy, electrotherapy/TENS (no evidence), hyperbaric oxygen therapy, laser therapy (potentially dangerous, e.g., high-energy laser > 4 W as used in sports medicine), magnetic field therapy, massage therapy, thermotherapy—cold therapy and transcranial current stimulation.[26,25,20,27,7]

Importance of Physiotherapy and Physical Approaches

Based on strong evidence by clinical trials, low-to-moderate intensity aerobic exercise and strength or resistance training are strongly recommended. Because of the effects of pain relief, spa therapy and balneo- or hydrotherapy are recommended, if they are available. No serious side effects were systematically recorded or reported, nor are those known from the literature or clinical experience. Based on low evidence, chiropractic/manual therapy, electrotherapy (e.g., TENS), hyperbaric oxygen therapy, laser therapy, magnetic field therapy, massage, and transcranial current stimulation are not recommended. The patient perspective should always be taken into account when selecting a suitable training. Guided physical therapy (e.g., guided by physiotherapists in a single patient or group setting) can increase motivation and confidence and encourage further self-management strategies, if information and explanations alone could not improve, for example, restrictions of activities in daily living or quality of life. Recommended physical exercise approaches or therapies with proven evidence of benefit should first be recommended and used. Second, self-management strategies, also without proven evidence of benefit, but with self-reported good benefits (e.g., local heat packs, distraction, stretching exercises), which are generally considered not to be harmful or dangerous and which can be easily implemented independently, can be used for the self-management of FMS. "Function first" as the overall management goal in FMS cannot be reached without physical approaches. Regular and long-term physical exercise training, adapted to the patients' capacity and preferences, is a cornerstone in the management approaches in FMS for best possible function in daily living, quality of life, and pain management.

REFERENCES

1. Ablin JN, Amital H, Ehrenfeld M, et al. Guidelines for the diagnosis and treatment of the fibromyalgia syndrome. Israeli Rheumatology Association. *Harefuah*. 2013;**152**(12):742–747, 751, 750. Hebrew.
2. Bennett RM, Jones J, Turk DC, Russell IJ, Matallana L. An internet survey of 2,596 people with fibromyalgia. *BMC Musculoskelet Disord*. 2007;**9**(8):27.
3. Bidonde J, Busch AJ, Webber SC, et al. Aquatic exercise training for fibromyalgia. *Coch Database Syst Rev*. 2014.**10**:CD011336.
4. Bidonde J, Busch AJ, Schachter CL, et al. Aerobic exercise training for adults with fibromyalgia. *Coch Database of Syst Rev*. 2017(6):CD012700.

5. Busch AJ, Webber SC, Richards RS, et al. Resistance exercise training for fibromyalgia. *Coch Database Syst Rev*. 2013.**12**:CD010884.
6. Collado-Mateo D, Adsuar JC, Olivares PR, et al. Effects of whole-body vibration therapy in patients with fibromyalgia: a systematic literature review. *Evid Based Complement Altern*. 2015; 2015:719082.
7. Efrati S, Golan H, Bechor Y, et al. Hyperbaric oxygen therapy can diminish fibromyalgia syndrome—prospective clinical trial. *PLoS ONE* 2015;**10**(5):e0127012. doi:10.1371/journal.pone.0127012.
8. Fitzcharles M-A, Ste-Marie PA, Goldenberg DL, et al; the National Fibromyalgia Guideline Advisory Panel. 2012 Canadian guidelines for the diagnosis and management of fibromyalgia syndrome: executive summary. *Pain Res Manag*. 2013;**18**(3):119–126.
9. Flodin P, Martinsen S, Mannerkorpi K, et al. Normalization of aberrant resting state functional connectivity in fibromyalgia patients following a three month physical exercise therapy. *NeuroImage: Clin*. 2015;**9**:134–139.
10. Fraioli A, Grassi M, Mennuni G, et al. Clinical researches on efficacy of spa therapy in fibromyalgia. A systematic review. *Ann Ist Super Sanità*. 2013;**49**(2):219–229. doi:10.4415/ANN_13_02_13.
11. Guidelli GM, Tenti S, De Nobili E, Fioravanti A. Fibromyalgia syndrome and spa therapy: myth or reality? *Clin Med Insights: Arthritis Musculoskelet Disord*. 2012;**5**: 19–26. doi:10.4137/CMAMD.S8797.
12. Häuser W, Jung E, Erbslöh-Möller B, et al. Der deutsche Fibromyalgieverbraucherbericht. *Schmerz*. 2012;**26**:150. doi:10.1007/s00482-012-1161-5.
13. Häuser W, Jung E, Erbslöh-Möller B, et al. The German fibromyalgia consumer reports—a cross-sectional survey. *BMC Musculoskelet Disord*. 2012;**13**:74.
14. Heilmittel der Ergotherapie. Erkrankungen des Stütz- und Bewegungssystems. http://www.heilmittelkatalog.de/files/hmk/ergo/kapitel1.htm. German. Accessed June 16, 2017.
15. Heilmittelkatalog. Heilmittel der physikalischen Therapie. Chronifiziertes Schmerzsyndrom. www.heilmittelkatalog.de/files/hmk/physio/cs.htm. German. Accessed June 16, 2017.
16. Jäkel A, von Hauenschild P. A systematic review to evaluate the clinical benefits of craniosacral therapy. *Compl Ther Med*. 2012;**20**:456–465.
17. Karagülle M, Kardeş S, Karagülle MZ. Real-life effectiveness of spa therapy in rheumatic and musculoskeletal diseases: a retrospective study of 819 patients. *Int J Biometeorol*. 2017;**61**(11):1945–1956.
18. Koçyiğit BA, Gür A, Altındağ Ö, Akyol A, Gürsoy S. Comparison of education and balneotherapy efficacy in patients with fibromyalgia syndrome: a randomized, controlled clinical study. *Agri*. 2016;**28**(2):72–78. doi:10.5505/agri.2015.77699.
19. Larsson A, Palstam A, Löfgren M, et al. Resistance exercise improves muscle function, health status and pain intensity in fibromyalgia—a randomized controlled trial. *Arthritis Res Ther*. 2015;**17**:161.
20. Li YH, Wang FY, Feng CQ, et al. Massage therapy for fibromyalgia: a systematic review and meta-analysis of randomized controlled trials. *PLOS ONE*. 2014;**9**:e89304.
21. Lorena SB, Lima Mdo C, Ranzolin A, et al. Effects of muscle stretching exercises in the treatment of fibromyalgia: a systematic review. *Rev Bras Reumatol*. 2015;**55**:167–173.
22. Macfarlane GJ, Kronisch C, Dean LE, et al. EULAR revised recommendations for the management of fibromyalgia. *Ann Rheum Dis*. 2017;**76**:318–328. doi:10.1136/annrheumdis-2016–209724.
23. Martinsen S, Flodin P, Berrebi J, et al. The role of long-term physical exercise on performance and brain activation during the Stroop Color Word Task in Fibromyalgia patients. *Clin Physiol Function Imag*. 2018;**38**:508–516.
24. Petzke F, Brückle W, Eidmann U, et al. General treatment principles, coordination of care and patient education in fibromyalgia syndrome: updated guidelines 2017 and overview of systematic review articles. *Schmerz*. 2017;**31**(3):246–254.
25. Winkelmann A, Bork H, Brückle W, et al. Physiotherapy, occupational therapy and physical therapy in fibromyalgia syndrome. Updated guidelines 2017 and overview of systematic review articles. *Schmerz*. 2017;**31**:255–265.

26. Winkelmann A, Häuser W, Friedel E, et al. Arbeitsgemeinschaft der Wissenschaftlichen Medizinischen Fachgesellschaften. Physiotherapy and physical therapies for fibromyalgia syndrome. Systematic review, meta-analysis and guideline. *Schmerz*. 2012;26:276–286.
27. Yuan SL, Matsutani LA, Marques AP. Effectiveness of different styles of massage therapy in fibromyalgia: a systematic review and meta-analysis. *Man Ther*. 2015; **20**:257–264.

CHAPTER 28

Noninvasive Brain Stimulation for the Treatment of Fibromyalgia Syndrome–Related Pain

Didier Bouhassira

Summary Points

- Repetitive transcranial magnetic stimulation (rTMS) and transcranial direct electrical stimulation (tDCS) are two noninvasive brain stimulation (NIBS) technics, which can induce at least short-term analgesic effects in fibromyalgia syndrome (FMS) patients.
- Long-lasting analgesic effects associated with an improvement of quality of life have been shown with rTMS, but not yet with tDCS.
- Both technics are safe in comparison with pharmacologic treatments, but there are still few long-lasting multicenter prospective studies to recommend their use in routine practice.

The clinical applications of NIBS consisting of rTMS and tDCS have rapidly expanded over the past few years.[8] This approach was initially proposed and has been most thoroughly studied for the treatment of depression.[11] However, recent studies have shown that NIBS of the primary motor cortex (M1) or dorsolateral prefrontal cortex (DLPFC) decreases pain perception in healthy volunteers under various experimental models and in various chronic pain conditions including FMS.[3,10,13,17,19]

The rationale for using NIBS in FMS was related to the fact that alterations of central pain processing affecting primarily pain modulatory systems have been described in these patients and that NIBS is supposed to act primarily on these systems.[15]

Here, we briefly summarize the main methodologic aspects, clinical results, and potential mechanisms of NIBS for the treatment of pain associated with FMS.

METHODOLOGIC ASPECTS

Transcranial magnetic stimulation involves a magnetic pulse produced by a coil placed close to the scalp over the cortical region to be modulated.[15] The magnetic field can penetrate the skull a few centimeters away from the coil to generate an electrical field in the brain, which depolarizes specific populations of the neurons. Parameters of stimulation include the intensity of the magnetic pulse, its direction, and the targeted cortical region. Most rTMS studies were performed with the "figure-of-eight" coil, which induces a relatively focal electric current. Clinical and experimental studies have generally concluded that relatively high frequencies (HFs; ≥5 Hz, frequently called "excitatory rTMS") are more effective than lower frequencies. Thus, typical stimulation paradigms consist of 10 to 20 series of 10-second trains of pulses with an intra-train frequency of 10 Hz and an interval of 50 seconds between each train, resulting in a total of 1,000 to 2,000 pulses per session, with an intensity of stimulation below than that of the motor threshold (typically 80%).

For the tDCS procedure, a weak current (1 to 2 mA) is directly applied to the scalp with anodal and cathodal electrodes. Usually, one electrode is placed over a specific site, and the other electrode used as a reference is placed in another location to complete the circuit. The electrode positioning is critical in determining direction and spatial distribution of the current flow and, ultimately, the effectiveness of the treatment.

For both technics, the primary motor cortex (M1) has been the most frequent target. This choice was related to the well-documented analgesic effects of invasive electrical epidural motor cortex stimulation (EMCS).[20] However, analgesic effects have also been reported with rTMS and tDCS of the DLPFC.

MECHANISMS OF ACTION

The mechanisms underlying the analgesic action of NIBS are still uncertain. It has been hypothesized that they depend on the changes in pain modulation systems, which may be related to changes in neuronal excitability with mechanisms related to classical long-term potentiation (LTP) and long-term depression (LTD) phenomena.[15] Consistent with this hypothesis, it has been shown that rTMs-induced analgesia involve opioidergic[6] and glutamatergic systems.[5]

CLINICAL RESULTS IN FIBROMYALGIA SYNDROME

Repetitive Transcranial Magnetic Stimulation

The study by Passard et al.[17] conducted in 30 patients was the first to show analgesic effects of rTMS in FMS patients. The treatment protocol of this double-blind, sham-controlled study consisted of one session per day for 10 consecutive working days of stimulation of the left primary motor cortex (M1) with a frequency of 10 Hz and an intensity at 80% of the motor threshold. The primary outcome measure was self-reported average pain intensity over the last 24 hours, measured at baseline, daily during the stimulation period and then 15, 30, and 60 days after the first stimulation. Other outcome measures included sensory and affective pain scores, quality of life and function (fibromyalgia impact questionnaire [FIQ]), mood, and anxiety. Active rTMS significantly reduced pain and improved several aspects of quality of life (including fatigue, morning tiredness, general activity, walking, and sleep) for up to 2 weeks after treatment had ended. The analgesic effects were observed from the fifth stimulation onward and were not related to changes in mood or anxiety. The effects of rTMS were more long-lasting for affective than for sensory pain, suggesting differential effects on brain structures involved in pain perception. Only few minor and transient side effects were reported during the stimulation period. Consistent with these results, two other studies confirmed the significant improvement of both pain and quality of life after 10 daily sessions of HF (10 Hz) stimulation of the left M1.[10,19] By contrast, negative results were reported in one study using HF stimulation of the left DLPFC[18] and in two studies using low-frequency stimulation (1 Hz) of the left M1[21] or the right DLPFC[14] in FMS and in a small study of patients with chronic widespread pain after stimulation of the left DLPFC.[1]

Although the results regarding the effects of HF stimulation (i.e., 10 Hz) of M1 in FMS were encouraging, their clinical relevance was uncertain, as it was not clear whether the effects could be maintained for long period of time (i.e., several months) in these patients. To address this question, we conducted a randomized, double-blind, sham-controlled parallel group study, aiming to analyze the long-term maintenance, for up to 25 weeks, of the effects of unilateral rTMS of M1 on pain, quality of life, mood, and anxiety, in patients with FMS.[13] Based on our previous results showing that the effects of rTMS lasted from 15 to 30 days after the stimulation and then subsided,[17] it was hypothesized that after an induction phase of five daily stimulations, a monthly periodicity would allow to maintain the analgesic effects over a long period of time. Two series of weekly and fortnightly stimulation sessions were added to the stimulation paradigm to test whether it was possible to reinforce the effects of the induction phase. This study was the first to show that the analgesic effects of rTMS of the primary motor cortex could be maintained for up to 6 months in patients with FMS. The decrease in pain intensity was associated with a long-term improvement in other clinical features including fatigue, catastrophizing, and several items related to quality of life. Interestingly, the effects of rTMS were also associated with changes in intracortical modulation, that is, short intracortical inhibition and intracortical facilitation. This finding, which was consistent with previous data showing significant alteration of intracortical modulation in these patients,[14] suggested that changes in intracortical modulation may be predictive of the efficacy of rTMS in patients with FMS. Another study including 14 stimulation sessions for more than 10 weeks (10 daily sessions and

4 weekly sessions) of the left M1 cortex[3] confirmed the long-term improvement of quality of life, although this was not associated with a significant improvement in pain intensity in these patients.

It is important to emphasize that these studies also confirmed that rTMS can be safely administered in an outpatient setting. The adverse events observed during the induction or maintenance phase were generally of mild-to-moderate severity and less than 5% discontinued treatment because of side effects (headache). This low incidence of adverse events and treatment discontinuation compare favorably with those for current pharmacologic treatments of FMS. Most issues related to the safety of rTMS concern the effects of the magnetic fields in the human body and especially the risk of seizures during the sessions and therefore rTMS is contraindicated in epileptic patients or in patients with a history of epilepsia. Other contraindications are related to the application of a magnetic field and include head or cochlear implants. Finally, it was shown in one recent study that long-term HF rTMS was not associated with alteration of cognitive functions.[2]

Transcranial Direct Electrical Stimulation

After a series of studies by Fregni et al.,[7] several over groups have reported positive results suggesting that anodal tDCS of the left M1[9,12] could induce analgesic effects in patients with FMS. The magnitude of the analgesic effects is variable ranging 14% to 58% with tDCS protocols including 5 to 10 stimulation sessions. In general, the analgesic effects were associated with more global effects on quality of life in the majority of these studies and the treatment was well tolerated. However, it has not clearly been determined whether the analgesic effects are related or not to changes in depression or anxiety. In addition, there is still no data regarding the possible maintenance of the effects over several months as it is the case for rTMS.

CONCLUSIONS

A series of studies conducted over the past decade have indicated that both rTMS and tDCS could induce not only analgesic effects, but also a more global improvement in quality of life of patients with FMS and that both technics are safe. In addition, it has been shown that the effects of rTMS can be maintained over long period of time with monthly stimulation, suggesting that it could represent a valid treatment option in these patients. However, there are still few multicenter studies, and most of the available data only concerned small cohorts of patients. Thus, confirmatory results are needed. Future progress in this field should also depend on new technologic developments and new stimulation paradigms such as theta-burst stimulation (TBS), which can induce better analgesic effects than "classical" rTMS with stimulation sessions lasting only 3 minutes.[16]

REFERENCES

1. Avery DH, Zarkowski P, Krashin D, et al. Transcranial magnetic stimulation in the treatment of chronic widespread pain: a randomized controlled study. *J ECT*. 2015;**31**(1):57–66.
2. Baudic S, Attal N, Mhalla A, Ciampi de Andrade D, Perrot S, Bouhassira D. Unilateral repetitive transcranial magnetic stimulation of the motor cortex does not affect cognition in patients with fibromyalgia. *J Psychiatr Res*. 2013;**47**(1):72–77.
3. Boyer L, Dousset A, Roussel P, et al. rTMS in fibromyalgia: a randomized trial evaluating QoL and its brain metabolic substrate. *Neurology*. 2014;**82**:1231–1238.
4. Carretero B, Martín MJ, Juan A, et al. Low-frequency transcranial magnetic stimulation in patients with fibromyalgia and major depression. *Pain Med*. 2009;**10**(4):748–753.
5. Ciampi de Andrade D, Mhalla A, Adam F, Texeira MJ, Bouhassira D. Repetitive transcranial magnetic stimulation induced analgesia depends on N-methyl-D-aspartate glutamate receptors. *Pain*. 2014;**155**:598–605.
6. de Andrade DC, Mhalla A, Adam F, Texeira MJ, Bouhassira D. Neuropharmacological basis of rTMS-induced analgesia: the role of endogenous opioids. *Pain*. 2011;**152**:320–326.
7. Fregni F, Gimenes R, Valle AC, et al. A randomized, sham-controlled, proof of principle study of transcranial direct current stimulation for the treatment of pain in fibromyalgia. *Arthritis Rheum*. 2006;**54**(12):3988–3998.
8. Galhardoni R, Correia GS, Araujo H, et al. Repetitive transcranial magnetic stimulation in chronic pain: a review of the literature. *Arch Phys Med Rehabil*. 2015;**96**(4 Suppl):S156–S172.
9. Knijnik LM, Dussán-Sarria JA, Rozisky JR, et al. Repetitive transcranial magnetic stimulation for fibromyalgia: systematic review and meta-analysis. *Pain Pract*. 2016;**16**(3):294–304.
10. Lee SJ, Kim DY, Chun MH, Kim YG. The effect of repetitive transcranial magnetic stimulation on fibromyalgia: a randomized sham-controlled trial with 1-mo follow-up. *Am J Phys Med Rehabil*. 2012;**91**(12):1077–1085.
11. Lefaucheur JP, André-Obadia N, Antal A, et al. Evidence-based guidelines on the therapeutic use of repetitive transcranial magnetic stimulation (rTMS). *Clin Neurophysiol*. 2014;**125**(11):2150–2206.
12. Lefaucheur JP, Antal A, Ayache SS, et al. Evidence-based guidelines on the therapeutic use of transcranial direct current stimulation (tDCS). *Clin Neurophysiol*. 2017;**128**(1):56–92.
13. Mhalla A, Baudic S, Ciampi de Andrade D, et al. Long-term maintenance of the analgesic effects of transcranial magnetic stimulation in fibromyalgia. *Pain*. 2011;**152**:1478–1485.
14. Mhalla A, de Andrade DC, Baudic S, Perrot S, Bouhassira D. Alteration of cortical excitability in patients with fibromyalgia. *Pain*. 2010;**149**:495–500.
15. Moisset X, de Andrade DC, Bouhassira D. From pulses to pain relief: an update on the mechanisms of rTMS-induced analgesic effects. *Eur J Pain*. 2016;**20**(5):689–700.
16. Moisset X, Goudeau S, Poindessous-Jazat F, Baudic S, Clavelou P, Bouhassira D. Prolonged continuous theta-burst stimulation is more analgesic than "classical" high frequency repetitive transcranial magnetic stimulation. *Brain Stimulat*. 2015;**8**:135–141.
17. Passard A, Attal N, Benadhira R, et al. Effects of unilateral repetitive transcranial magnetic stimulation of the motor cortex on chronic widespread pain in fibromyalgia. *Brain*. 2007;**130**:2661–2670.
18. Short EB, Borckardt JJ, Anderson BS, et al. Ten sessions of adjunctive left prefrontal rTMS significantly reduces fibromyalgia pain: a randomized, controlled pilot study. *Pain*. 2011;**152**:2477–2484.
19. Tekin A, Ozdil E, Guleken MD, et al. Efficacy of high frequency [10Hz] repetitive transcranial magnetic stimulation of the primary motor cortex in patients with fibromyalgia syndrome: a randomized, double blind, sham-controlled trial. *J Musculoskeletal Pain*. 2014;**22**:20–26.
20. Tsubokawa T, Katayama Y, Yamamoto T, Hirayama T, Koyama S. Treatment of thalamic pain by chronic motor cortex stimulation. *Pacing Clin Electrophysiol PACE*. 1991;**14**:131–134.
21. Yagci I, Agirman M, Ozturk D, Eren B. Is the transcranial magnetic stimulation an adjunctive treatment in fibromyalgia patients? *Turk J Phys Med Rehab*. 2014;**60**:206–211.

CHAPTER 29

Complementary or Integrative Medicine for Fibromyalgia Syndrome

Jost Langhorst and Anna K. Koch

Summary Points

- Complementary or integrative medicine (CIM) use is high among patients with fibromyalgia syndrome (FMS).
- Meditative movement therapies (MMT) like Qigong, Tai Chi, or yoga can reduce sleep disturbances, depression, and heighten health-related quality of life.
- Spa and hydrotherapy yield potential to reduce pain and improve health-related quality of life.
- Exercise has beneficial effects on physical function, pain, and stiffness.
- CIM can be a useful supplement within the framework of a multimodal therapeutic concept, but there is a need for further high-quality clinical trials.

The use of CIM is high among patients particularly with chronic diseases such as FMS. According to an internet sample of 2,596 people with FMS from the National Fibromyalgia Association (NFA),[3] patients reported the use of heat modalities (warm water, hot packs; 74%), relaxation/meditation (47%), massage/reflexology (43%), non-aerobic exercise (stretching, yoga, Tai Chi; 24%), acupuncture (15%), biofeedback (6%), and hypnosis (3%). Patients rated the effectiveness of these interventions from 6.3 (heat modalities) to 2.5 (hypnosis) on a scale of 0 to 10. This survey has been conducted 10 years ago. A more recent survey also concludes that non-pharmacologic therapies like self-management strategies and aerobic exercise are important in the long-term management of FMS.[14] Especially, young female patients with high overall disease burden seem to make use of CIM.[23,25] Hence, CIM use is high among patients with FMS and might be a promising treatment alternative to cope with the disease. Table 29.1 shows the most frequently used CIM therapies by the United States and German patients, and their effectiveness as rated by the patients.

TABLE 29.1 **Use and effectiveness of complementary and alternative therapies most frequently used by United States and German patients**

	United States		Germany	
Nutritional supplements	68%	3.8 ± 2.8	30%	4.0 ± 3.0
Relaxation/meditation	47%	5.1 ± 5.5	65%	5.1 ± 2.9
Massage/reflexology	43%	6.1 ± 2.8	23%	5.4 ± 2.9
Chiropractic manipulation	30%	5.1 ± 3.0	29%	4.7 ± 2.8
Non-aerobic exercise (stretching, yoga, Tai Chi)	40%	4.8 ± 3.0	24%	5.1 ± 2.9
Pilates	8%	4.6 ± 3.3		
Energy healing (e.g., reiki)	7%	4.0 ± 3.2	12%	4.8 ± 3.1
Hypnosis	3%	2.5 ± 2.9	4%	4.1 ± 2.3
Homeopathy			31%	4.5 ± 3.1

Note: Effectiveness was rated on an 11-point scale, with 10 being most effective.

Despite the frequent use and high patient request, only limited research has been conducted on complementary and integrative therapies so far. To judge their value in the treatment of FMS, data on efficacy and safety are indispensable and without those data, therapies that might benefit FMS patients will not be included in standard care. Recently, several studies on the therapy of FMS with CIM is growing. Therefore, complementary therapies have been introduced to German evidence-based guidelines on the management of FMS.[12,18,30] Systematic reviews and meta-analyses now can be considered to ensure a high-quality basis for treatment recommendations for at least some of the available CIM treatments. This chapter aims to give patients and physicians an evidence-based orientation on the management of FMS with CIM. We summarize CIM treatment modalities for FMS following the proposed categorization system by Wieland et al.[29] for the Cochrane Collaboration: mind–body medicine (MBM), whole medical systems, natural product-based therapies, manipulative and body-based practices, and energy medicine. Due to the limited space, we will not be able to give a full review on each available treatment modality.

MIND–BODY MEDICINE

According to the National Center for Complementary and Integrative Health (NCCIH) MBM "focuses on the interactions among the brain, mind, body, and behavior, and the powerful ways in which emotional, mental, social, spiritual, and behavioral factors can directly affect health. It regards as fundamental an approach that respects and enhances each person's capacity for self-knowledge and self-care, and it emphasizes techniques that are grounded in this approach," cited after Paul and Dobos.[26] This includes, for example, lifestyle modification, mindfulness interventions, relaxation techniques, hypnotherapy, and MMTs.

Meditative Movement Therapies (Qigong, Tai Chi, and Yoga)

MMT is a category of exercise defined by some form of movement or body positioning, a focus on breathing and a calm state of mind with meditative aspects and a goal of relaxation. Mostly Qigong, Tai Chi, and yoga are subsumed as MMT. Qigong is a Chinese medical exercise. It combines physical exercises, breathing exercises, and meditation and aims to increase the energy flow through the body, the so-called qi. It is effective for physical conditions and for psychologic well-being. Like Qigong, Tai Chi is also a traditional Chinese medicine (TCM) technique that incorporates physical exercises, breathing exercises, and attentional training with the goal of improving disease symptoms and maintain health. In contrast to Qigong, Tai Chi is a form of martial arts with a focus on self-defense. Yoga is an ancient Indian form of physical movement. It consists of body postures, breathing techniques, and meditation and has been shown to have beneficial effects on quality of life and mental health for various health-related aspects. A meta-analysis on the efficacy and safety of MMT in FMS showed that MMT reduced sleep disturbances, depression, and health-related quality of life compared to controls at final treatment. However, there was no significant effect on pain. At follow-up, MMT still did not reduce pain and depression, but had beneficial effects on sleep disturbances and health-related quality of life.[19] Furthermore, there seem to be differences regarding the efficacy of the different MMT modalities. Subgroup analyses showed that especially yoga might be most beneficial.[19] A meta-analysis regarding Qigong in specific has shown that there is low-quality evidence for short-term improvement of pain, quality of life, and sleep quality and very low-quality evidence for improvement of fatigue compared to usual care. No evidence was found for superiority of Qigong compared to active treatments.[22] Regarding the treatment of FMS, Qigong, Tai Chi, and yoga are some of the few complementary therapies with sufficient data to allow recommendation. Therefore, MMTs have recently been included into evidence-based guidelines on the management of FMS with a positive recommendation (EL1a, low-quality evidence, strong consensus).[12,18,30]

Biofeedback

During a biofeedback, patients' bodily responses like heart rate, muscle tension, or skin temperature are measured and reported through an auditory or visual modality. Biofeedback's efficacy can be explained by increases of self-efficacy and coping strategies.[27] Regarding the treatment of FMS, biofeedback has been shown to have beneficial short-term effects in pain reduction, physical functioning, and mood.[28,13] The poor methodologic studies' quality, however, limits the credibility of these effects and therefore biofeedback has been included into evidence-based guidelines with an open recommendation (EL2a, low-quality evidence, strong consensus).[12,18,30]

Mindfulness-Based Stress Reduction

Mindfulness-based stress reduction (MBSR) is a treatment modality that has been used for various chronic pain conditions. Originally, it has been developed as a behavioral medical intervention for patients who suffer from chronic pain conditions and stress-related disorders.[17] Regarding the treatment of FMS, it has been shown to have beneficial short-term effects on quality of life and pain when compared to usual care and on quality of life and pain when compared to active control interventions.[21] However, it should not be applied as a monotherapy because the quality of evidence is not sufficient to allow positive recommendations within the guidelines (EL1a, moderate quality of evidence, strong consensus).[12,18,30]

RELAXATION

Relaxation techniques like muscle relaxation or autogenic training help people to attain a calm state of mind and body. Because FMS is reported to be associated with heightened levels of stress, stress-management approaches might be beneficial for FMS patients. However, no conclusive evidence was found regarding the effectiveness of relaxation formats like muscle relaxation or autogenic training. Further studies are required[24] and relaxation techniques should not be used as monotherapy (EL1a, low-quality evidence, strong consensus).[12,18,30]

Hypnosis and Guided Imagery

Hypnosis is a mental state like sleep that can be used for hypnotherapy, which is an alternative curative healing method. Hypnosis and guided imagery show promising effects for the treatment of FMS[4,32] and therefore have been recommended as an adjunct to efficacious pharmacologic and non-pharmacologic treatments by the German evidence-based guidelines on the management of FMS (EL2a, low-quality evidence, strong consensus).[12,18,30]

WHOLE MEDICAL SYSTEMS

Whole medical systems are complete systems of diagnosis and practice. Major Eastern whole medical systems include, for example, TCM and Ayurveda. Homeopathy is a Western whole medical system.

Homeopathy

The idea behind homeopathy is that minute doses of natural substances that cause symptoms of a disease in healthy people treat those diseases in sick people. Regarding homeopathy, amount of data and data quality are very limited, but results do not preclude the possibility of some benefit.[7] However, because of its low-evidence quality, no evidence-based recommendation can be given (EL2a, low quality of evidence, no consensus).[12,18,30]

Acupuncture

Acupuncture is a part of TCM. "Acupuncture" literally means to puncture with a needle. Needling may be combined with moxibustion—the burning on or over the skin of selected herbs—or other kinds of stimulation, for example, electrical stimulation. Regarding the treatment of FMS, there is low-to-moderate-level evidence that acupuncture improves pain and stiffness compared with no treatment and standard therapy.[10] But those beneficial effects seem not to differ from sham acupuncture (where the needles do not go as deep and are not used at the same points) regarding reductions of fatigue or pain, or improving sleep or global well-being. Furthermore, there is evidence that electroacupuncture is more efficacious than manual acupuncture. Electroacupuncture has been included into German evidence-based guidelines on the management of FMS with an open degree of recommendation (EL2a, moderate quality of evidence, consensus).[12,18,30]

NATURAL PRODUCT–BASED THERAPIES

Herbal Medicine

Pharmacologic therapy is often used for FMS patients. However, a high percentage does not respond well to drug therapy with, for example, nonsteroidal anti-inflammatory drugs (NSAIDs), muscle-relaxing medications, or painkillers. Herbal medicines are a promising treatment option. Regarding the treatment of FMS especially *topical capsaicin* (the main active ingredient of chili peppers, so-called *Capsicum annuum)* and *O24* (consisting of white camphor oil, eucalyptus oil, aloe vera oil, peppermint oil, rosemary oil, lemon oil, and orange oil) have been evaluated within clinical trials and demonstrated positive effects in pain relief due to their analgesic effects, and also beneficial influences on quality of life, anxiety, sleep disruption, and physical function in comparison to placebo.[9]

Dietary Intervention

Because there is a high prevalence of obesity and overweight among FMS patients, dietary interventions like a vegetarian diet, elimination diet, or therapeutic fasting might be an effective approach to improve symptoms. However, the empirical evidence regarding this topic is scarce. Today, no systematic review or meta-analysis is available. Three studies on this topic found that (a) a vegetarian diet resulted in pain reduction, but amitriptyline was more effective at the completion of therapy,[2] (b) a 3-month low-salt uncooked vegetarian diet was superior to a normal diet in reducing pain and improving function,[16] and (c) patients receiving exclusion diet (e.g., of wheat, nutritional supplements) based on immunologic tests reported a 50% reduction in pain, whereas the controls who continued their normal diets reported no changes.[11] Consensus guidelines conclude that weight reduction should be recommended for patients with obesity (EL2b, recommendation, strong consensus).[12,18,30]

Spa and Hydrotherapy

The use of water as a medical therapy is a body-based practice and dates back to ancient cultures from China, Japan, and Europe. There are different forms of hydrotherapy. Balneotherapy, for example, means drinking of and/or bathing in medicinal water, bathing in warm or cold water or mud. Spa therapy means drinking of and/or bathing in thermal or mineral water. Regarding the treatment of FMS, a meta-analysis has shown moderate evidence for a reduction of pain and improved health-related quality of life at the end of therapy.[20] At follow-up, there was also moderate evidence for a reduction of pain and improved health-related quality of life. Hydrotherapy has been included into evidence-based guidelines with a positive recommendation (EL2a, low quality of evidence).[12,18,30]

MANIPULATIVE AND BODY-BASED PRACTICES

Exercise

Exercise is a promising treatment modality for patients with FMS. Activities like walking and cycling for at least half an hour twice or three times weekly can have beneficial effects on pain, quality of life, and tiredness.[5,31] To obtain maximum benefit, exercise should be done on a regular basis because this might heighten the chance of long-term efficacy. Especially low- and middle-frequency exercise is recommended for the treatment of FMS within evidence-based guidelines (EL1a, moderate quality of evidence, strong consensus).[12,18,30]

Aquatic Exercise

Aquatic exercise is an exercise that takes place in the water. Regarding the treatment of FMS, aquatic exercise has beneficial effects, for example, on physical function, pain, and stiffness[6] and has been included into evidence-based guidelines with a positive recommendation (EL1a, moderate quality of evidence, strong recommendation).[12,18,30]

Bio-Sauna and Infrared Cabin

Even though there are no randomized controlled trials (RCTs) on the use of bio-sauna and infrared cabin, the application of warmth to the whole body is a well-used self-management strategy of FMS patients.[15] Because patients rate whole body warmth therapy to be first place among the top 10 most effective management strategies, those treatment approaches have been included into German FMS guidelines (strong clinical consensus).[12,18,30]

Water-Filtered Near-Infrared Whole-Body Hyperthermia

Water-filtered near-infrared whole-body hyperthermia has been tested as an adjunct to standard rehabilitation practices. One RCT testing the effects of infrared whole-body hyperthermia is available.[8] The results showed significant differences between groups for affective and sensory pain in favor of infrared whole-body hyperthermia. Therefore, it might serve as a useful adjunct, but the current data do not allow any recommendations in this case (strong consensus).[12,18,30]

ENERGY MEDICINE

The approaches of energy medicine vary widely and include a great amount of diverse treatment approaches. However, most of them have not been studied adequately.

Reiki

One of the few energy medicine approaches that has been studied within RCTs regarding the treatment of FMS is reiki. Reiki is a practice where energy is supposed to be transferred through the palms of the practitioner to the patient to encourage emotional or physical healing. One trial that evaluated the effects of either direct or distant reiki treatment on 25 patients did not find a significant effect on pain, fatigue, sleep, or quality of life.[1] Hence, there is a negative recommendation for the use of reiki in the treatment of FMS (EL2b, strong consensus).[12,18,30]

Table 29.2 shows an overview on the efficacy and safety of complementary and alternative therapies in FMS discussed in this chapter.

CONCLUSION

Alternative and complementary therapies provide promising approaches for the treatment of FMS that offer the hope to be beneficial with only few side effects. However, as many of these trials of CIM in FMS tend to be single center studies and relatively small, the efficacy has not been fully proven. Furthermore, the safety has

TABLE 29.2 **Overview on the efficacy and safety of complementary and alternative therapies in fibromyalgia syndrome at the end of therapy**

	Quality of life SMD (95% CI)	Pain SMD (95% CI)	Sleep problems SMD (95% CI)	Fatigue SMD (95% CI)	Safety
Dietary interventions	i.d.	i.d.	i.d.	i.d.	
Meditative movement therapies[a,19]	−0.59 (−0.93, −0.24)	−0.35 (−0.80, 0.11)	−0.61 (−0.95, −0.27)	−0.66 (−0.99, −0.34)	No serious adverse events known
Biofeedback[13]	0.62 (−0.77, −2.02)	0.79 (0.22, 1.36)	0.23 (−0.20, 0.65)	0.38 (−0.46, 1.08)	
Mindfulness[b,21]	−0.35 (−0.57, −0.12)	−0.23 (−0.46, −0.01)	−0.07 (−0.33, 0.20)	i.d.	No serious adverse events known
Relaxation	i.d.	i.d.	i.d.	i.d.	
Hypnosis[4]	−0.19 (−0.62, 0.24)	−1.12 (−1.97, −0.28)	−0.91 (−1.51, −0.11)	−0.46 (−0.91, 0.00)	No serious adverse events known
Acupuncture[c,10]	i.d.	−0.14 (−0.53, 0.25)	0.16 (−0.29, 0.61)	−0.10; (−0.81, 0.61)	Rare serious adverse events
Homeopathy[d,7]	i.d.	−0.54 (−0.97, −0.10	i.d.	0.47 (−0.90, −0.05)	No serious adverse events known
Phytotherapy	i.d.	i.d.	i.d.	i.d.	

(Continued)

TABLE 29.2 **Overview on the efficacy and safety of complementary and alternative therapies in fibromyalgia syndrome at the end of therapy** *(Continued)*

	Quality of life SMD (95% CI)	Pain SMD (95% CI)	Sleep problems SMD (95% CI)	Fatigue SMD (95% CI)	Safety
(Aerobic) Exercise[31]	−0.38 (−0.52, −0.24)	−0.40 (−0.55, −0.26)	−0.15 (−0.38, 0.09)	−0.37 (−0.58, −0.17)	
Hydrotherapy[a,20]	−1.67 (−2.91, −0.43)	−0.78 (−1.42, −0.13)	i.d.	i.d.	No serious adverse events known
Bio-sauna and infrared cabin	i.d.	i.d.	i.d.	i.d.	
Hyperthermia	i.d.	i.d.	i.d.	i.d.	
Reiki	i.d.	i.d.	i.d.	i.d.	

CI, confidence interval; i.d., insufficient data; SMD, standardized mean difference.

[a]Compared to mixed controls.

[b]Compared to usual care.

[c]Compared to sham or placebo.

[d]Compared to placebo.

not been completely established. Most convincing evidence for FMS management is present for treatment approaches like MMT, exercise, and acupuncture. Those treatment approaches frequently constitute a useful supplement within the framework of a multimodal therapeutic concept that patients can apply as self-help strategies (e.g., MBSR, yoga, or qigong). However, there is a need for further high-quality clinical trials.

REFERENCES

1. Assefi N, Bogart A, Goldberg J, Buchwald D. Reiki for the treatment of fibromyalgia: a randomized controlled trial. *J Alt Compl Med.* 2008;**14**(9):1115–1122.
2. Azad KA, Alam MN, Haq SA, et al. Vegetarian diet in the treatment of fibromyalgia. *Bang Med Res Coun Bull.* 2000;**26**(2):41–47.
3. Bennett RM, Jones J, Turk DC, Russell IJ, Matallana L. An internet survey of 2,596 people with fibromyalgia. *BMC Musculoskelet Disord.* 2007;**8**:27.
4. Bernardy K, Fuber N, Klose P, Hauser W. Efficacy of hypnosis/guided imagery in fibromyalgia syndrome—a systematic review and meta-analysis of controlled trials. *BMC Musculoskelet Disord.* 2011;**12**:133.
5. Bidonde J, Busch AJ, Schachter CL, et al. Aerobic exercise training for adults with fibromyalgia. *Coch Database Syst Rev.* 2017;**6**:CD012700.
6. Bidonde J, Busch AJ, Webber SC, et al. Aquatic exercise training for fibromyalgia. *Coch Database Syst Rev.* 2014(10):CD011336.
7. Boehm K, Raak C, Cramer H, Lauche R, Ostermann T. Homeopathy in the treatment of fibromyalgia—a comprehensive literature-review and meta-analysis. *Compl Ther Med.* 2014;**22**(4):731–742.
8. Brockow T, Wagner A, Franke A, Offenbacher M, Resch KL. A randomized controlled trial on the effectiveness of mild water-filtered near infrared whole-body hyperthermia as an adjunct to a standard multimodal rehabilitation in the treatment of fibromyalgia. *Clin J Pain.* 2007;**23**(1):67–75.
9. de Souza Nascimento S, Desantana JM, Nampo FK, et al. Efficacy and safety of medicinal plants or related natural products for fibromyalgia: a systematic review. *Evidence Based Compl Alt Med.* 2013;**2013**:149468.
10. Deare JC, Zheng Z, Xue CC, et al. Acupuncture for treating fibromyalgia. *Coch Database Syst Rev.* 2013(5):CD007070.
11. Deuster PA, Jaffe RM. A novel treatment for fibromyalgia improves clinical outcomes in a community-based study. *J Musculoskelet Pain.* 1998;**6**(2):133–149.
12. Eich W, Bar KJ, Bernateck M, et al. Definition, classification, clinical diagnosis and prognosis of fibromyalgia syndrome: updated guidelines 2017 and overview of systematic review articles. *Schmerz.* 2017;**31**(3):231–238.
13. Glombiewski JA, Bernardy K, Häuser W. Efficacy of EMG- and EEG-biofeedback in fibromyalgia syndrome: a meta-analysis and a systematic review of randomized controlled trials. *Evidence Based Compl Alt Med.* 2013;**2013**:962741.
14. Hauser W, Jung E, Erbsloh-Moller B, et al. The German fibromyalgia consumer reports—a cross-sectional survey. *BMC Musculoskelet Disord.* 2012;**13**:74.
15. Hauser W, Jung E, Erbsloh-Moller B, et al. German fibromyalgia consumer reports. Benefits and harms of fibromyalgia syndrome therapies. *Schmerz.* 2012;**26**(2):150–159.
16. Kaartinen K, Lammi K, Hypen M, Nenonen M, Hanninen O, Rauma AL. Vegan diet alleviates fibromyalgia symptoms. *Scand J Rheumatol.* 2000;**29**(5):308–313.
17. Kabat-Zinn J. An outpatient program in behavioral medicine for chronic pain patients based on the practice of mindfulness meditation: theoretical considerations and preliminary results. *Gen Hosp Psychiat.* 1982;**4**(1):33–47.

18. Langhorst J, Heldmann P, Henningsen P, et al. Complementary and alternative procedures for fibromyalgia syndrome: updated guidelines 2017 and overview of systematic review articles. *Schmerz.* 2017;**31**(3):289–295.
19. Langhorst J, Klose P, Dobos GJ, Bernardy K, Hauser W. Efficacy and safety of meditative movement therapies in fibromyalgia syndrome: a systematic review and meta-analysis of randomized controlled trials. *Rheumatol Int.* 2013;**33**(1):193–207.
20. Langhorst J, Musial F, Klose P, Hauser W. Efficacy of hydrotherapy in fibromyalgia syndrome—a meta-analysis of randomized controlled clinical trials. *Rheumatology.* 2009;**48**(9):1155–1159.
21. Lauche R, Cramer H, Dobos G, Langhorst J, Schmidt S. A systematic review and meta-analysis of mindfulness-based stress reduction for the fibromyalgia syndrome. *J Psychosomat Res.* 2013;**75**(6):500–510.
22. Lauche R, Cramer H, Hauser W, Dobos G, Langhorst J. A systematic review and meta-analysis of qigong for the fibromyalgia syndrome. *Evidence Based Compl Alt Med.* 2013;**2013**:635182.
23. Lind BK, Lafferty WE, Tyree PT, Diehr PK, Grembowski DE. Use of complementary and alternative medicine providers by fibromyalgia patients under insurance coverage. *Arthritis Rheumat.* 2007;**57**(1):71–76.
24. Meeus M, Nijs J, Vanderheiden T, Baert I, Descheemaeker F, Struyf F. The effect of relaxation therapy on autonomic functioning, symptoms and daily functioning, in patients with chronic fatigue syndrome or fibromyalgia: a systematic review. *Clin Rehabilitat.* 2015;**29**(3):221–233.
25. Nicassio PM, Schuman C, Kim J, Cordova A, Weisman MH. Psychosocial factors associated with complementary treatment use in fibromyalgia. *J Rheumatol.* 1997;**24**(10):2008–2013.
26. Paul A, Dobos GJ. *Mind-body-Medizin—Die moderne Ordnungstherapie in Theorie und Praxis.* München: Urban & Fischer Verlag/ Elsevier GmbH; 2011.
27. Rains JC. Change mechanisms in EMG biofeedback training: cognitive changes underlying improvements in tension headache. *Headache.* 2008;**48**(5):735–736; discussion 736–737.
28. Theadom A, Cropley M, Smith HE, Feigin VL, McPherson K. Mind and body therapy for fibromyalgia. *Coch Database Syst Rev.* 2015;**4**:CD001980.
29. Wieland LS, Manheimer E, Berman BM. Development and classification of an operational definition of complementary and alternative medicine for the Cochrane collaboration. *Alt Ther Health Med.* 2011;**17**(2):50–59.
30. Winkelmann A, Bork H, Bruckle W, et al. Physiotherapy, occupational therapy and physical therapy in fibromyalgia syndrome: updated guidelines 2017 and overview of systematic review articles. *Schmerz.* 2017;**31**(3):255–265.
31. Winkelmann A, Hauser W, Friedel E, et al. Physiotherapy and physical therapies for fibromyalgia syndrome. Systematic review, meta-analysis and guideline. *Schmerz.* 2012;**26**(3):276–286.
32. Zech N, Hansen E, Bernardy K, Hauser W. Efficacy, acceptability and safety of guided imagery/hypnosis in fibromyalgia—a systematic review and meta-analysis of randomized controlled trials. *Eur J Pain.* 2017;**21**(2):217–227.

CHAPTER 30

Psychological Aspects and Psychological Approaches

Christine Cedraschi and Anne-Françoise Allaz

Summary Points

- Fibromyalgia syndrome (FMS) should be understood within a biopsychosocial model where the search for a single explanatory cause should be replaced by considering the interaction between factors that would predispose, precipitate, or perpetuate the symptoms. Among psychological factors, traumatic experiences have been linked with long-standing affect regulation disorder, associated with difficulties in emotional disclosure and expression.
- Affect regulation disorder associated with somatization and trauma is correlated with difficulties in interpersonal relationships, manifested as an "insecure attachment style." This insecure attachment style, and high sensitivity to neglect or abandonment associated with little ability to create trusting bonds is often observed in the clinical practice.
- The reported effect sizes of psychological approaches used in the context of FMS often remain in the low or medium range. Thus, integration of alternative treatment approaches might add to improve the outcome, thus making the exploration of the efficacy of different forms of psychotherapy of clear clinical relevance.

Discussions about psychological treatments of FMS patients are often entangled with questions about the importance of psychological contributions to this syndrome. In fact, FMS has been long classified within the field of chronic pain syndromes; whereas it has been largely discussed whether or not it should be assimilated to a somatoform disorder in the debates about the new classification systems for pain disorders of the *Diagnostic and Statistical Manual of Mental Disorders*—Fifth edition (*DSM-5*) and the *International Statistical Classification of Diseases and Related Health Problems—10th Revision* (*ICD-10*),[19,45] it is still widely acknowledged that it should be understood within a biopsychosocial model where the search for a single explanatory cause should be replaced by considering the interaction between factors that would predispose, precipitate, or perpetuate the symptoms.[18]

Among these factors, psychological and psychosocial dimensions play an important part. This comes as no surprise because chronic pain is inserted in a dynamic process resulting from a constant interaction between somatic and psychologic aspects. Considering psychological factors is by no means a way to deny the role of somatic aspects—central sensitization[15,49] as well as a neurogenic implication[39] have often been called upon—which are often mentioned when discussing the FMS.[6,13]

It is in any case extremely difficult, and even counterproductive to attempt a distinction between symptoms that would be labeled as "somatogenic" as opposed to others that would be termed "psychogenic" in a chronic pain syndrome where both the somatic component and the psychological distress could be involved in producing physical symptoms. Taking into account and legitimizing the experience of pain and suffering in these patients is thus in the foreground. The focus needs to be on the representations these patients may have regarding the causes and consequences of their pain problem, the treatment they may consider as acceptable and useful, and their views about a future is often seen as threatened by a loss of point in time and identity benchmarks.

Various psychological conditions have been described as associated with FMS. In their review for clinicians, Arnold et al.[6] indicate that mood or anxiety disorders have high lifetime prevalence in FMS patients, with lifetime anxiety disorder reported in as much as 35% to 62% of patients, and lifetime major depressive disorder in 58% to 86% of the patients. However, although symptom overlap is obvious, FMS should not be confused with mood and anxiety disorders,[6,47] pointing to the necessity to focus treatment on both physical and emotional dysfunction.[47]

TRAUMA AND FIBROMYALGIA SYNDROME

Among the psychological factors accounting for this emotional dysfunction, traumatic experiences during childhood (such as emotional neglect, physical and sexual abuse, death of a relative, prolonged hospitalization, or accident) play a major role.[10] A prospective cohort study has shown a link between early violent experiences and chronic pain diseases—not only FMS.[23] Such traumatic events could result in relational and attachment problems, in the form of fear of being abandoned with individuals struggling to keep a high degree of independence while trying at the same time to adapt as closely as possible to some relationships.[33]

Trauma is defined by an experience that is emotionally painful, distressful, or shocking, which may result in acute or lasting mental and physical effects. A traumatic event involves a single experience or enduring or repeated events, which overwhelm the individual's ability to cope with the thoughts and emotions involved with that experience.[40] The association between traumatic experience and FMS has been often discussed and remains debated.[11] The debate around this association discussion refers to the hypothesis that it is the subjective experience rather than the objective reality of the trauma, whether physical or emotional, that has the most important impact on the severity of symptoms.

A qualitative study of the discourse of women suffering from FMS and investigating their principal attributions related to perceived pain onset indicated that these attributions often referred to the psychological dimension of the reported events (e.g., relational problems or death of a relative), even when the events also had a clear somatic dimension, such as violence during childhood, accident, or gynecologic/obstetric problems.[9] These attributions thus often pointed to distressful experiences or were expressed as a series of disruptive events. Sexual abuse, violence, the threat, or the witnessing of either, which have been mentioned in some of the respondents have also been described as causes of psychological trauma.

A secondary analysis of these patient narratives considered from the perspective of clinicians familiar with FMS who were asked to provide their own appraisal of the affective load of the patients' narratives showed that these clinicians perceived and emphasized the salience and pervasiveness of distressful illness perceptions in the patient narratives regarding pain onset.[10]

Therefore, the salience of a traumatic load in the patient narratives as considered from the clinicians' perspective questions not only the way patients cope with pain problems associated with highly distressing emotions, but also the resonance of these emotions in the clinicians. These findings may be related to recent research indicating that patients suffering from FMS and other pain conditions are often raised in emotional avoidance cultures, in which traumatic events are not positively processed verbally, and have therefore learned to avoid expressions of traumatic and stressful events.[27] These events are thus not transformed into a coherent narrative. Furthermore, consistent with earlier negative experiences and by avoiding to tell others of their emotionally difficult experiences, these patients may not receive either social support or stress relief from the related affective load by verbalizing their concerns and related distress.

Traumatic experience such as child abuse or neglect has been linked with long-standing affect regulation disorder itself associated with difficulties with emotional disclosure and expression.[25,38] In the clinical encounter, reluctance to talk about personal history and difficulties in creating trusting relationships may point to the existence of such traumatic experiences, especially when a seemingly minor event leads to a perplexing intractable pain or disability.

Since Engel's description of the "pain-prone-patient" about five decades ago, chronic refractory pain has often been associated with a history of abuse, neglect, or childhood trauma. Epidemiologic data associating pain and abuse point to a notable issue.[14] It is particularly prevalent in patients suffering from chronic pain syndromes like FMS,[22] or chronic pelvic pain.[24] Recently, however, interest has shifted from abuse per se to an emphasis on the central importance of the dimension of neglect or abandonment.[25] The importance of chronic stress has also been emphasized in this context.[48]

ATTACHMENT AND SOMATIZATION

Bowlby's[8] conceptual developments about the role of early experiences with caregivers in forming models of relationships later reproduced throughout life have gained wide recognition as "attachment theory." The dimension of attachment has recently attracted renewed interest in the field of pain and has been the subject of recent reviews.[25,32,37] A recent book edited by two consultation–liaison psychiatrists[21] also called attention on attachment theory, both in primary and specialized care. In their presentation of the theory, the authors emphasize that:

> *There is a surprising degree of consistency in patterns of attachment behaviour as children grow into adolescents and then adults. As we mature, we turn to new people to serve our attachment needs, first peers and then, typically, romantic partners. But the functions that attachment figures serve remain the same [...]. Patterns of adult attachment can be understood in different ways, as 'states of mind' about attachment phenomena or as clusters of attitudes, behaviour and emotional expression in close relationships. We can describe [...] patterns of attachment, which we can locate on two dimensions of attachment insecurity: attachment anxiety and attachment avoidance. In this system of classification, the X-axis refers to attachment anxiety, which is the degree of discomfort one feels with separation. The Y-axis is attachment avoidance, which is the extent to which one is distressed by crowding or closeness. Every individual person has an attachment style, and in this model, each style can be located in this two-dimensional space, depending on the degree to which he or she is prone to attachment anxiety and attachment avoidance.*

Not unexpectedly, affect regulation disorder associated with somatization and trauma is correlated with difficulties in interpersonal relationships, manifested as an "insecure attachment style."[25] This insecure attachment style is marked by feelings of defenselessness in interpersonal encounters, and high sensitivity to neglect or abandonment associated with little ability to create trusting bonds, as observed in the clinical practice with chronic pain patients,[12] but also in the romantic relationships of these patients.[35] Neumann et al.[35] have investigated relations between adult romantic attachment and somatization, starting from the hypothesis that the inhibition of emotions (in cases of high avoidance, where attachment-related emotions are suppressed) and emotional confusion (in cases of high anxiety, where nuanced awareness of feelings is missing, leading to difficulties to set apart emotional arousal into specific emotions) might foster the tendency to experience and express intrapersonal and interpersonal conflicts in the form of somatic complaints. The results showed that both attachment anxiety and avoidance are associated with somatization—with depression and general anxiety as moderating variables—and a stronger association for attachment anxiety.[35] As the authors indicate, these patients tend to feel neglected in their relationships with others, and this shows not only with their partner, as the most important attachment figure, but also with other significant others, such as their care providers. Indeed, difficulties in creating interpersonal relationships can in turn contribute to further difficulties in constructing and developing a therapeutic alliance.[4]

An insecure attachment style has been identified as contributing to high pain intensity and disability, to single out pain as a threat and to increase the degree of pain-related distress.[33,25] Insecure attachment is also correlated to high levels of depression, anxiety, and catastrophism and to a tendency to present express distress in a somatic way, in children as well as in adults.[25,37] Globally, attachment disorders represent a strong vulnerability for difficult adjustment to pain as described in the attachment–diathesis model of chronic pain.[33,32]

The association between affect regulation disorder and the tendency to express distress by means of somatic symptoms has also been linked with the concept of "alexithymia," that is, an absence of words to express emotions, a concept related to the model of somatization.[29,44] Pain is a prevailing form of somatization in primary care and specialized consultations alike, throughout different cultures.[17]

The process of somatization continues to challenge clinicians and researchers. The neurobiologic and neuropsychological entanglement between pain and emotions is now largely supported.[5]

To summarize this section, the preferred expression of distress through bodily symptoms may be related to several factors. Psychological dimensions are of major importance with alexithymia as a central phenomenon. The association of traumatic experiences during childhood with the presentation of multiple somatic symptoms and alexithymia has been discussed earlier.[38] There is growing evidence that epigenetic factors—that is the modulation of gene expression by environmental factors such as affective deprivation or trauma—can be at stake.[31] The presentation of distress through a bodily channel can be subjected to reinforcement. In this view, somatization may correspond to learned attitudes and behaviors or to a reinforcement from the social environment, leading to the entry in the health care system to try and comply with biomedical classifications that have the symbolic effect of stabilizing identity and restoring coherence.[34] This can be paralleled with the emotional avoidance discussed earlier, in which traumatic events are not positively processed verbally, and not transformed into a coherent narrative, hence often precluding these patients from getting support and stress relief by verbalizing their distress.[28] In an anthropologic view, somatization can be identified as a culture-bound mode of communication. Psychodynamic theories have proposed to refer to somatization as a kind of "short cut of the psyche" acting as a protection or a defense against an unbearable suffering like grief or melancholy.[30] To avoid the suffering related to a loss (whether real or symbolic), the individual unconsciously overinvests a body space that becomes difficult to cure.[36] In summary, the various models trying to account for the process of somatization point to painful symptoms and pain behaviors as messages of distress.[3]

PSYCHOLOGICAL APPROACHES

Psychological approaches used in the context of FMS (often entrenched within the context of somatic disorders or multisomatoform disorder) are various and some have been presented elsewhere in this book (see Chapter 26). The efficacy of psychological interventions such as *cognitive behavioral therapy (CBT)* on a range of symptoms has been clearly established although the reported effect sizes are in the low or medium range.[16] Integration of other treatment approaches might add to improve the outcome, thus making the exploration of the efficacy of different forms of psychotherapy of clear clinical relevance.[43]

The possible contribution of *hypnosis and guided imagery*, two techniques that aim to promote changes in subjective experience, alterations in perception, sensation, emotion, thought, or behavior by suggestion and/or imagination, in FMS has been acknowledged in a recently published systematic review and meta-analysis. This review found low-quality evidence of a clinically relevant benefit of guided imagery/hypnosis as compared to controls on ≥50% pain relief and psychological distress at the end of therapy, and of a clinically relevant benefit by hypnosis compared to controls in ≥30% pain relief, reduction of mean pain and sleep problems at 3-month follow-up. There was low-quality evidence that hypnosis combined with CBT was superior to CBT alone in reducing psychological distress at the end of therapy. As Zech et al.[50] note, hypnosis and guided imagery are categorized as "*mind-body therapies*" by the US National Center for Complementary and Integrative Health. An earlier systematic overview of reviews for *complementary and alternative treatments of FMS* also noted the overall low quality and the numerous methodologic flaws that hamper definite conclusions drawn from the reviews that could be retrieved in this domain. Yet, consistently positive results (on pain or other key symptoms of FMS) were found for *mind/body interventions, including meditation- or mindfulness-based techniques*, but also *biofeedback, and hypnosis/guided imagery.*[26] Although patient expectations are often oriented toward relaxation techniques, the benefit of these approaches remains to be demonstrated.[46]

A systematic review and meta-analysis of clinical trials[1] showed that *short-term psychodynamic psychotherapies* (STPPs) appear to contribute improving physical and psychological symptoms, social–occupational function, and health care utilization. STPPs are brief alternatives to the prior long-term psychodynamic therapies. STPPs have been developed "to work with unconscious impulses, feelings and processes, often related to losses and traumas in the past that can underpin or perpetuate symptoms."[2] Another review stressed that the severity of such losses and traumas (e.g., childhood maltreatment including emotional abuse and emotional neglect) may have a graded relationship with poor psychological outcomes in adulthood, pain complaints, and medical utilization.[7]

Psychodynamic psychotherapy, with its emphasis on resolving old trauma and its damaging effect on relationships, may be more or less focused on emotional mobilization and experiencing versus insight into processes.[2] Indeed, although some STPP methods aim for "insight into various unconscious phenomena, others seek to address alexithymia, or difficulty identifying and experiencing emotions. They share the common goals of making unconscious phenomena conscious and working through underlying conflicts."[1] A Cochrane review[2] indicated that treatment effect sized tended to be greater in long-term than in short-term follow-up suggesting accrued gains over time; study quality was highly variable, however. Furthermore, the authors stressed that it remains to be determined whether the outcomes are better explained through common (e.g., adherence, therapist training) or specific (e.g., emotional experiencing, intellectual insight) effects.[2]

Three recent randomized controlled trials (RCTs) provide additional information underlining the importance of the various *aspects of the patient–therapist relationship*. Sattel et al.[41] investigated the effects of *brief psychodynamic interpersonal psychotherapy (PIT)* as compared to enhanced medical care (EMC), including education, counseling, and symptom management. The results suggest that clinically significant improvements can be achieved using a short-term intervention consisting of sessions in patients who experience chronic and disabling bodily symptoms. In particular, this RCT showed that, in comparison with EMC, brief PIT provides greater improvement in physical quality of life at follow-up for those with multiple chronic and disabling symptoms and a high rate of comorbid depression and anxiety. It is noteworthy that the authors indicate that they were not able to show a significant improvement in depression for PIT compared to EMC, and they also comment on this finding as suggesting that "the assumption that an improvement in bodily function is solely or primarily related to an improvement in depression is incorrect."[41] Scheidt et al.[43] conducted an RCT exploring the effectiveness of brief psychodynamic psychotherapy in patients with FMS with concurrent depression as compared to standard primary care including advice concerning medication and health behavior (i.e., physical activity and stretching exercises). Contrary to the authors' expectations, the results did not allow to demonstrate a superior outcome of FMS symptoms and depression in the group receiving STPP as compared to high-standard routine primary care treatment.[43] A third trial[42] investigated the *combination of competence in family medicine and competence in the assessment and management of psychosomatic illness*, using a group intervention conducted by their general practitioner and a psychosomatic specialist in the general practitioner's office, as compared to guideline-based general practitioner training. Patients were invited to participate if they suffered persistent somatic symptoms corresponding to "somatic symptom disorders," but patients with illness anxiety in the absence of somatic symptoms were not included. The intervention was based on the rationale that empowering interpersonal factors through group work and building a strong therapeutic relationship and stable relationships between the group members would allow for "building a better understanding of the symptoms in a biopsychosocial perspective; physical and mental stabilization along with establishing active coping skills; strengthening the patient's self-functioning, affective communication and regulation of relationships; and enabling a new awareness of the interaction of symptoms with interpersonal and intrapsychic conflicts," based on the assumption of the importance of an interpersonal approach in a context where insecure attachment and interpersonal difficulties play a significant role.[42] The results showed that the collaborative intervention resulted in a clinically meaningful change in patients' mental quality of life, without improving physical quality of life at a 1-year follow-up.

It is noteworthy that the last two trials[43,42] both stressed the benefits of a multicomponent approach considering the integration of different treatment components and thus indicated the addition of some components of CBT (e.g., dealing with maladaptive beliefs, pain behavior, or dysfunctional coping) to the STPP.

CONCLUSION

Progress has been made in the past 20 years in the field of psychotherapy for FMS patients. Research offers a better understanding of the benefits and limits of psychotherapy in an evidence-based paradigm.

However, the discrepancy between patient representations and expectations, personal experience of pain, and the results of current research remains an area of concern. The issues of alexithymia, somatization as well as the wish for passive body-oriented treatments may contribute to problematic patients' commitment to psychotherapy. These issues need renewed attention.

The positive impact of a strong therapeutic alliance is to be underlined as it is known to be one of the major components of psychotherapy's benefits in alleviating suffering.

REFERENCES

1. Abbass A, Kisely S, Kroenke K. Short-term psychodynamic psychotherapy for somatic disorders. Systematic review and meta-analysis of clinical trials. *Psychother Psychosom*. 2009;**78**:265–74. doi:10.1159/000228247.
2. Abbass AA, Kisely, SR, Town JM, et al. Short-term psychodynamic psychotherapies for common mental disorders (review). *Coch Database Syst Rev*. 2014;(7):Art No: CD004687. doi:10.1002/14651858.CD004687.pub4.
3. Allaz AF, Piguet V, Kossovsky M, Desmeules J, Besson M, Cedraschi C. Extreme pain intensity as a message of global distress. *J Psychosom Res*. 2017. doi:10.1016/j.jpsychres.2017.03.214.
4. Allaz AF. Le messager boiteux: approche pratique des douleurs chroniques rebelles. Genève: Médecine & Hygiène; 2003.
5. Apkarian AV, Bushnell MC, Treede RD, Zubieta JK. Human brain mechanisms of pain perception and regulation in health and disease. *Eur J Pain*. 2005;**9**:463–484.
6. Arnold LM, Clauw DJ, McCarberg BH; FibroCollaborative. Improving the recognition and diagnosis of fibromyalgia. *Mayo Clin Proc*. 2011;**86**:457–464.
7. Arnow BA. Relationships between childhood maltreatment, adult health and psychiatric outcomes, and medical utilization. *J Clin Psychiat*. 2004;**65**(Suppl 12):10–15.

8. Bowlby J. *Attachment and Loss: vol 2: separation: Anxiety and Anger.* New York: Basic Books; 1973.
9. Cedraschi C, Girard E, Luthy C, Kossovsky M, Desmeules J, Allaz AF. Primary attributions in women suffering fibromyalgia emphasize the perception of a disruptive onset for a long-lasting pain problem. *J Psychosomat Res.* 2013;**74**:265–269.
10. Cedraschi C, Girard E, Piguet V, Desmeules J, Allaz AF. Assessing the affective load in the narratives of women suffering from fibromyalgia: the clinicians' appraisal. *Health Expect.* 2015;**18**:3325–35. doi:10.1111/hex.12323.
11. Ciccone DS, Elliott DK, Chandler HK, Nayak A, Raphael KG. Sexual and physical abuse in women with fibromyalgia syndrome, a test of the trauma hypothesis. *Clin J Pain.* 2005;**21**:378–386.
12. Ciechanowski PS, Walker EA, Katon J, Russo JE. Attachment theory: a model for health care utilization and somatization. *Psychosom Med.* 2002;**84**:660–667.
13. Clauw DJ, Arnold LM, McCarberg BH; FibroCollaborative. The science of fibromyalgia. *Mayo Clin Proc.* 2011;**86**:907–911.
14. Davis DA, Luecken LJ, Zautra AJ. Are reports of childhood abuse related to the experience of chronic pain in adulthood? A meta-analytic review of the literature. *Clin J Pain.* 2005:**21**:398–405.
15. Desmeules JA, Cedraschi C, Rapiti E, et al. Neurophysiologic evidence for a central sensitization in patients with fibromyalgia. *Arthritis Rheum.* 2003;**48**(5):1420–1429.
16. Glombiewski JA, Sawyer AT, Gutermann J, Koenig K, Rief W, Hofmann SG. Psychological treatments for fibromyalgia: a meta-analysis. *Pain.* 2010;**151**:280–295. doi:10.1016/j.pain.2010.06.011.
17. Gureje O, Simon GE, Von Korff M. A cross-national study of the course of persistent pain in primary care. *Pain.* 2001;**92**:195–200.
18. Häuser W, Burgmer M, Köllner V, et al. Fibromyalgia as a psychosomatic disorder—diagnosis and therapy according to current evidence-based guidelines. *Z Psychosom Psychother.* 2013;**59**:132–152.
19. Häuser W, Hennigsen P. Fibromyalgia syndrome: a somatoform disorder? *Eur J Pain.* 2014;**18**:1052–1059.
20. Häuser W, Kosseva M, Üceyler N, Klose P, Sommer C. Emotional, physical, and sexual abuse in fibromyalgia syndrome: a systematic review with meta-analysis. *Arthritis Care Res.* 2011;**63**(6):808–820.
21. Hunter J, Maunder R, Lan Le T. Fundamentals of attachment theory In: Hunter J, Maunder R, eds. *Improving Patient Treatment with Attachment Theory: A Guide for Primary Care Practitioners and Specialists.* Switzerland: Springer International Publishing; 2016:9–26. doi:10.1007/978-3-319-23300-0_5.
22. Imbierowicz K, Egle UT. Childhood adversities in patients with fibromyalgia and somatoform pain disorder. *Eur J Pain.* 2003;**7**:113–119.
23. Jones G, Power C, Macfarlane GJ. Adverse event in childhood and chronic widespread pain in adult life: results from the 1958 British Birth Cohort Study. *Pain.* 2009;**143**:92–96.
24. Lampe A, Doering S, Rumpold G, et al. Chronic pain syndromes and their relation to childhood abuse and stressful life events. *J Psychosom Res.* 2003;**54**:361–367.
25. Landa A, Peterson BS, Fallon BA. Somatoform pain: a developmental theory and translational research review. *Psychosom Med.* 2012;**74**:717–727.
26. Lauche R, Cramer H, Häuser W, Dobos G, Langhorst J. A systematic overview of reviews for complementary and alternative therapies in the treatment of the fibromyalgia syndrome. *Evid Based Compl Alt Med.* 2015;**2015**:610615. doi:0.1155/2015/610615.
27. Lind AB, Delmar C, Nielsen K. Struggling in an emotional avoidance culture: a qualitative study of stress as a predisposing factor for somatoform disorders. *J Psychosomat Res.* 2014;**76**:94–98.
28. Lind AB, Risoer MB, Nielsen K, Delmar C, Christensen MB, Lomborg K. Longing for existential recognition: a qualitative study of everyday concerns for people with somatoform disorders. *J Psychosomat Res.* 2014;**76**:99–104.
29. Mattila AK, Kronholm E, Jula A, et al. Alexithymia and somatization in general population. *Psychosom Med.* 2008;**70**:716–722.
30. McDougall J. *Theaters of the Body: A Psychoanalytic Approach to :sychosomatic Illness.* New York: W.W Norton; 1989.

31. Mehta D, Klengel T, Conneely KN, et al. Childhood maltreatment is associated with distinct genomic and epigenetic profiles in posttraumatic stress disorder. *Proc Natl Acad Sci USA*. 2013;**110**:8302–8307.
32. Meredith P, Ownsworth T, Strong J. A review of the evidence linking adult attachment theory and chronic pain: presenting a conceptual model. *Clin Psychol Rev*. 2008;**28**:407–429.
33. Meredith PJ. Attachment theory and pain. In: Hunter J, Maunder R, eds. *Improving Patient Treatment with Attachment Theory: A Guide for Primary Care Practitioners and Specialists*. Cham Heidelberg New-York Dordrecht London: Springer International Publishing; 2016:55–73. doi:10.1007/978-3-319-23300-0_5.
34. Nettleton S. "I just want permission to be ill": towards a sociology of medically unexplained symptoms. *Soc Sci Med*. 2006;**62**:1167–1178.
35. Neumann E, Sattel H, Gündel H, Henningsen P, Kruse J. Attachment in romantic relationships and somatization. *J Nerv Ment Dis*. 2015;**203**:101–106.
36. Nissen B. Hypochondria: a tentative approach. *Int J Psychoanal*. 2000;**81**:651–666.
37. Porter LS, Davis D, Keefe FJ. Attachment and pain: recent findings and future directions. *Pain*. 2007;**128**:195–198.
38. Raphael KG, Widom CS, Lange G. Childhood victimization and pain in adulthood: a prospective investigation. *Pain*. 2001;**92**:283–293.
39. Russell IL, Larson AA. Neurophysiopathogenesis of fibromyalgia syndrome: a unified hypothesis. *Rheum Dis Clin North Am*. 2009;**35**:421–435.
40. Sack M, Lahmann C, Jaeger B, Henningsen P. Trauma prevalence and somatoform symptoms: are there specific somatoform symptoms related to traumatic experiences? *J Nerv Ment Dis*. 2007;**195**:928–933.
41. Sattel H, Lahmann C, Gündel H, et al. Brief psychodynamic interpersonal psychotherapy for patients with multisomatoform disorder: randomised controlled trial. *Br J Psychiat*. 2012;**200**:60–67. doi:10.1192/bjp.bp.111.093526.
42. Schaefert R, Kaufmann C, Wild B, et al. Specific collaborative group intervention for patients with medically unexplained symptoms in general practice: a cluster randomized controlled trial. *Psychother Psychosom*. 2013;**82**:106–119. doi:10.1159/000343652.
43. Scheidt CE, Waller E, Endorf K, et al. Is brief psychodynamic psychotherapy in primary fibromyalgia syndrome with concurrent depression an effective treatment? A randomized controlled trial. *Gen Hosp Psychiat*. 2013;**35**:160–167. doi:10.1016/j.genhosppsych.2012.10.013.
44. Sifneos PE. The prevalence of 'alexithymic' characteristics in psychosomatic patients. *Psychother Psychosom*. 1973;**22**:255–262.
45. Tavel ME. Somatic symptom disorders without know physical causes: one disease with many names? *Am J Med*. 2015;**128**:1054–1058.
46. Thieme K, Häuser W, Batra A, et al. Psychotherapie bein Patienten mit Fibromyalgiesyndrom. [Psychotherapy in patients with fibomyalgia syndrome]. *Schmerz*. 2008;**22**:295–302.
47. Thieme K, Turk DC, Flor H. Comorbid depression and anxiety in fibromyalgia syndrome: relationship to somatic and psychosocial variables. *Psychosom Med*. 2004;**66**:837–844.
48. Van Houdenhove B, Luyten P. Beyond dualism: the role of life stress in chronic pain. *Pain*. 2005;**113**:238–239.
49. Yunus MB. Central sensitivity syndromes: a new paradigm and group nosology for fibromyalgia and overlapping conditions, and the related issue of disease versus illness. *Semin Arthritis Rheum*. 2008;**37**:339–352.
50. Zech N, Hansen E, Bernardy K, Häuser W. Efficacy, acceptability and safety of guided imagery/hypnosis in fibromyalgia—a systematic review and meta-analysis of randomized controlled trials. *Eur J Pain*. 2017;**21**:217–227. doi:10.1002/ejp.933.

SECTION 7

Conclusion and Future Research Agenda

CHAPTER 31

Conclusions and Future Perspectives

Serge Perrot and Winfried Häuser

With this book, we hope that all readers, from different fields, understand the complexity of fibromyalgia syndrome (FMS) and catch the recent progresses in the knowledge of pathophysiology, the relevance of clinical descriptions, and the validity of treatment approaches. Far from controversies, this book has integrated different views, different concepts, and tried to provide a comprehensive overview of current FMS scientific literature. We are also happy that several renowned authors agreed to participate in this project, gently interacting with both of us, to provide the most relevant articles for colleagues, not only for pain specialists, but also for other health care professions.

The International Association for the Study of Pain (IASP) is committed to promote pain awareness, all over the world, not only to all health care professionals, but also to politicians, mostly for the benefit of patients. With this book on FMS, officially supported by IASP, we do hope that FMS should not be considered anymore as an artificial condition, created by few clinicians, or something that does not exist at all, but as a widely accepted scientific entity, based on high-quality research.

This book should not represent an end, we hope that it should be an important step for future research, involving numerous specialties and researchers. In this line, we may suggest future axes of research and a research agenda:

- Fundamental research in longitudinal studies should investigate links between brain and body, and dynamic changes not only on pain but also on sleep, fatigue, and cognition triggered by numerous stressors implicated in FMS pathophysiology.
- Clinical research should develop the FMS subclassifications, as it has been proposed in headaches, because FMS is not a homogeneous condition. A better interpretation of clinical features may help to propose adapted therapeutic management.
- Therapeutic research should discuss the role of complementary approaches in pain management and efficacy of all pain modulatory techniques.
- Societal analyses should discuss the recognition of FMS and how conditions that are related to the new third descriptor of pain mechanism classification are accepted by health care systems.

FMS is an emblematic chronic pain condition, considering not only pathophysiologic discussions but also therapeutic and socio-legal issues. We believe that all findings and approaches developed in FMS and proposed in this book increase knowledge of pain pathophysiology and globally improve pain care for several patients, all over the world.

INDEX

Note: Page numbers followed by *f* and *t* refer to figures and tables, respectively.

A

B

C

N

O

P

Q

R

U

V

W

Y